AF771561

Nano- and Microencapsulation - Techniques and Applications

Edited by Nedal Abu-Thabit

Published in London, United Kingdom

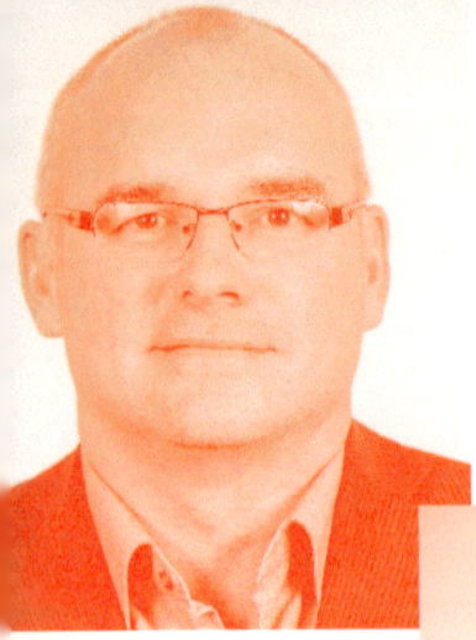
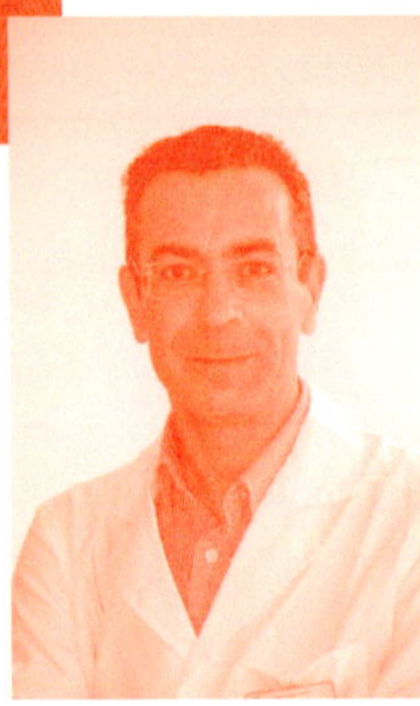
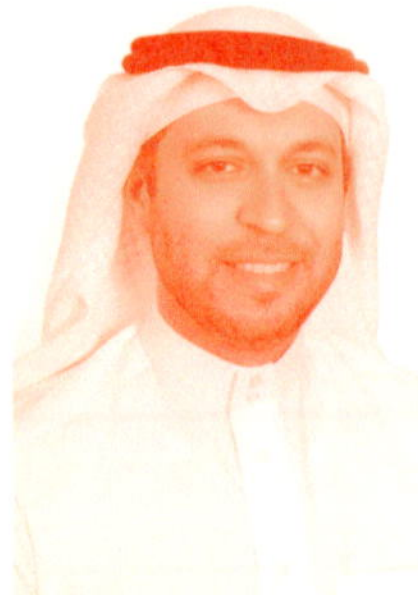
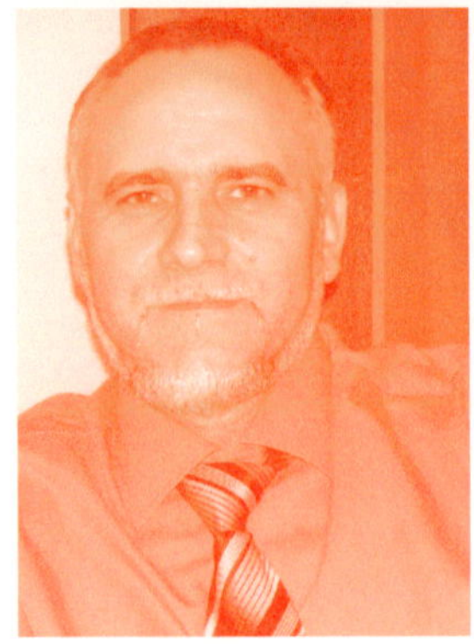
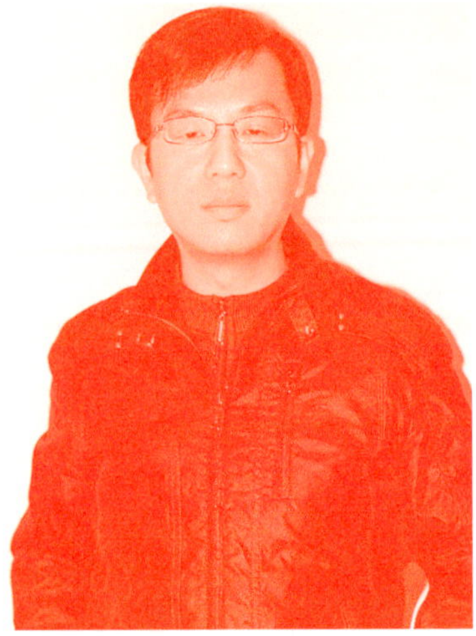
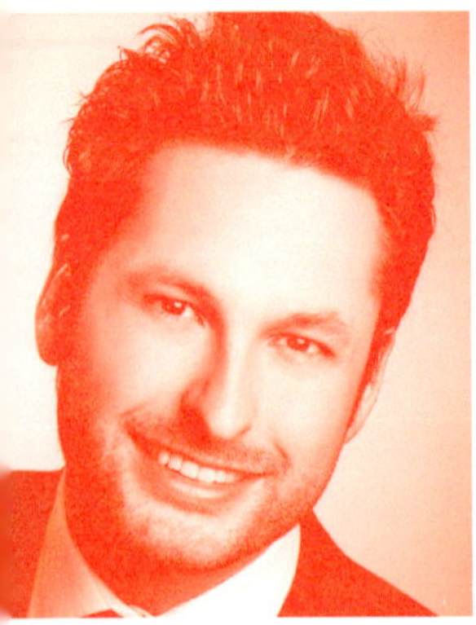
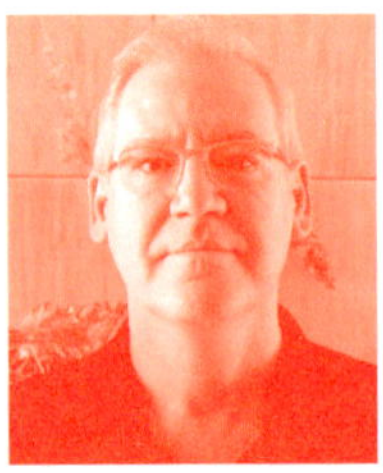

IntechOpen

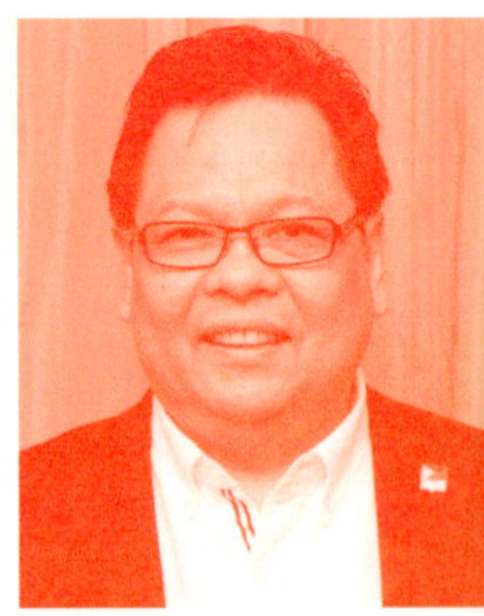
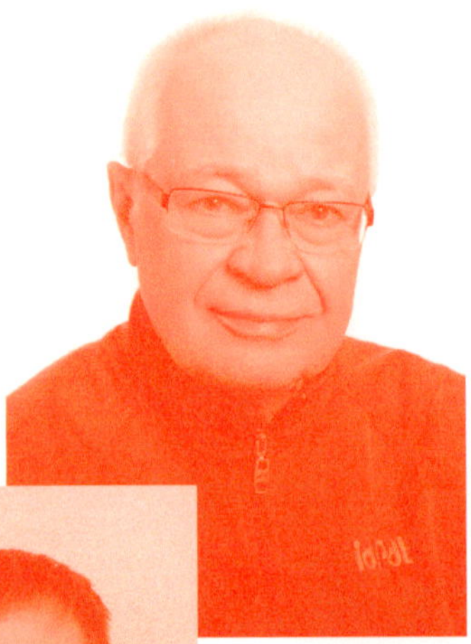
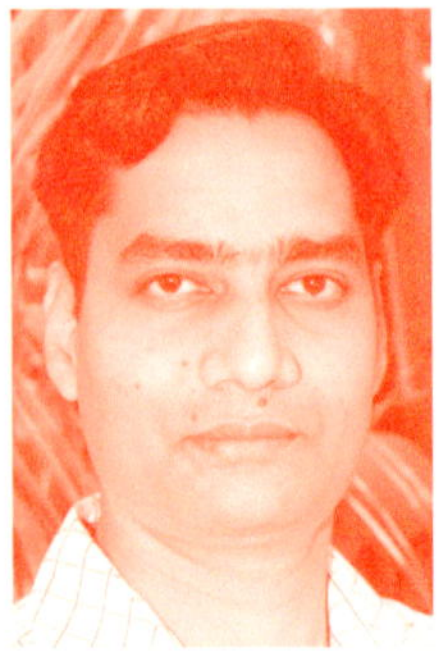
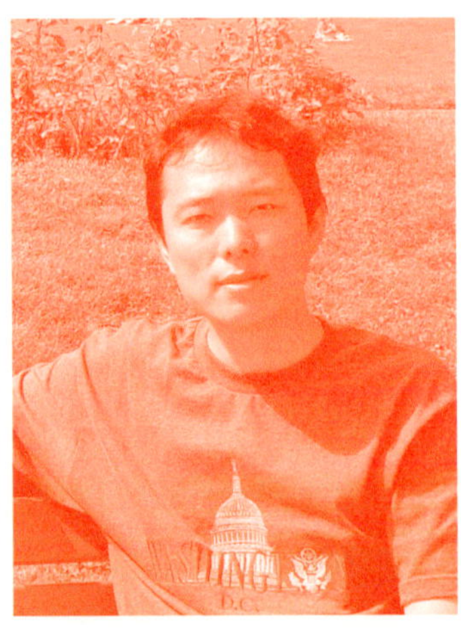
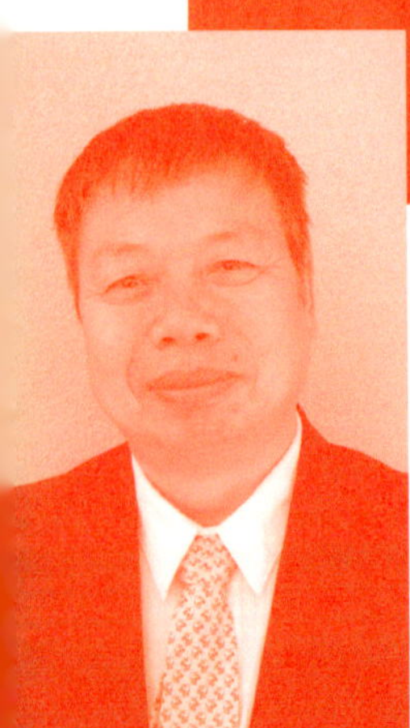
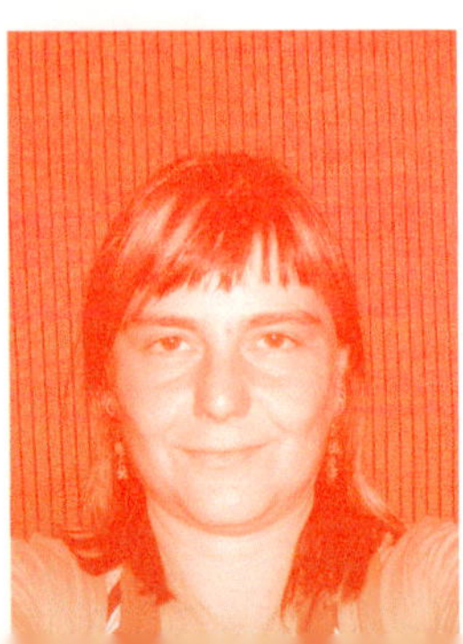

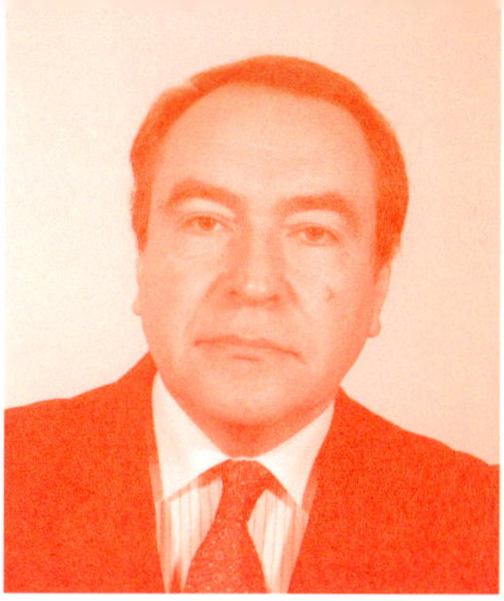
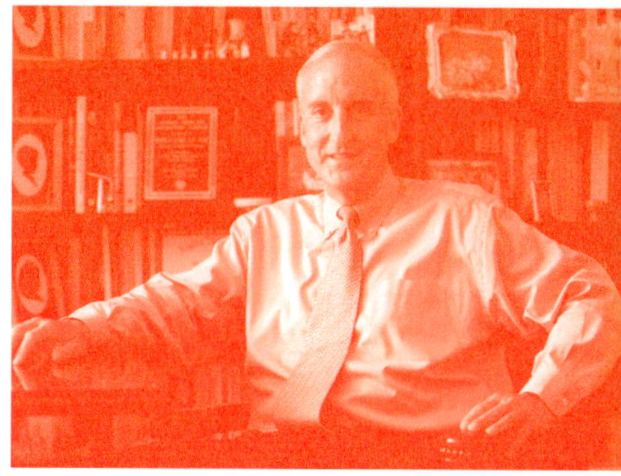
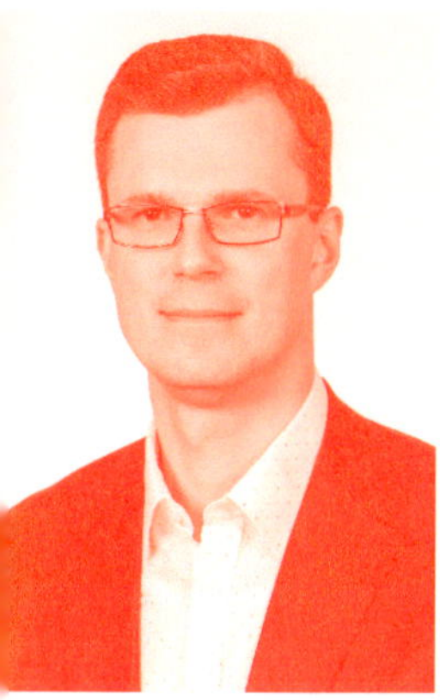
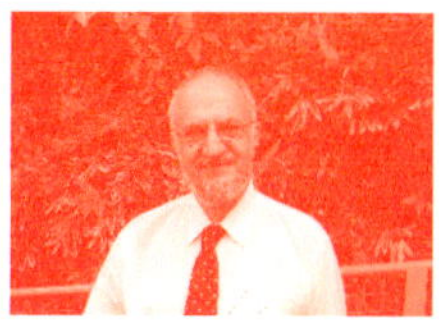
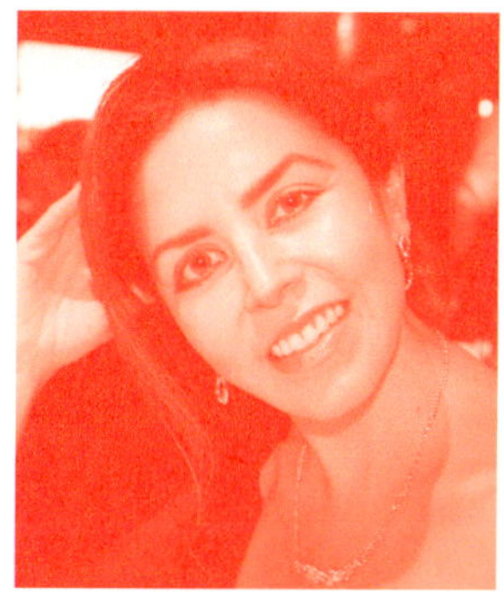

Supporting open minds since 2005

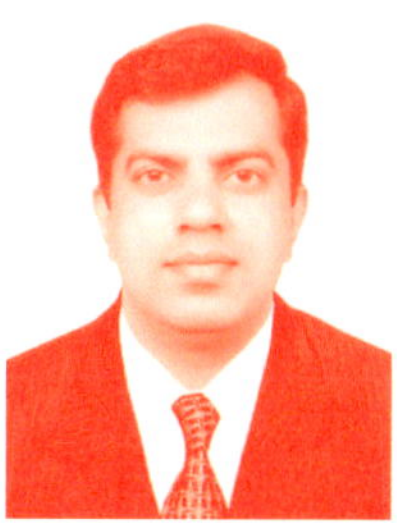
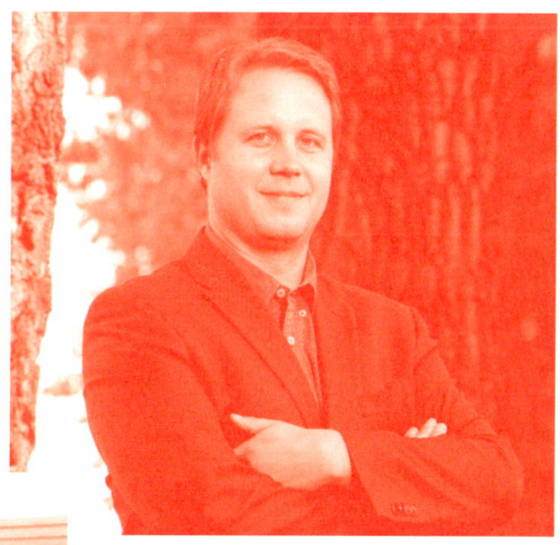
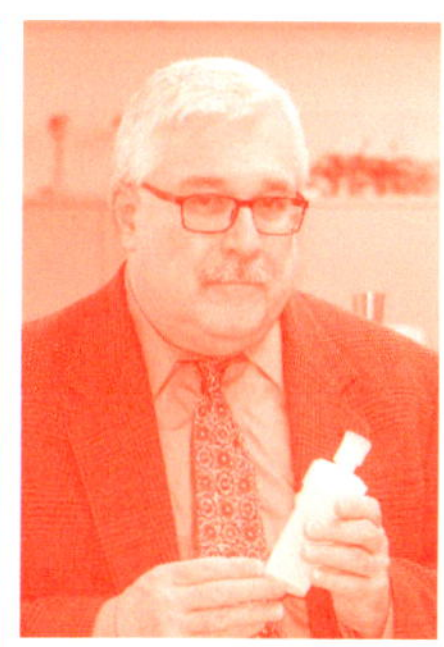
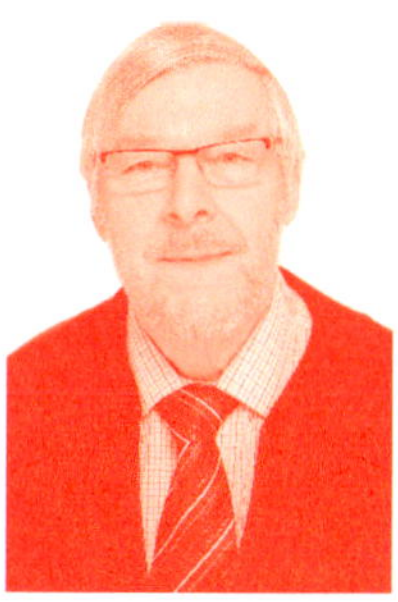
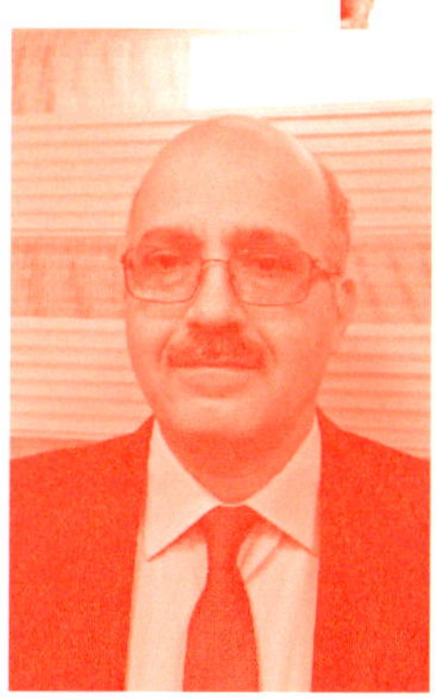
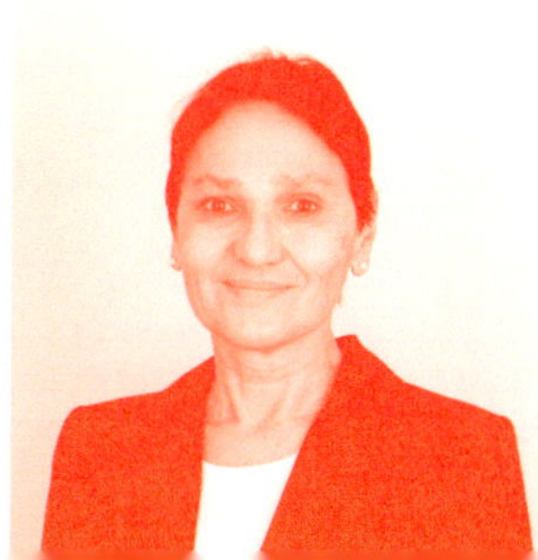
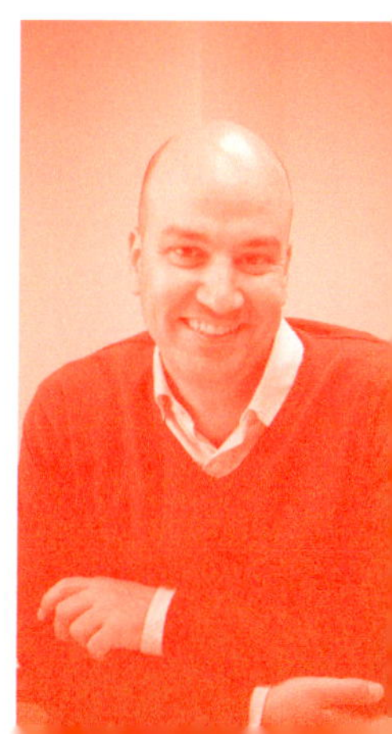

Nano- and Microencapsulation - Techniques and Applications
http://dx.doi.org/10.5772/intechopen.88590
Edited by Nedal Abu-Thabit

Contributors
Dwi Hudiyanti, Febriani Kusuma Wardani, Khairul Anam, Nur Kamila, Abhishek Sharma, Saurabh Dubey, Nusrat Iqbal, Emrah Yucesan, Beyza Goncu, Siti Rohaida Mohd Shafian, Ismail Mohd Saaid, Norzafirah Razali, Ahmad Fadhil Jahari, Sonny Irawan, Manaf Rizvan Manafov, Dilgam Taghiyev, Gudret Isfandiyar Kelbaliev, Nedal Abu-Thabit, Noura A.A. Ebrahim, Mahmoud Abu Elella, Soliman M.A. Soliman, Riham Mohamed, Joan Erebor, Margaret O. Ilomuanya, Onyinye Uwaezuoke, Ndidi C. Ngwuluka, Calvin Andeve, Edith Amuhaya, Victoria Fasiku, Kingo Rajab, Claudia Elizabeth Mora Huertas, Luis Fernando Ospina Giraldo, Oscar Iván Martínez Muñoz

© The Editor(s) and the Author(s) 2021
The rights of the editor(s) and the author(s) have been asserted in accordance with the Copyright, Designs and Patents Act 1988. All rights to the book as a whole are reserved by INTECHOPEN LIMITED. The book as a whole (compilation) cannot be reproduced, distributed or used for commercial or non-commercial purposes without INTECHOPEN LIMITED's written permission. Enquiries concerning the use of the book should be directed to INTECHOPEN LIMITED rights and permissions department (permissions@intechopen.com).
Violations are liable to prosecution under the governing Copyright Law.

Individual chapters of this publication are distributed under the terms of the Creative Commons Attribution 3.0 Unported License which permits commercial use, distribution and reproduction of the individual chapters, provided the original author(s) and source publication are appropriately acknowledged. If so indicated, certain images may not be included under the Creative Commons license. In such cases users will need to obtain permission from the license holder to reproduce the material. More details and guidelines concerning content reuse and adaptation can be found at http://www.intechopen.com/copyright-policy.html.

Notice
Statements and opinions expressed in the chapters are these of the individual contributors and not necessarily those of the editors or publisher. No responsibility is accepted for the accuracy of information contained in the published chapters. The publisher assumes no responsibility for any damage or injury to persons or property arising out of the use of any materials, instructions, methods or ideas contained in the book.

First published in London, United Kingdom, 2021 by IntechOpen
IntechOpen is the global imprint of INTECHOPEN LIMITED, registered in England and Wales, registration number: 11086078, 5 Princes Gate Court, London, SW7 2QJ, United Kingdom
Printed in Croatia

British Library Cataloguing-in-Publication Data
A catalogue record for this book is available from the British Library

Additional hard and PDF copies can be obtained from orders@intechopen.com

Nano- and Microencapsulation - Techniques and Applications
Edited by Nedal Abu-Thabit
p. cm.
Print ISBN 978-1-83968-348-0
Online ISBN 978-1-83968-349-7
eBook (PDF) ISBN 978-1-83968-350-3

For EU product safety concerns:
IN TECH d.o.o., Prolaz Marije Krucifikse Kozulić 3, 51000 Rijeka, Croatia, info@intechopen.com or visit our website at intechopen.com.

We are IntechOpen, the world's leading publisher of Open Access books

Built by scientists, for scientists

5,200+
Open access books available

127,000+
International authors and editors

150M+
Downloads

156
Countries delivered to

Our authors are among the

Top 1%
most cited scientists

12.2%
Contributors from top 500 universities

CLARIVATE ANALYTICS BOOK CITATION INDEX INDEXED

WEB OF SCIENCE™

Selection of our books indexed in the Book Citation Index in Web of Science™ Core Collection (BKCI)

Interested in publishing with us?
Contact book.department@intechopen.com

Numbers displayed above are based on latest data collected.
For more information visit www.intechopen.com

Meet the editor

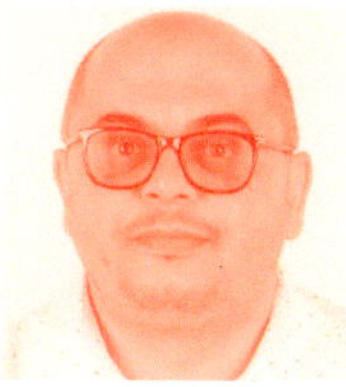

Dr. Nedal Abu-Thabit holds a Ph.D. in Chemistry with a specialization in polymer chemistry from King Fahd University of Petroleum and Minerals (KFUPM). Currently, Dr. Nedal is an associate professor in the Chemical & Process Engineering Technology department at Jubail Industrial College. During the period 2013–2018, Dr. Nedal held the position of program director for the Polymer Engineering Technology major. Dr. Nedal has published more than forty research articles and reviews in refereed journals, fifteen book chapters, four books, and two patents. His research interests are related to polymer synthesis, preparation of nanocomposites, nanomaterials, and electrically conducting polymers for water sterilization and sensing applications, and isolation of biopolymers from renewable and sustainable resources. Dr. Nedal has contributed many articles to educational polymer chemistry.

Contents

Preface

Encapsulation is a process in which an active ingredient that forms the core material (e.g. pharmaceutical drugs, diagnostics, biologics, antibacterial agents, self-healing agents, enzymes, microorganisms, etc.) is entrapped within a carrier (capsule, shell, coating material, or matrix). Encapsulation offers advantages such as safe handling of hazardous but useful materials; controlled release; stimuli-responsive release; taste, odor, and color masking; site-specific delivery; and solidifying of liquid droplets. In the past, micro-carriers (1 μm–1 mm) have been used for various applications including pharmaceuticals, biotechnology, agrochemicals, environmental remediation, food safety, and cosmetics. However, recent advancements in nanotechnology have opened the door for nano-encapsulation using different materials at the nanoscale level (1–300 nm), especially for drug delivery applications. Nano-encapsulation offers advantages such as enhanced drug solubility, greater encapsulation efficiency, and selective targeting.

This book is divided into three parts. The first part discusses various techniques of nano-/micro- encapsulation for drug delivery applications using different natural carriers. Chapters 1 and 2 provide a comprehensive overview of various chemical, physical, and physicochemical encapsulation techniques using biopolymers, proteins, and lipids, with a focus on their recent advanced therapeutic and diagnostic applications. Chapter 3 discusses the nanoprecipitation technique for nano-/micro-encapsulation of active pharmaceutical ingredients. Chapter 4 provides a detailed description related to nano-/micro-encapsulation via covalent drug conjugation. Chapter 5 discusses the clinical and transplantation applications of micro-encapsulated alginates. Finally, Chapter 6 discusses the use of phospholipids derived from coconut for preparing liposomes and encapsulating vitamin C.

The second part of the book discusses the rheology of micro-emulsions. Chapter 7 discusses the rheology of crude oil emulsions and Chapter 8 discusses the aggregation of silica nanoparticles in a porous medium with potential application for enhanced oil recovery.

The third part of the book examines diverse applications of micro-emulsion formulations. Chapter 9 discusses the formulations of botanical oil micro-emulsions for extended and controlled release of biopesticides as a sustainable agro-ecosystem.

Nedal Abu-Thabit
Department of Chemical and Process Engineering Technology,
Jubail Industrial College,
Jubail Industrial City,
Saudi Arabia

Section 1

Encapsulation Techniques for Drug Delivery Applications

Chapter 1

Natural Polymers in Micro- and Nanoencapsulation for Therapeutic and Diagnostic Applications: Part I: Lipids and Fabrication Techniques

Ndidi C. Ngwuluka, Nedal Y. Abu-Thabit, Onyinye J. Uwaezuoke, Joan O. Erebor, Margaret O. Ilomuanya, Riham R. Mohamed, Soliman M.A. Soliman, Mahmoud H. Abu Elella and Noura A.A. Ebrahim

Abstract

Encapsulation, specifically microencapsulation is an old technology with increasing applications in pharmaceutical, agrochemical, environmental, food, and cosmetic spaces. In the past two decades, the advancements in the field of nanotechnology opened the door for applying the encapsulation technology at the nanoscale level. Nanoencapsulation is highly utilized in designing effective drug delivery systems (DDSs) due to the fact that delivery of the encapsulated therapeutic/diagnostic agents to various sites in the human body depends on the size of the nanoparticles. Compared to microencapsulation, nanoencapsulation has superior performance which can improve bioavailability, increase drug solubility, delay or control drug release and enhance active/passive targeting of bioactive agents to the sites of action. Encapsulation, either micro- or nanoencapsulation is employed for the conventional pharmaceuticals, biopharmaceuticals, biologics, or bioactive drugs from natural sources as well as for diagnostics such as biomarkers. The outcome of any encapsulation process depends on the technique employed and the encapsulating material. This chapter discusses in details (1) various physical, mechanical, thermal, chemical, and physicochemical encapsulation techniques, (2) types and classifications of natural polymers (polysaccharides, proteins, and lipids) as safer, biocompatible and biodegradable encapsulating materials, and (3) the recent advances in using lipids for therapeutic and diagnostic applications. Polysaccharides and proteins are covered in the second part of this chapter.

Keywords: natural polymers, biopolymers, drug delivery, nanoencapsulation, microencapsulation, lipids, therapeutic, diagnostic, polysaccharides, proteins

1. Introduction

Encapsulation, a process involving entrapment of an active ingredient or diagnostic tool within a carrier (capsule, shell, coating material or a matrix) is an old technology that has gained traction over the years with advances in polymer science and encapsulation technologies. The applications of encapsulation span pharmaceuticals, biotechnology, agrochemical, environmental, food and cosmetic spaces with immense benefits found in the pharmaceutical and biotechnology spaces. Encapsulation is used for immobilization of volatile compounds, enzymes, and microorganisms; protection and stabilization from environmental factors; safe handling of hazardous but useful materials; controlled release; taste, odor and color masking; site-specific delivery and solidifying of liquid droplets. Encapsulation improves on the challenges of conventional dosage forms in enhancing stability, taste, bioavailability and biodistribution. Some drugs such as insulin are not given orally because of degradation in the GIT before absorption. Encapsulation may be an approach to change route of administration from intravenous to oral.

The parameters for encapsulation of active ingredients depend on the physicochemical properties of the active ingredient such as solubility, thermal and redox stability; however, the release of the active is then modulated by mechanical process, pH variations, enzymatic actions or other external stimuli [1]. The encapsulation methods classified as chemical, physicochemical and physicomechanical methods are used to encapsulate an active ingredient with the specific method chosen based on application and desired outcomes. The choice of materials to be used for encapsulation to accommodate the physicochemical behavior of the active in order to produce the desire encapsulation efficiency, shell or capsule size, surface morphology and functionalities of the capsule and the behavior of encapsulated active ingredient are fundamental preformulation studies before a new encapsulated product is developed. The bioavailability of existing poorly soluble drugs and those in the development pipeline can be significantly enhanced by encapsulation with the right encapsulating material(s).

Natural polymers are choice materials for encapsulation. Natural polymers are macromolecules of large molecular weights obtained from nature and are preferred due to their flexibility to modification, biocompatibility, biodegradability, renewability, and low toxicity [2]. Being of natural origins such as plants, animals and microorganisms, they are able to interact with tissues and cells displaying some properties the body identifies with and as a result do not treat them as foreign bodies [3]. Natural polymers such as proteins, polysaccharides and lipids have been employed as encapsulation materials for encapsulating hydrophilic or hydrophobic active ingredients which may be in liquid, solid and gaseous states for transport and delivery to the sites they are needed. The chapter reviews fabrication techniques, lipids, and their applications in micro- and nanoencapsulation elucidating their functionalities which enable them to be utilized for encapsulation of therapeutics and diagnostics producing delivery systems with the desired outcomes. Polysaccharides and proteins are covered in part (II) of this chapter.

2. Encapsulation

Encapsulation is the process of enclosing, entrapping, coating, or surrounding a liquid, solid or gas active compound within a material to achieve a more controlled/sustained release, protect the active compound/active pharmaceutical ingredient from degradation before reaching the site of absorption or before reaching the site of action as well as reducing the associated adverse effects that go along with some non-encapsulated compounds like NSAIDS [4, 5]. Research on encapsulation utilizing natural polymers and their derivatives (semi-synthetic polymers) has evolved over time with the particle size as the main difference. Encapsulation on the micro scale is referred to as microencapsulation while when encapsulation is done on the nanoscale it is referred to as nanoencapsulation [6].

2.1 Microencapsulation

Microencapsulation refers to the formulation process of encapsulating a bioactive compound in a particle size that is 1–1000 μm in diameter for the purpose of controlled and sustained delivery as well as protection of the encapsulated bioactive compound from the surrounding environment [7, 8]. Microencapsulation technology came into existence with the focus of achieving controlled and extended release profiles. Due to the size of micro carriers, encapsulation of macromolecules with large molecular weight such as proteins for controlled release can be encapsulated. Bochenek *et al.,* [9] utilized chemically modified alginate microsphere formulations to encapsulate allogeneic pancreatic islet cells for transient islet-graft function that have reached clinical trial stage for management insulin deficiency in diabetic populations. This was due to the fact that the immune-modulating alginate copolymer employed had controlled release profile that caused encapsulated islet cells to remain viable after transplantation into the general intraperitoneal (IP) space of human subjects, while also exhibiting lowered foreign-body reaction (FBR) compared to previous formulations. Chitosan-alginate microcapsules encapsulating biologically active compounds from aqueous extracts of *Garcinia kola* (GK) and *Hunteria umbellata* (HU) seeds, have also been shown to have selective release patterns depending on the pH of the medium [10]. Slower release of the GK and HU microcapsules of the active compounds was observed at pH 1.2, but increased controlled extended release profiles were observed to occur at pH 6.8 unlike conventional tablets that did not show controlled extended release profiles [10].

2.2 Nanoencapsulation

Nanoencapsulation can be defined as the entrapment, enclosure, or coating of a bioactive compound within a carrier that is on the nanoscale dimension [5]. Nanoscale dimension is seen as particle sizes 1–100 nm [6]. However more recent definitions have given room for 1–300 nm and others 1–1000 nm [11]. The advancement of encapsulation from the micro scale to the nano scale was driven by the need for more site selective targeting purposes such as the use of chemotherapeutics in cancer. The main draw back in cancer chemotherapeutics has been that severe adverse effects occur due to toxicity caused by the non-selective action on both cancer cells and healthy cells at therapeutic doses. Hence, the inception of nanomedicines that could achieve active targeting was born. Nanoencapsulation in drug delivery has the merit of having a higher encapsulation efficiency, due to enhanced drug solubility of bioactive molecules in the core [12].

Silk fibroin nanoparticles encapsulating curcumin were found to demonstrate selective cytotoxicity for cancer therapy in neuroblastoma cells and hepatocarcinoma cells while not adversely affecting the healthy cells [13]. Diagnostics are also gaining from the merits of encapsulation. This was demonstrated in the simultaneous co-encapsulation of MRI contrast agent Gd-DTPA and fluorescent label ATTO488 in multimodal PEG – crosslinked hyaluronic acid nanoparticles (PEG-cHANPs) to formulate a probe for diagnostic purposes [14]. The PEG-cHANPs were observed to improve MR signals while concurrently magnifying the relaxation time, T_1 5 times due to the presence of the ATTO 488 in the human glioma U87 MG cell line. Tammaro *et al.,* [14] implied that this could lead to the decrease in the administered dose of the probe, thereby resulting in a better resolution and higher quality images.

3. Merits and demerits of encapsulation

The merits and demerits of encapsulation are viewed from the expected outcomes of encapsulation and are based on physicochemical properties of core materials (small molecules, biologics, or diagnostics), encapsulating techniques and materials. Encapsulating materials such as natural and semi-synthetic polymers have many advantages because they are obtained from natural sources. Immunogenicity issues when natural polymers are used as the encapsulating materials are greatly reduced compared to synthetic polymers. Encapsulation using natural polymers can be done without high temperatures thus preventing degradation due to high temperatures as seen in alginate–chitosan micro/nanoparticles which were successfully fabricated at room temperature excluding the utilization of organic solvents [4].

Encapsulation of an active compound using pegylated phospholipids also known as lipopolymers such as 2000 Da PEG-DSPE have demonstrated the merit of prolonging circulation time of active compounds when administered as nanoliposomes. This led to a reduction in the dosage frequency and reduction in uptake by the RES, thus leading to an increase in patient compliance as was observed in the first FDA approved nanomedicine; liposomal doxorubicin Doxil® in 1995 [15].

Efficacious poorly water-soluble drug candidates for therapeutics before now posed a challenge in formulation due to their low solubility profile and pharmacokinetic characteristics [16]. Micro- and nanoencapsulation technologies such as supramolecular hydrogels formulated with natural cyclic oligosaccharides also called cyclodextrins have successfully been able to encapsulate and deliver such drug candidates. This was demonstrated when lipophilic non-hydroxylated coumarins were encapsulated in the core of β-cyclodextrin hydrogels for trypanocidal activity via mitochondrial membrane potential studies for Chagas disease caused by the protozoan parasite, *Trypanosoma cruzi*. Trypanocidal activity was increased by 10% with the Supramolecular hydrogels of β-cyclodextrin linked to calcium homopoly-L-guluronate as compared to the free corresponding amidocoumarins [17, 18].

Demerits of natural and semi-synthetic polymers in micro- and nanoencapsulation mainly depends on the individual materials. However, a major drawback observed with natural polymers and their derivatives is batch to batch variation depending on regions/environments that these polymers were sourced from. Plant and animals of the same species have been found to have some slight differences in their composition based on factors such as type of soil or geographical regions [19, 20]. Low mechanical strength leading to weak wall formation, susceptibility to change in pH causing a reduction in stability, highly hygroscopic leading to denaturation are challenges that are observed with such polymers as alginate, gelatin and sodium hyaluronate [8].

To overcome the demerits of these polymers, physical and chemical modifications are undertaken. Extra care should be taken during storage of natural polymers to reduce degradation and denaturation that occur during storage. Despite any demerits that natural polymers and their derivatives may have, the application of natural polymers and their derivatives for micro- and nanoencapsulation will continue to increase because of their immense merits in therapeutics and diagnostics.

4. Encapsulation techniques

The process of enclosing vesicles in a thin continuous film of a natural or semi synthetic polymer has been accomplished using a variety of both physical and chemical methods or a combination of both depending on the size of the targeted capsules either in the nanometer, micrometer or millimeter range. Over the years and as a result of continuous innovation, these techniques have evolved from the earliest relatively simple coacervation phase separation used for making only microcapsules to current comparatively complex techniques capable of making both microcapsules and nanocapsules with a careful tuning of process parameters. The choice of a technique not only determines the size but also the morphology and probably the stability expected of the targeted capsules [21]. The choice of technique stems from other parameters such as the physicochemical fingerprint of both shell and core material, the objective of the encapsulation process, the expected release profile/mechanism, the intended application of the final capsules, need for scale up, and of course, processing cost for large scale manufacture. An ideal technique aims at achieving monodispersed capsules with great stability to aggregation, adherence and other destabilizing factors, and high loading and encapsulation efficiency for the cargo. The changing landscape of expectations for drug delivery and other applications is driving the application of more than one encapsulation technique towards achieving goals such as in theragnostic applications. Bazylińska and colleagues [22] combined two encapsulation techniques (**Figure 1**), emulsion solvent evaporation and Layer by layer assembly (LbL) to engineer nanocapsules for dual fluorescence bioimaging and drug delivery.

Encapsulation processes have been classified broadly into physical and chemical techniques. There is no consensus over the third class, physicochemical techniques, and may be because the techniques only take the mechanism of capsule formation into consideration. However, each encapsulation technique involves processing that may involve mechanism not inherent in the name. For instance, emulsion solvent evaporation or in situ polymerization techniques are core chemical techniques but may involve physical processes such as mechanical stirring, homogenization, and sonication in achieving solvent evaporation. **Table 1** outlines the different classification of encapsulation techniques.

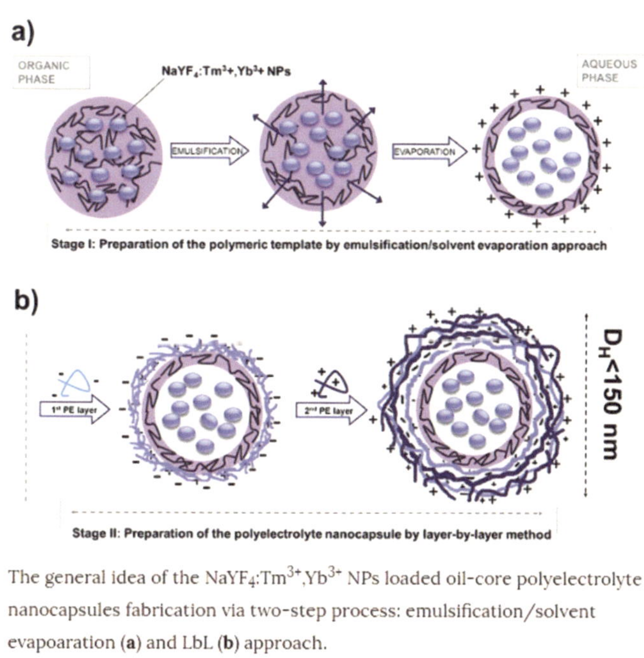

Figure 1.
Combination of two encapsulation techniques for microcapsule formation [22].

Physical/mechanical/thermal techniques				Physicochemical techniques	Chemical techniques
Coating	**Atomization**	**Extrusion**	**Thermal**	**Coacervation**	**Polymerization**
• Pan Coating • Fluid bed coating	• Spinning disc	• Stationary nozzle • Centrifugal extrusion • Vibrating nozzle/annular jet (Coextrusion) • Electrohydrodynamics • Microextrusion • Single or twin screwed extrusion	• Spray drying • Spray chilling • Spray congealing • Phase inversion	• Layer by Layer deposition • Solvent evaporation • Solvent extraction • Molecular inclusion • Sol–gel	• Suspension • Emulsion • Interfacial

Table 1.
Classification of encapsulation techniques.

4.1 Physical encapsulation techniques

Physical/mechanical encapsulation techniques involve formation of micro or nanocapsules by a transformation in the physical attributes of a droplet such as its size or a change from a liquid droplet to a solid droplet. Some steps as discussed below are common to most physical encapsulation techniques.

Atomization: This a process whereby tiny droplets are created from a liquid by dispersion in a gas phase. A range of atomization methods are available and can be adapted to various techniques. These are pressure nozzles, vibrating nozzles, and spinning disc atomizers. There are a variety of archetypes for each.

4.1.1 Spray drying

Spray drying is a widely used encapsulation method that dates to the early fifties. It also serves as a means of microcapsule recovery for many other encapsulation methods. The process involves dispersion of the core material in a solution of the shell material (most commonly water or cosolvents) to form a dispersion, emulsion or suspension [23]. The resulting liquid is fed into the drying chamber at the same time atomized with hot air (nitrogen in rare gases) coming from sonic energy, pressure nozzle, two-fluid nozzle or veined wheel. The solvent is flash evaporated in the hot air stream leaving a free flowing solid of core encapsulated in the shell. It is a simple, flexible encapsulation method that yields consistently distributed particles size between 10 and 40 μm range and is amenable to automation [24]. The first step in the process is to dissolve the shell material in a solvent, most commonly water, and homogenize with the core active ingredient, most commonly hydrophobic. The film forming materials predominantly used in spray drying are hydrophilic natural polymers such as modified starch, gelatin, gum Arabic and maltodextrin. It is not uncommon to use blends of these polymers. The second step is to feed this dispersion into the drying chamber using a sprayer that atomizes it to droplets. Hot air fed into the chamber quickly evaporates the solvent leaving a deposit of the shell forming material around the core droplet. The encapsulated material is then collected through a separator that separates the product from the exhaust air. Even though spray coating is one of the most common and industrialized encapsulation methods particularly for lipids, flavors, aromas and pigment, the process is beset with low thermal efficiency, nozzle clogging, high maintenance cost and product loss [21]. Optimization of process parameters such as inlet temperature, nozzle diameter, liquid feed viscosity and flow rate, gas flow rate, atomization pressure, temperature distribution efficiency and drying rate can minimize negative outcomes in terms of morphology, size and size distribution of the product [25]. Zang and coworkers [26] explored the influence of process parameters on the physical characteristics of tea tree oil microcapsules. They found that there is a need to strike a balance in inlet temperature as an extremely high temperature cracked the microcapsules while an extremely low temperature led to the formation of droplets instead of microcapsules. More recently, Wei and colleagues [27] studied the influence of inlet temperature and precursor concentration among other parameters on the physicochemical properties of theophylline loaded chitosan-triphosphate particles prepared by spray drying. They showed that particle size increased with precursor concentration. In their study, the optimum temperature for making the targeted size of microcapsules was 130° C. Zhang and coworkers [26] found the optimum temperature for their targeted application in the range of 210°C - 215° C buttressing the need for personalizing each process.

4.1.2 Prilling (spray congealing/spray chilling/spray cooling)

This is an encapsulation technique in which a homogenized dispersion of core material in a molten shell material (spray congealing, Prilling) or thermally gelling matrix (spray chilling) is atomized by suspension in a gas phase at ambient or low temperature (usually air or nitrogen (gas or liquid) that causes rapid solidification of the shell material around the core material [28, 29]. When the melting point of the lipophilic matrix is above 45° C, solidification is brought about at ambient temperature in a spray cooling process but for matrixes with lower melting point, frozen gases are used, and the process known as two major steps are involved firstly of which is creating free falling drops from molten solid, strong solutions or slurries using spinning discs and baskets. The second is solidifying the drops individually in a countercurrent of cold air. The size of each droplet determines the final size of each sphere. The resulting encapsulates of this high productivity, grossly monodispersity technique are microspheres with sizes in the range of 60 to 2000 μm [28]. Prilling is a high throughput, relatively inexpensive, easy-to-operate technique that has found extensive use in the fertilizer industry. When used for food encapsulation, the process is limited by the possibility of granule agglomeration due to high temperatures. Most used shell materials are lipids, waxes, fats and gelling hydrocolloids. Russo and colleagues [30] recently explored the possibility of combining Zn and Ca cations as an ionic gelation agents for prednisolone encapsulated alginate beads developed with the Prilling technique. The calcium carbonate decomposed internally in the acidic environment releasing a gas that increased porosity of the microcapsules ultimately translating to buoyancy in the gastrointestinal fluid and extended hours of anti-inflammatory effect.

4.1.3 Coating

Coating as an encapsulation technique involves the deposition of a thin film of membrane around a solid particle or a liquid adsorbed onto a solid. Two approaches have been used. The traditional older pan coating and the air suspension coating or fluid bed coating.

Pan coating: Pan coating is old coating technique that dates to the 18th century and traditionally used for applying sugar and film coats to tablets and pellets measuring several millimeters. In encapsulation, it is generally used for core material measuring above 600 μm [31]. The process involves the application of a coating solution through a spray unto the granule bed in a rotating coating pan inclined at an angle and fitted on the inside with anti-slip bars or angled blade that enable circulation of the core material. Warm or room temperature air is continually introduced and removed through exhaust pipes to facilitate the drying of the coating solution. Coating pans can be conventional or vented with perforations that allow for the escape of the drying air through the powder bed [32].

Air suspension technique: This technique also known as fluid bed coating is the gold standard in coating. The core material is suspended in a stream of hot or ambient air (depending on the coating solution) in relation to a coating spray that can be applied in the same direction as the fluidized air, tangentially or in opposite direction. **Figure 2** shows the application from the bottom of the chamber also known as the Wurster set up. The air suspension technique has also been used for both drying and granulation. For encapsulation purposes, a powder bed is initially fluidized by a jet of hot or ambient air. Subsequently, a coating solution of the shell material is sprayed through an atomizing nozzle onto the fluidized particles depositing a coat, consequent to the evaporation of the solvent, on individual particles

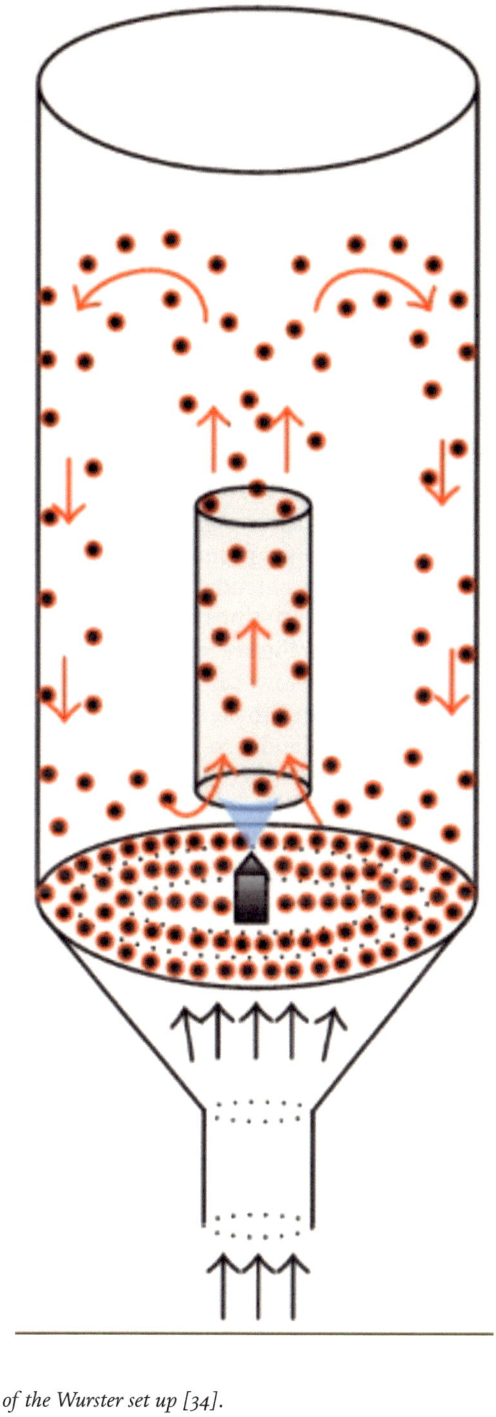

Figure 2.
Schematic representation of the Wurster set up [34].

as they get to the top of the chamber. The exhaust air passes through a filter to the outside while the particles recycle to the base of the chamber and the coating cycle continues till adequately coated. Almost any type of wall material can be applied in the Wurster process [33]. The particle size ranges from less than 100 μm to 150 μm [24]. Uniformity of the coat and the size of the capsules depend on the size and type of spraying nozzle. The viscosity of the coating liquid, air inlet temperature and flow rate must be optimized for each application.

4.1.4 Extrusion

Generally, extrusion is a process in which a material is subjected to some form of compression that bring about a change in its physical properties as it is pushed through the orifice or die of an extruder, that is made up of one or two screws, under controlled conditions [35]. The core material is blended with the polymeric shell material in a molecular mixing to form a solid dispersion or solution. The solid dispersion is then passed through extruders to produce submicron capsules. A variety of extruders and nozzles configuration exists for different applications.

Extrusion-spheronisation: In this technique, the core material is intimately combined with the shell material and extruded into cylindrical mass that is subsequently broken up and rounded into spheres [36]. Muley and coworkers [36] described a variety of extruders to include sieve, basket, ram, screw and roll extruders.

Hot melt extrusion (HME): This continuous process technique originated for the food, plastic and rubber industries in the early nineteenth century but was applied much later in the pharmaceutical industry for product development and manufacturing of poorly soluble drugs. It involves pumping polymeric material that serves as the shell and the API through screw extruders at temperatures above their glass transition or gelling (and sometimes, melting) temperature to achieve molecular mixing of the component as shown in **Figure 3** [37].

The rotating screw pushes the feed towards the orifice whilst generating frictional heat that increases the viscosity of the feed as it melts. The extrudate is shaped by passing through a flake forming calendar roll or a pellet forming rotary knives, traveling shears or saws as it leaves the orifice. Materials capable of HME processing must be capable of deformation inside the extruder and individually capable of physically and chemically withstanding high temperatures. Waxes find extensive use as inert carrier materials for HME process. Starches, sugars, and sugar alcohols have also been used. Plasticizers such as acetic acid, stearic acid, citric acid, salicylic acid and triethyl citrate are used to alleviate the temperature effects in the HME process.

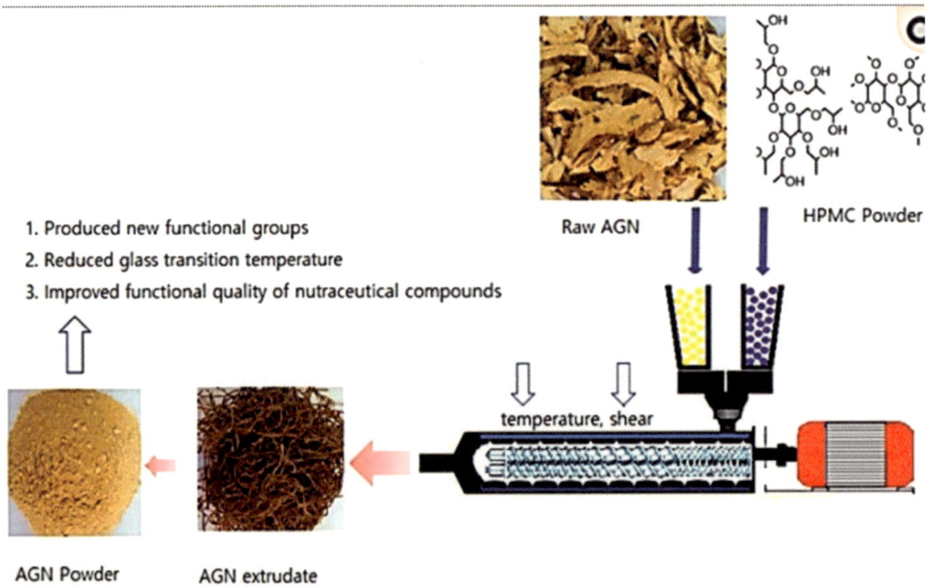

Figure 3.
A schematic diagram of the hot melt extrusion process used in the encapsulation of Angelica gigas Nakai (AGN) [38].

Gately and colleague [39] explored the possibility of using a natural polymer, shellac as a low temperature extrudable polymer in the encapsulation of a probiotic powder. They found that not only was it possible, but the probiotic powder had an additional plasticizing effect on the extrudates. Melt extrusion and its earlier variant, melt injection has found extensive use as an encapsulation technique especially for fragrances and flavors due to the lower energy requirement, minimal emission of odor fouled exhaust, no requirement for solvent, and possibility for large volume encapsulation [40]. In addition, extrusion encapsulations impart longer stability on flavors and lower degradation for enzymes, when compared to other encapsulation methods like spray drying [39]. Glassy carbohydrates, polysaccharides, proteins and their blends have all been used as carrier polymers for melt extrusion encapsulated flavors [41]. Carnauba wax was also recently used for melt encapsulation of Quercetin [42].

4.1.5 Coextrusion

Coextrusion is a variation of the extrusion technique that involves two concentric nozzles through which the core and shell material are extruded individually and exiting the nozzle as a single drop of core material encapsulated in the shell. It is designed primarily for liquid materials and the process schematically represented in **Figure 4**. The core material and the shell material do not mix unlike in the extrusion technique. The liquid shell material is pumped through the outer nozzle while the core material is extruded through the inner nozzle. The stream of liquid forms a laminar that is broken into discrete drops of the core enveloped by the shell. The drops are received in a curing liquid that hardens the encapsulated product [43]. It has been shown that coextrusion encapsulation technique offers better protection against instability in encapsulated aroma oils than extrusion technique [44].

Additionally, extrusion yields matrix spheres in which there is an intimate mixture between the shell and the core. Whereas in coextrusion, the core is separated from and covered by the shell. Sodium alginate has extensively been used as a shell

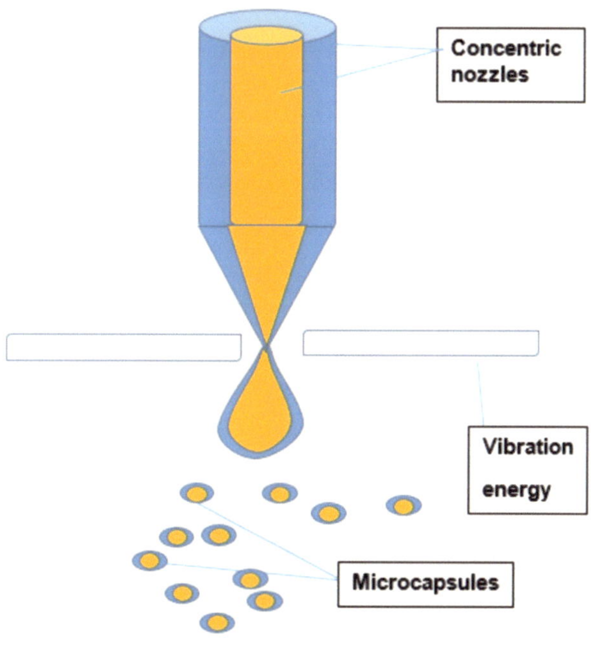

Figure 4.
Schematic representation of the co-extrusion technique.

forming polymer which is usually cured by ionic interactions with divalent cations. Silva and colleagues [44] compared the extrusion technique with co-extrusion for the encapsulation of probiotic, *Lactobacillus acidophilus* LA3 using a blend of alginate and shellac. They found that co-extrusion using sunflower oil as a carrier for the probiotic provided additional stability.

Centrifugal extrusion: This variation of co-extrusion is a liquid extrusion technique that makes use of a spinning extrusion head that carries the concentric nozzles. The concentric feeding tube serves as a tributary to the many concentric nozzles located at the surface of the device. As the spinning head rotates, the inner core and the outer shell material are extruded in flow that break into droplets as it makes its way from the nozzles (**Figure 5**). The particle size of extrudates can be as small as 150 μm. The particles harden by solvent evaporation as they take flight from the device.

4.1.6 Techniques based on drop generation method

Mechanical means are used for droplets generation during co-extrusion and has given rise to many modern encapsulation techniques. These all depend on the dripping and jet break up principle for droplet generation at an orifice or from a laminar jet. A droplet that forms at an orifice and is discharged is a result of a formation process that depends on the interplay of surface tension of the extruded liquid, velocity of extrusion, gravitational force, impulse and frictional forces. Configurations for droplet generation are based on five mechanisms.

A. At extremely low velocity, single droplet form at the orifice. The drop detaches under gravity as gravity overcomes surface tension and frictional forces.

B. As the velocity increases, the number of drops ejected from the orifice increases marginally, leading to increased coalescence and polydispersity of the drops.

C. Co-axial flow: A higher increase in velocity results in the formation of a continuous liquid laminar jet that breaks by surface tension and axial symmetrical vibration.

D. Further increase in velocity causes normal distribution of droplets because of spiral symmetrical vibrations.

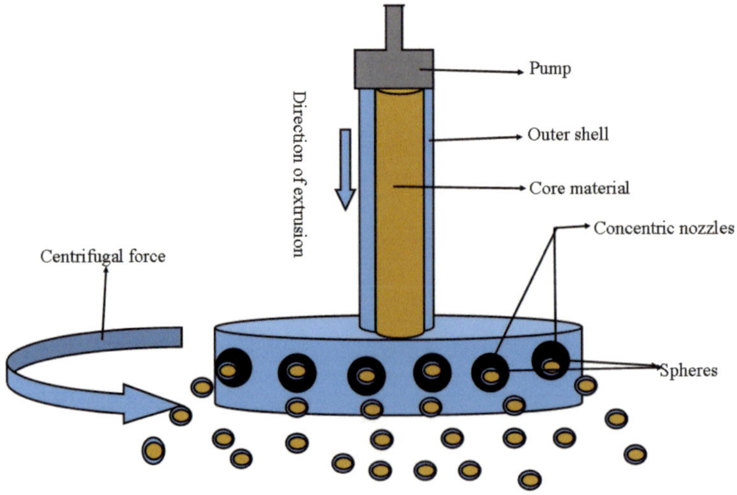

Figure 5.
A schematic representation of the centrifugal extrusion device.

E. C could also result in droplet formation because of high frictional forces when a jet is sprayed.

Encapsulation methods based on these mechanisms and on the droplet generation method are elucidated below.

Vibrating nozzle/jet: This encapsulation technique, commercialized by Inotech Biotechnoly Ltd. and Nisco Ltd., makes use of permanent vibrational or sinusoidal frequencies of definite amplitude to break up a laminar jet into equally sized droplets stabilized by electrostatic repulsion and achieved by application of an electric field [45]. Two variations are the vibrating nozzle and the vibrating chamber techniques. The size distribution of the droplets is narrow and the size generated with a given amplitude is in the range of 0.10–1.50 mm and depends on the nozzle diameter, jet velocity, rheology and surface tension of the liquid [46]. It is predominantly used in cell immobilization with Newtonian systems. Dorati and coworkers undertook an assessment of the vibrating nozzle technique combined with freeze drying technique in the encapsulation of a model hydrophilic molecules in a hydrophilic polymer, alginate. They concluded that vibrating nozzle technique is an easy and scalable process for microencapsulation of hydrophilic drugs [47].

Simple dripping: This simple method involves the free formation of a droplet at the orifice. The drop continues to increase in volume until the weight of the liquid just exceed the capillary force. The drop detaches and forms a sphere due to surface tension. This method of low droplet production rate is mostly applicable to laboratory encapsulation with droplets sizes approximately 1000 μm. It has found use in microfluidic devices and in porous membranes such as Shirasu porous glass in which high pressure is applied to cause the droplet generation of a disperse phase directly into the continuous phase held in the membrane [48]. These membranes are used for generation of emulsions and mini emulsions on a lab scale. The membrane pore size directly controls the droplet size. The membranes are hydrophilic and therefore, favors oil-in- water emulsions formation. For an oil continuous phase, there may be a need to coat the membrane using silicone resins [46].

Generally, in microfluidic devices, several configurations are obtainable for droplet generation and include co-flowing, T-junction and fluid focusing [49]. The fluid focusing configuration is particularly advantageous since it is passive and droplet generation and cell encapsulation depends on hydrodynamically pumping fluid adjacent to an outflowing cell and can therefore prove useful for sensitive materials such as living cells for probiotics [46, 50]. In fluid focusing, the focused fluid (disperse phase) is introduced into a capillary tube enclosed in a chamber containing the focusing fluid (carrier/continuous phase) which exerts pressure on the focused fluid as it exits the orifice facing the feeding tube. The pressure exerted on the disperse phase, compounded by fluid instabilities, is sufficient to cause it to break into droplets as it squeezes pass the orifice [51]. The droplet size of the internal phase does not depend on the orifice diameter. Device geometry, fluid properties and the process parameters such as flow rate and pressure drop determine what happens as the internal phase emerges.

For microencapsulation applications requiring the generation of microsized droplets of narrow size distribution, it is important that these parameters be tuned such that the carrier phase acts as micro tweezers that pressure the tip of the disperse phase meniscus at the orifice causing it to break into a microjet that eventually breaks into homogenous small droplets [52]. Microfluidic devices have found application in the facile preparation of double emulsions.

Spinning disc: In this technique, also known as centrifugal suspension separation, drops are generated when coated particles are flung off a rotating disc by the generated centrifugal force. The core material usually in solid form is suspended in a viscous coating liquid and poured on top of the rotating disc. The suspension spreads out to form a thin film on the disc and subsequently gathers momentum as it moves towards the edge of the disc. At the edge, the droplets hold unto the rim due to interfacial tension and viscosity. It is detached when the centrifugal force overcomes the interfacial tension. The drop is detached an angle to the disc and to a distance from the disc depending on their size. This separation by distance traveled as per size is used to sort different size ranges enabling the collection of monodispersed capsules in the solidifying chamber. The rotary speed and geometry of the disc, alongside the viscosity of the suspension and the feed flow rate determine the size of the droplet which usually ranges from 1 to 200 μm [45].

Spinning disc method represented in **Figure 6**, is an easily scalable method for producing large quantities of spherical beads with a narrow size distribution, using liquids of varying viscosities, in minutes. However, product recovery usually requires large space for the gelling bath which makes sterilization difficult. Even though it is amenable to continuous manufacturing, it is expensive comparatively. The coating materials are usually meltable waxes, diglycerides that solidify on cooling.

Electrospraying (Electrohydrodynamic atomization)/Electrospinning: This technique of droplet generation depends on electrohydrodynamics which deals with interaction of fluid and electric field. Electrospraying depends on the principle of charged droplet which states that when an electric field is applied to a drop of liquid, it acquires an electrostatic force which competes with the cohesive force due to surface tension. If this coulomb force is large enough to overcome the surface tension force, the drop detaches and breaks up into submicron droplets which quickly solidify into self-dispersing nano and micro capsules with limited agglomeration and

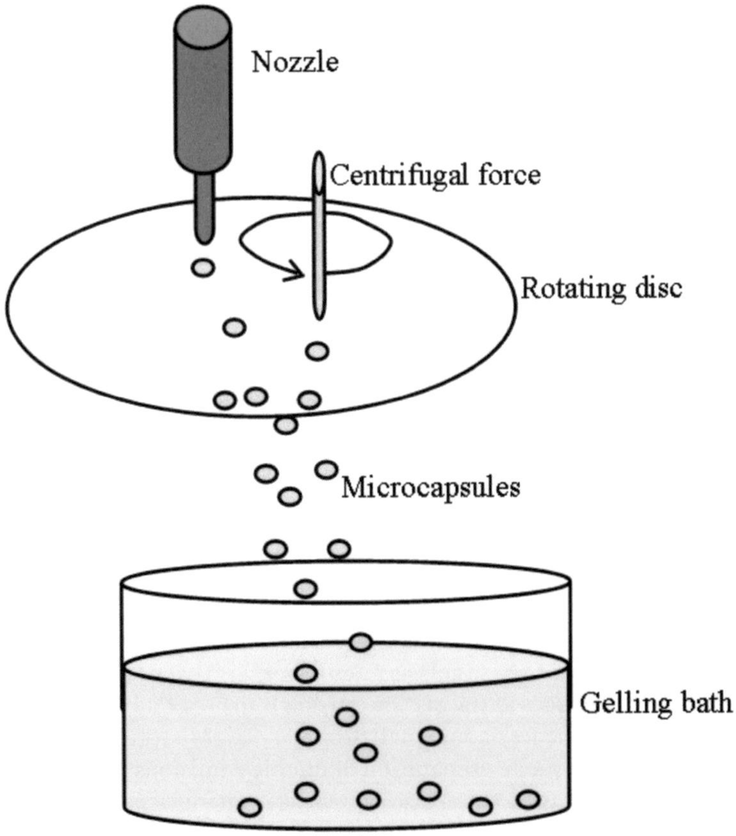

Figure 6.
Schematic representation of the spinning disc assembly.

coagulation. The technique just like its better applied counterpart, electrospinning, is a facile relatively inexpensive, flexible, easy-to set-up and versatile (in terms of processable materials, set up configuration) process that is amenable to continuous manufacture of tunable compositions, and customized properties of size, and morphology [53]. Droplet generation starts with pushing the liquid in the syringe to flow through the nozzle to the metallic capillary which is connected to the collector through a voltage generating unit. As the liquid passes the electric field, electric charges are inducted leading to the formation of a conically shaped lower meniscus (also known as the Taylor's cone) at which tip the acquired charges are concentrated as a result of equilibrium between capillary forces and electrodynamics [54]. The liquid then accelerates away from the nozzle in a tiny thread tip leading to formation of a jet with high charge density. What happens next determines whether electrospinning or electrospraying will occur. The former occurs if the jet experiences sufficiently high axial tension such that the jet undergoes a whipping instability and elongates to reach the collector instead of breaking up. This high axial tension usually results from a high concentration of high molecular weight polymers. Alternatively, the liquid jet breaks up into primary droplets that could experience the so-called Coulombs fission on their way to the collector. This occurs due to solvent evaporation, droplet shrinkage and subsequent break up again into submicron encapsulation due to charge density. Subsequent break ups that could lead to polydispersity could be prevented by a secondary voltage set up known as corona neutralizer.

Other electrospraying modes, other than the Taylor's cone, is possible as the applied voltage gradually increases. The dripping mode gives way to micro dripping, then spindle, Taylor cone jet, and multiplet mode. Obtaining a continuous jet is important for determining the droplet size and morphology which depends on interplay of factors related to the polymer liquid such as density, concentration, surface tension, conductivity [55], molecular weight, viscosity and solvent; and process parameters such as gravity, applied voltage, flow rate, capillary diameter, and distance of the collector from the capillary tip [56]. Among natural polymers that have been applied in electrospraying are chitosan, cellulose and alginate [57].

Different configurations have been used in electrospraying due to the wide range of factors that needs optimization for droplet size and morphology. One of these is the coaxial assembly which uses two concentric capillaries, the inner and the outer for pushing two different liquid compositions. A typical coaxial set up is shown in **Figure 7**. Shams and colleagues [58] developed pH responsive prednisolone loaded Eudragit L100–55 microparticles for colon specific delivery using single and coaxial electrospraying. In vitro assessment of the five developed formulations showed that careful selection of polymeric system alongside process parameters in electrospraying technique can yield site specific delivery.

Yuan and colleagues [59] also used the coaxial electrospray assembly in the fabrication of curcumin-loaded microcapsules aimed at improving the release profile of curcumin. The improved coaxial electrospray was able to generate stable Taylor's cone mode under a variety of operating condition that yielded an obvious core-shell structure of targeted size and morphology [59]. Likewise, Gómez-Mascaraque and colleagues [60], for the first time, encapsulated probiotic, *Lactobacillus plantarium* with a whey protein inner core and a gelatin outer shell using acetic acid as an external gelling agent. They found that the application of high voltage alongside the presence of acetic acid negatively impacted the viability of the probiotic [60].

Another configuration that has been explored to overcome the low throughput of the stable Taylor's cone mode in electrospray is the multiple capillary assembly. Though not without challenges, Parhizkar and colleagues [55] designed and tested two multiple needle electrospraying geometries with each consisting of four needles. The challenge was to operate all four needles at stable cone mode. Higher particles

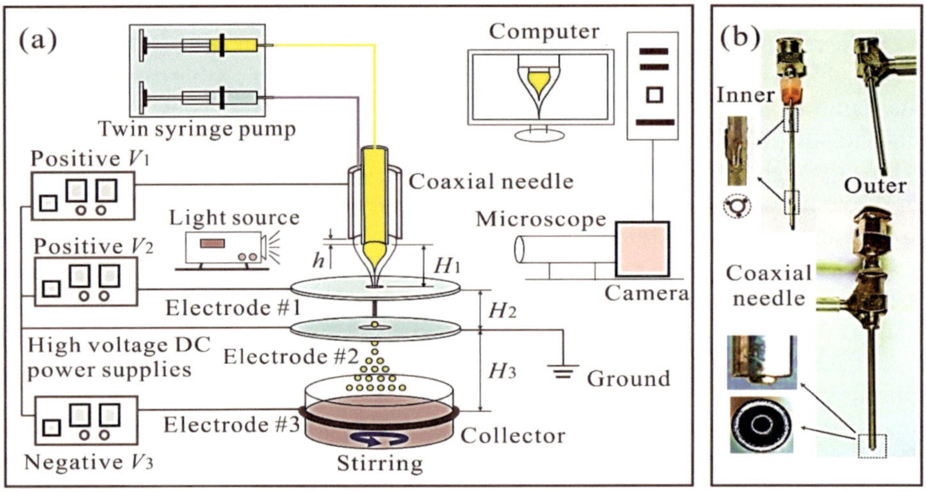

Figure 7.
(a) Coaxial assembly for electrospraying. (b) Inner and outer coaxial needles [59].

recovery rate was recorded for the assemble comparatively for the same collection time with no significant changes in size and morphology [55]. Also, Lee and coworkers [61] designed functionable poly-styrene-random-glycidyl methacrylate that was used to fabricate microparticles via electrospraying. They further studied the influence of both polymer factors and process parameters on the size and morphology of the fabricated microparticles. Their results showed that polymer structure and properties can be used to tune the structural parameters of the capsules [61].

Jet cutting method for droplet generation: This technique commercialized by geniaLab is a rarely used but cost effective technique that depends on a set of cutting wires that serve as a cutting tool for a jet of liquid as it rotates about its axis to generate uniformly sized droplets that is shaped as a result of surface tension. It is suited for cutting high viscosity liquids that harden on cooling or by ionotropic gelation. The drops generated are generally in the size range of 120 μm to 3 mm. Paulo and colleagues [62] recently x-rayed the process parameters requisite for the generation of optimally suited calcium alginate beads using the jet cutter. A maximum flow rate of 49 mL/minute yielded beads of about 2 mm size. Increasing the rotational speed of the cutter decreased the bead size by 50% though increased the tangential velocity of the droplets leading to a larger space requirement for product collection [62]. Other parameters such as gravitational force, surface tension, viscosity and flow rate were also noted. A major limitation is the cutting loss occurring with each cut of the liquid jet.

4.1.7 Phase inversion

Phase inversion and separation occurs in a system due to mass transfer. Usually, for phase inversion to be induced, a polymer solution is exposed to a miscible non-solvent. When a polymer solution is exposed to its non-solvent, the solvent molecules would move out of the polymer while the non-solvent will move in. The first step in the process is to dissolve a polymer in its solvent. The second step is to cast the polymer solution. The third step is to initiate phase separation by immersion of the cast polymer in a coagulation bath containing the non-solvent. Other methods that have been used to induce phase separation is non-solvent vapor [63]. Ammendola and colleagues [63] used the phase inversion technique to prepare fragrance loaded cellulose acetate microcapsules. They then compared the vapor induced phase separation with immersion induced phase separation. Their study showed that the relatively uncommon vapor induced phase separation yielded microcapsules with more controllable characteristics in terms of structure.

4.2 Encapsulation techniques based on chemical mechanisms

Chemical methods of encapsulation generally depend on chemical interactions for encapsulation to occur. These involve predominantly polymerization reactions involving monomer dispersions. The major chemical methods are interfacial polymerization, interfacial polycondensation polymerization, emulsion polymerization and in-situ polymerization.

4.2.1 Interfacial polymerization

In this technique, the wall material is made to form at the oil-in-water interface of dispersed oil drops. Monomers of the wall forming polymer (usually multi-functional) is first dissolved in the core material and then emulsified in the aqueous continuous phase containing other polymerization reactant. Polymerization ensues right after on both sides of the interface of the dispersed oil drops with water leading to the formation of rigid capsule walls [64]. Particle sizes as low as 3 μm can be achieved though most commercialized capsules from this technique are in the range of 20–60 μm. This technique can also be employed for reverse emulsions. The polymerization occurs across the interface of the droplets. Four major groups of polymers have been employed and include polyamides, polyurea, polyurethane and polyesters in applications that spans the fields of agriculture, pharmaceutics, cosmetics, and energy storage materials. Interfacial polymerization is a well-controlled technique capable of delivering targeted sizes and morphology. An interfacial polymerization approach has been developed that makes use of safer polymers for cosmetic and internal use is the transacylation interfacial polymerization. In this approach, biodegradable oligosaccharides, polysaccharides such as acacia; and polyethylene glycol, and alginate are used in the internal and external phases respectively or vice versa. On mixing the two phases, acacia reacts with the carboxylic acid group of the propylene glycol leading to the overall attachment of alginate and release of polyethylene glycol. The operational shell material is made up of acacia-alginate polymer that does not require further crosslinking [65].

4.2.2 In-situ polymerization

This technique is very much like interfacial polymerization. The difference is that the polymerization occurs entirely in the one phase. This term includes suspension polymerization, emulsion polymerization, and dispersion polymerization. In a typical process, the wall forming monomer or pre-polymer is dissolved in the continuous phase and used to emulsify the external phase under high pressure homogenization. Thereafter, an initiator for polycondensation soluble in the continuous phase is added to initiate polycondensation. Acids are normally added to reduce pH and trigger polycondensation which leads to crosslinking and the deposition of crosslinked wall material round the oil drops [66]. Material used, stirring speed, pH, and curing temperature are some of the factors for optimization. Urea-formaldehyde and melamine—formaldehyde are well known examples developed with this method. Ishizuka and colleagues [67] recently prepared microcapsules by this technique with an amphiphilic macro RAFT wall material they synthesized. Their procedure eliminated the use of toxic solvents. The wall monomer was introduced into the rice bran oil continuous phase which was then emulsified with the aqueous phase containing sodium chloride in a shirasu porous glass membrane.

The crosslinkers, ethyleneglycoldimethacrylate, was added to the formed emulsion to bring about polymerization [67].

Emulsion polymerization: In this procedure, the core material is dissolved in a surfactant. The monomer solution is then added to it dropwise.

Dispersion polycondensation: In the category, all the components including the monomer, the dispersant and the initiator are present in a solvent in which the polymer to be formed is insoluble. Here, swelling of the polymer occur leading to growth of microcapsules which is sustained by continued addition of monomer and oligomer [68]. Jiang and colleagues [69] used this method to prepare a core shell for site specific delivery of a small molecule, doxorubicin and a protein drug, TRAIL, for cancer therapy.

Suspension polymerization: In this approach, the monomers used are insoluble in the continuous phase hence, they are dispersed as liquid droplets, in the aqueous phase, in the presence of a stabilizer using high pressure homogenization. The polymer is obtained as dispersed solid in the continuous phase. Racoti and coworkers [70] recently used suspension polymerization for the microencapsulation of ginger oil in polymethyl methacrylate shell using triethyleneglycol dimethachrylate as a monomer and Azobisisobutyronitrile (AIBN) as initiator. Their study showed that particle size increased with initiator concentration while encapsulation efficiency decreased with increasing oil concentration.

4.3 Physicochemical techniques

The physicochemical techniques discussed here are classified as chemical methods by some authors. However, they are classified as physicochemical techniques here because each technique involves one or two physical steps. Such techniques are solvent evaporation, coacervation, layer by layer deposition and liposomes.

4.3.1 Solvent evaporation

The first step is the dispersion of the core material in the coating solution to form an oil-in-water emulsion. The mixture is then homogenized in the presence of stabilizers such as polyvinyl alcohol (PVA), tween 80 and span 80 to obtain appropriately sized microcapsules. The last step is to evaporate the solvent off either at ambient or elevated temperatures depending on the solvent. For double emulsion solvent evaporation, the formed oil-in-water emulsion is emulsified again, homogenized before solvent evaporation [71]. The type of emulsion chosen will be dependent on the lipophilicity or hydrophilicity of the core material. Double emulsions of the w/o/w type are usually used for highly hydrophilic materials in order to improve their encapsulation efficiency and limit their diffusion out of the capsule into the continuous phase of oil-in-water emulsions [71]. Another approach that has been used for hydrophilic payloads is the suspension in organic phase template [72]. Solvent evaporation is the common method for preparing nanoparticles. Hoa and coworkers [73] prepared PVA stabilized ketoprofen loaded Eudragit E100-Eudragit RS nanoparticles using the solvent evaporation method. They studied effect of process and formulation parameters on the properties of the nanoparticles. They confirmed that the size and morphology of the particles depended on polymer and surfactant concentration, power and duration of applied energy, and volume ratio of water to oil phases. More recently, Jiang and colleagues [74] developed nanoparticles of Ginkoglide using solvent evaporation method. Likewise, Urbaniak and Musial [72], using solvent evaporation technique, prepared submicron sized capsules from lamivudine conjugated poly-ε-caprolactone polymer and studied the influencing parameters such as concentration and type, homogenization time and rate on the particle size. Surfactant concentration and homogenization rate were identified as the most important factors affecting particle size. Solvent evaporation method is advantageous in that it limits the use of toxic solvents, proceeds rapidly yielding particles in the size range of 10–100 nm.

4.3.2 Nanoprecipitation

This technique also known as solvent displacement technique was patented by Fessi in 1989 [75] for making nanospheres and nanocapsules. It has close resemblance to solvent evaporation technique. Here, the solvent phase containing the film forming polymer, and the drug to be encapsulated is a water miscible solvent such as acetone or methanol, and the non-solvent phase which is a water immiscible solvent such as chloroform or dichloromethane, also called the oil phase, are mixed under stirring. Thereafter, the solvent is removed to yield nanoparticles suspension or nanocapsules if a mineral oil was added. Centrifuging and freeze drying will yield the powder. Chitosan, starch, and gelatin are among the commonly used natural polymer film formers. Many studies have tried to analyze the difference in nanoparticles generated by solvent evaporation and solvent displacement. Hernández-Giottonini and colleagues [76] evaluated the effect of process parameters and formulation parameters on polylactic-co-glycolic acid (PLGA) nanoparticles prepared by both techniques. While particle size was dominantly affected by PLGA and PVA concentrations for the nanoprecipitation method, solvent fraction had the most effect of the particle size for the solvent evaporation technique. However, the influence of agitation speed in both techniques was the same- a decrease in average particle diameter [76].

4.3.3 Coacervation

This technique involves the phase separation of one or more hydrocolloids from its initial solution brought about by changes such as pH, ionic strength, temperature, solvent type or polarity and the subsequent deposition of the separated coacervate on the core droplets in the solution [77]. The lower particle diameter obtainable from simple coacervation is 20 μm while that for complex coacervation is 1 μm; and 500 μm capsules are also possible from both [33]. Generally, the first step in any coacervation process is the dispersion of the oil phase in the solution of the hydrocolloid (formation of oil-in-water emulsion). The next step involves the precipitation of the hydrocolloid by temperature, polarity, pH, or ionic strength change (polyelectrolyte complex formation). This is usually achieved by addition of a salt such as sodium sulphate, or desolvation with water miscible non-solvent, in simple coacervation [78]. Induction of polymer-polymer gelling by addition of a second oppositely charged hydrocolloid happens only in complex coacervation. The resulting complex is stabilized by cross-linking (usually glutaraldehyde, transglutaminase, calcium ions or tripolyphosphate) and the harvested microcapsules washed and dried. Complex coacervation is advantageous due to the high loading of payload up to 99%. From the relatively simple and early use of pork skin gelatin and gum arabic, many other variations have emerged including patented deviations. Majority of the polymers used are natural polysaccharides such as starches, maltodextrins, and gum arabic; and proteins such as albumin, gelatin, and casein; and lipids such as diglycerides [77].

Brito de Souza and coworkers [79] used complex coacervation as a tool to protect the phenolic compounds and mask the astringent taste of spray dried hydrophilic proanthocyanidins-rich cinnamon using a combination of various polysaccharides and gelatin as the coacervate wall material. They also evaluated the stability of the microcapsules under various storage conditions. Their study showed that gelatin/k-carrageenan and gelatin/cashew tree gum were exceptional in maintaining the stability of the microcapsules as wall material. Complex coacervation using these combinations enabled the efficient use of proanthocyanidins-rich cinnamon extract in ice cream formulation while keeping the taste masked [79]. Lemos and colleagues [80] evaluated the effect of homogenizing speed and the hydrodynamics int. coacervation medium on the carotenoid rich Buriti oil microcapsules formulated using gelatin-alginate wall material. They found that as the Reynold number increased beyond 70,000, the particle size reduced to 200 μm. With about 80% encapsulation efficiency, the hydrodynamic conditions affected the particle size of the complex coacervates [80].

4.3.4 Layer by layer (LbL) deposition

This encapsulation technique is a straightforward versatile technique that involves the serial alternate deposition of oppositely charged polyelectrolytes films on a colloidal particle used commonly as a sacrificial template that is later eliminated or calcined. The technique permits the assembly of different compounds that interact through primary electrostatic interactions, though other bonds such as dipole–dipole moment, hydrogen bonds, host-guest interaction, acid–base interaction, and Van der Waals forces are possible. In the preparation of LbL capsules, layers have been deposited by dipping, spraying, and spin coating with the polyelectrolyte [81]. It is important to wash with distilled water after each layer deposition to minimize cross contamination by polyelectrolytes. Parameters that require monitoring include number of deposition cycles, ionic strength, pH, polyelectrolyte concentration to tune the thickness, roughness and porosity of the product [82]. Both nanocapsules and microcapsules can be prepared by this technique. The availability of wide permeability coefficient spectrum permits tuning to achieve specific application targets which could be biosensing, drug delivery, bioreactor, or biogenic application. With careful selection of the layering material, and assembly conditions final properties of the capsule can be determined. A major drawback is the lengthy fabrication process though this has drastically been reduced by the spraying approach [81]. Piccinino and colleagues [83] prepared micro- and nanocapsules of mixed polyphenols, tannic acid and sulfonate lignin using Manganese carbonate ($MnCO_3$) and organosolv lignin nanoparticles as a template and polydiallyldimethylammonium chloride and chitosan as supporting layers. The prepared nano and microcapsules displayed good antioxidant activity and photo-shielding and electrochemical responsiveness that was higher than that possible from the individual homopolymers. Rochín-Wong and coworkers [84] recently developed a LbL assembly of two natural polymers, κ-carrageenan and chitosan on diflunisal nanoemulsion droplets with the aim of studying the release properties. They reported the formation of stable 300 nm-sized particles that demonstrated controlled released of diflunisal in proportion to the number of adsorbed layers. Paşcalău and colleagues [85] recently developed Sorafenib nanocapsules using the LbL deposition. They initially co-precipitated bovine serum, BSA, with the sacrificial calcium carbonate ($CaCO_3$) porous templates to form the BSA gel core microtemplate. The microtemplate was then coated Ca^{2+} crosslinked hyaluronic acid hydrogel and subsequently alternated with chitosan in a multilayer assembly. Subsequently, the sacrificial template was removed through a semipermeable membrane and the BSA thermo-gelled. The sorafenib was then loaded into the microcapsule by diffusion to yield a delivery system that was thermo-responsive.

4.3.5 Supercritical fluids (SCF)

This technique involves the use of SCFs which are substances that exist above their critical temperature and pressure (at this point they exist in single phase and exhibit properties of both gases and liquids) and therefore can diffuse through solids like a gas would and dissolve solids and liquids like a liquid. They exhibit densities close to that of a liquid but with viscosities and diffusion coefficients like that of a gas as shown in **Figure 8**. Supercritical carbon dioxide is the commonly used SCF for encapsulation because it is cheap, easily available, inert, non-toxic, uninflammable, with low critical temperature of 31.06°C. The technique may involve supercritical CO_2 ($SCCO_2$) as a solvent, antisolvent, co-solvent, or nebulizer. The process generally involves dissolution of both the core material and wall material in the SCF. Then, the solution is released through a small nozzle and the rapid reduction in pressure caused desolvation and deposition of polymer material shell on the core.

Approaches using $SCCO_2$ as a solvent involves rapid expansion of a supercritical solution (RESS) as shown in **Figure 9**. In this process, components are dissolved in $SCCO_2$ and the solution is then released into a collector through tiny nozzles at atmospheric pressure. The rapid decrease in pressure brings about the desolvation of $SCCO_2$

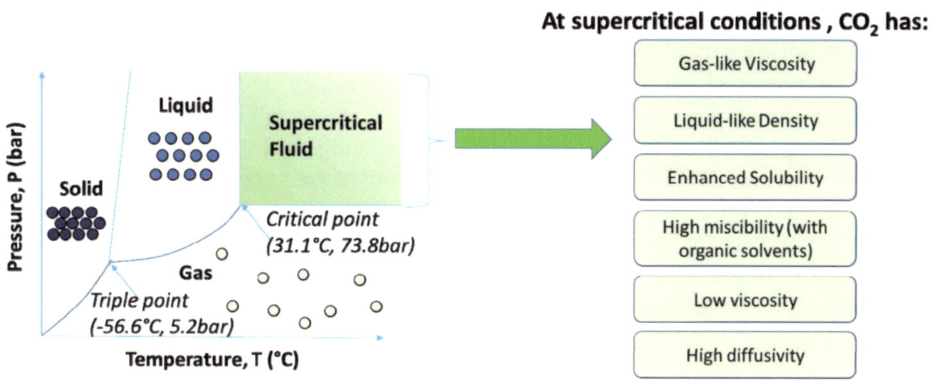

Figure 8.
Phase diagram of $SCCO_2$ (not to scale) [86].

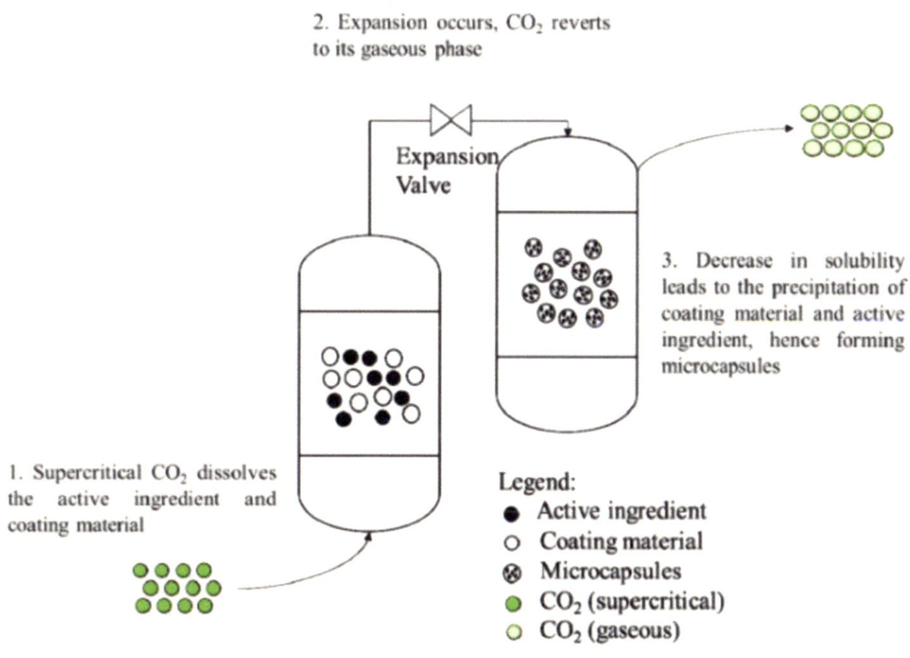

Figure 9.
Schematic representation of the RESS process [86].

and the solution components deposited as submicron particles. The major setback is that many polymer materials, fats, and encapsulants are poorly soluble in $SCCO_2$.

Another approach is the antisolvent gas, GAS approach (**Figure 10**). In this approach, the components of microcapsules are dissolved in a suitable (primary) organic solvent and then introduced into $SCCO_2$ which reduces the solubility of the components in the organic solvent. $SCCO_2$ does this by rapidly permeating through the solution due to its high diffusion coefficient effecting a mass transfer process that is evidenced by increase in volume, decrease in viscosity and density. Decrease in density significantly reduces the solubility of the components in the solvent, producing a supersaturated solution from which the components precipitate as micro and nano particles. The solutes used in this process must have minimal solubility in $SCCO_2$. The GAS technique is advantageous for the encapsulation of polar compounds and compounds not soluble in $SCCO_2$ using organic solvents may leave worrisome traces in the capsules.

The third approach is particles from gas saturated solution, PGSS, (**Figure 11**) that depends on the high solubility of $SCCO_2$ in materials such as molten fats, lipids and polymers at relatively low pressures, and the cooling effect of depressurization (Joule- Thompson effect). In this procedure, $SCCO_2$ is introduced into a substrate, its suspension or solution in an organic solvent at high pressure. The resulting saturated solution is rapidly expanded through a tiny nozzle using moderate pressure which leads to reduction in temperature and the formation of particles due to the cooling effect. Zhu and colleagues [87] encapsulated menthol in beeswax using the PGSS.

Equipment required for SCF encapsulation include a compressed $SCCO_2$ cylinder, two high pressure liquid pumps for $SCCO_2$ and the other solvents, high pressure chambers, product separation units, liquefying units, recirculating pumps, manometers, in-line filters, thermocouples, and a host of others. Parameters that needs to be optimized for each application include temperature, pressure, and feed emulsion rate. Karim and coworkers [88] used the GAS process to microencapsulate fish oil using a semi synthetic polymer, ethyl cellulose.

4.3.6 Sol: Gel technique

Translated literally means solution gelling and basically refers to an encapsulation method involving solutions (sol) that transform to a gel in response to alternating

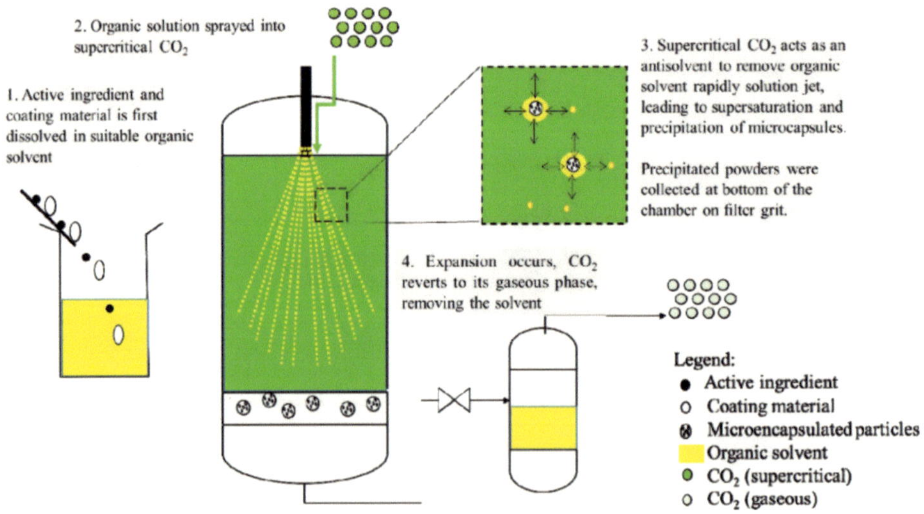

Figure 10.
Schematic representation of the GAS process [86].

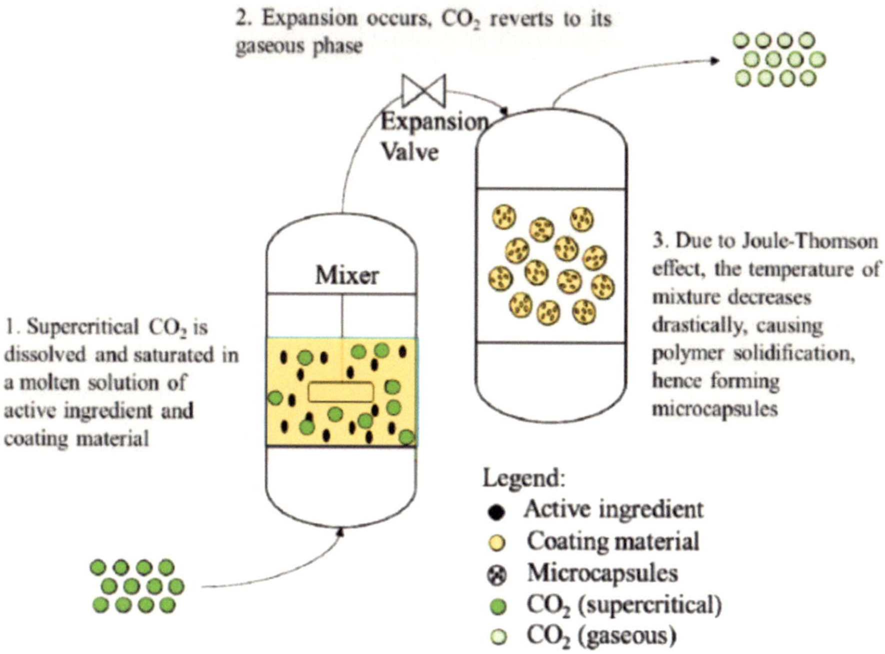

Figure 11.
Schematic representation of the PGSS approach [86].

physicochemical changes. In this process, the sol precursor is added to water which gels or hardens to capsules enclosing any included cargo. Generally, the steps involved are hydrolysis, condensation, gelling, aging, drying and densification. Organosilanes are the most commonly used encapsulation sols in contemporary times [89]. Their properties including surface functionalities, biocompatibility with many drugs and biomolecules, mild processing conditions of temperature and pH. This technique is commonly used for encapsulation of biomolecules, enzymes, and drugs. The alkoxysilanes precursors such as tetraethyl orthosilicate, triethoxysilane, trimethoxysiliane, methyltrimethoxysilane, tetraethylorthosilicate are insoluble in water so their dispersion in water in the presence of a surfactant and possibly a hydrophobic cargo results in the formation of emulsion droplets that serve as templates from which hydrolysis, condensation and polycondensation occurs at room temperature in the presence of water and an acid to form silanol groups which subsequently condense at basic pH to form organosillane matrixes or cages of different porosity and size ranging from 1 to 40 μm [90]. The general equation is given in Eq. (1).

$$\text{Precursor} + \text{Si(OR)}_4 + 2\text{H}_2\text{O} \rightarrow \text{Active} + \text{SiO}_2 + 2\text{ROH} \tag{1}$$

One byproduct of that reaction is ethanol which acts as a preservative for enclosed biomolecules. The matrix can be dried to form xerogels and can serves as a container for the enclosed biomolecule since there is no covalent relationship between them. Although rotation and unfolding movements are restricted for proteins, their inclusions can still be detected in appropriate setting by the target receptors.

4.3.7 Liposomes

Liposomes are lipid bilayer phospholipid vesicles with diameters ranging from 25 nm to 10 μm. They form spontaneously when disrupted in water. They can encapsulate polar materials in their core while keeping hydrophobic materials in their lipid bilayer. Liposomes are traditionally made by the film hydration method with constituents like lipid, cholesterol, and solvent. Film hydration involves the dissolution of the lipid components in a suitable solvent most commonly ethanol and chloroform. The solvent is removed in a rotary evaporator leaving behind a thin film which is rehydrated to yield large multilamellar vesicles liposomes. The size of the liposomes can be reduced by passing through successively smaller sized polycarbonate filters. Ultrasonication method of preparing liposomes involves an aqueous dispersion of lipids using a strong sonicator probe and usually yields small unilamellar vesicles. Reverse phase evaporation is another method for liposome preparation [91]. In this method, a mixture of lipids and cholesterol dissolved in an appropriate solvent is subjected to the rotary evaporator for solvent removal. The residue is dried with hydrogen and resuspended in an organic solvent usually diethyl ether. An aqueous solution of the drug to be encapsulated is added to the lipid solution and sonicated under nitrogen until a homogenous mixture result. The solvent is then removed to yield large unilamelar vesicles usually used to encapsulate large molecular weight biomolecules. Ether vaporization method involves a mixture of lipids dissolved in an organic solvent such as ether and subsequently injected into a hot aqueous solution resulting in osmotic liposomes [92].

Major instability issues with liposomes is related to hydrolysis, oxidation, aggregation, and fusion. Appropriate buffer inclusion is necessary to limit oxidation of liposome phospholipids. Freeze drying has also been used to overcome the effect of temperature on liposomes. Such proliposomes are then reconstituted in water just before use. Research by Gomez and coworkers [91] showed that the encapsulation efficiency of any liposome preparation depend on the encapsulated molecule.

4.3.8 Molecular inclusion complexes

Inclusion complexes are microcapsules made by including a material to be encapsulated into the cavity of cyclodextrin molecule. Cyclodextrins are a family of cyclic oligosaccharides made up of glucopyranosyl linked by α (1,4) bonds. The most common members of the family are α-, β-, and γ- cyclodextrins consisting of 6, 7, and 8 glucopyranose units respectively. The most frequently used is β-cyclodextrin. The unique nature of a cyclodextrin molecule with a hydrophobic cavity enclosed by a hydrophilic container makes them targets for encapsulation of hydrophobic molecules. They serve as host to a great variety of hydrophobic compounds. Materials are enclosed into their cavity through different means.

Physical mixing through a kneading action of a solution of guest molecule with a slurry of cyclodextrin. The kneaded paste is dried and washed with a solvent. This is usually reserved for very poorly soluble materials and unsuitable for large scale production. In co-precipitation method, the guest molecule is dissolved is a suitable organic solvent such as diethyl ether, chloroform. Then, an aqueous solution of the cyclodextrin is added under agitation. The complex formed is precipitated out of solution using temperature reduction. The crystals are collected, washed with organic solvent and dried at 50°C. This method is usually reserved for payloads not too soluble in water [93].

Heating can also be used for inclusion complex formation. For this procedure, the physical mixture of the guest and the host can adsorb water and thereafter is heated in an enclosed vessel at a temperature of 40–145°C. This process yields crystalline complexes but can only be used for payloads stable at such temperature range [93]. Freeze drying is usually reserved for heat labile water-soluble cargoes. The required quantities of both guest and host materials are dissolved in water with stirring and then freeze dried. The obtained crystals are then washed with an organic solvent and dried in vacuum. This method is scalable and gives good yields [93].

Spray drying has also been used to obtain host-guest complexes. The host and guest molecules are dissolved in deionized water under agitation and subsequently dried in a spray dryer. There is need to optimize the operation conditions and this process may be unsuitable for heat labile materials [93].

5. Natural polymers in encapsulation

In 1953, Hermann Staudinger was awarded the Nobel Prize in chemistry for demonstrating the existence of "*Makromoleküle*" macromolecules which led to the birth of the polymer chemistry field [94]. In the past 50 years, various natural, synthetic and semi-synthetic polymers have been investigated for developing diverse nano-, micro-, and macroscale drug delivery system (DDSs) for various therapeutic and diagnostic applications [94–96]. Natural polymers along with their derivatives (semi-synthetic polymers) are the safest micro- and nanocarriers due to their low toxicity, biocompatibility and intrinsic biodegradability by enzymes [97, 98]. This section highlights the main types of natural polysaccharides, proteins and lipids that have been employed as nanocarriers for therapeutic and theranostic applications.

5.1 Polysaccharides

Polysaccharides are the most abundant natural biopolymers derived from diverse bioresources, **Figure 12**. Polysaccharides are different from proteins, nucleic acids,

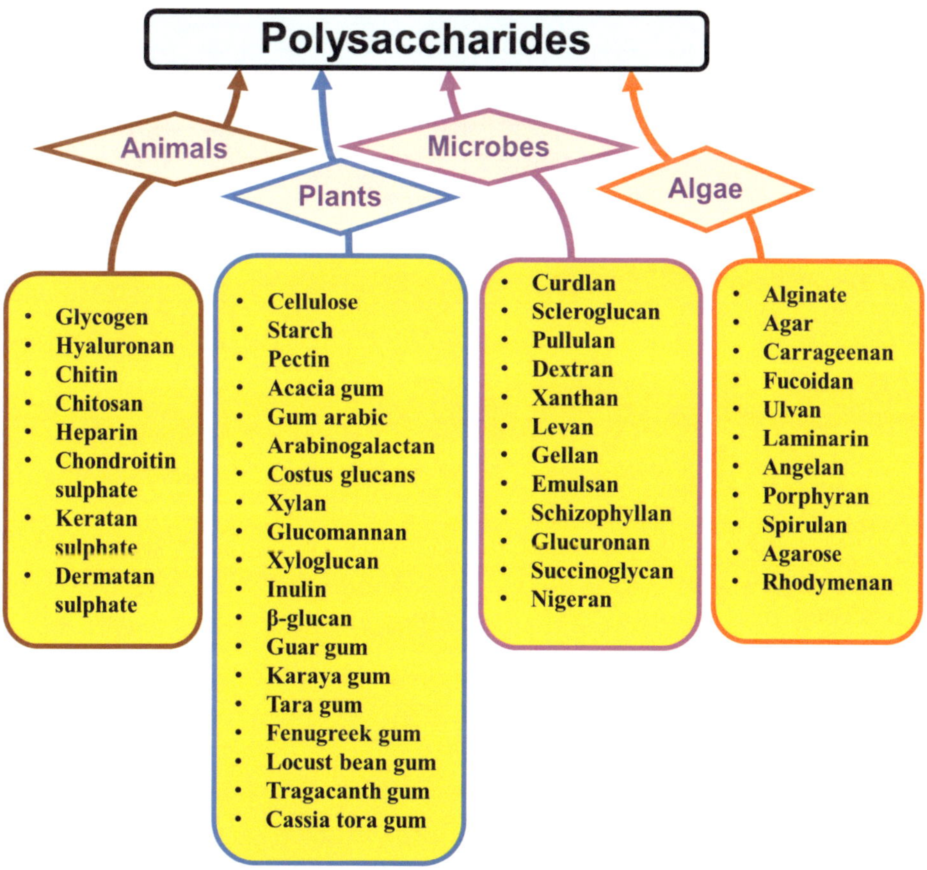

Figure 12.
Classification of polysaccharides based on their origin [100].

glycoproteins and glycolipids, in that they contain repetitive structural features [99]. Polysaccharides have been employed as responsive nanocarriers for targeted and controlled gene delivery and drug delivery of small molecules, proteins, peptides, nucleic acids, and antibiotics [100]. Among various polysaccharides, cellulose is the most abundant renewable natural polymer on earth, which is unbranched, linear homopolysaccharide, composed of repeating β-(1 → 4) linked D-glucose units [101]. However, since cellulose is water-insoluble, various water-soluble and hydrophilic cellulose-based derivatives have been used for creating macroscale DDSs and devices for oral drug delivery to the gastrointestinal (GI) tract due to their good compression characteristics and adequate water-swelling property which allows for controlled release drugs through rapid formation of an external gel layer [102]. Examples of commercialized macroscale DDSs based on cellulose acetate and hydroxypropyl methylcellulose (HPMC) are shown in **Figure 13** (I, II). The details about the former DDSs/devices and the mechanisms of drug release are described by Abu-Thabit and Makhlouf [94].

Another important polysaccharide is starch. Starches are made from 300 to 1000 glucose monomeric units. The main components of starch are amylose (~20%) and amylopectin (~80%) macromolecules. Amylose is unbranched, linear homopolysaccharide, composed of repeating α-(1 → 4) linked D-glucose units. Amylose adapts helical structure due to the formation of hydrogen bonding among D-glucose monomeric units. The helical conformation of amylose provides room to accommodate the iodine molecules in its core, and results in the formation of iodine-amylose complex with the characteristic blue-violet color as a strong indication for the presence of tiny amounts of starch. Amylopectin is a branched polysaccharide that is composed of repeating

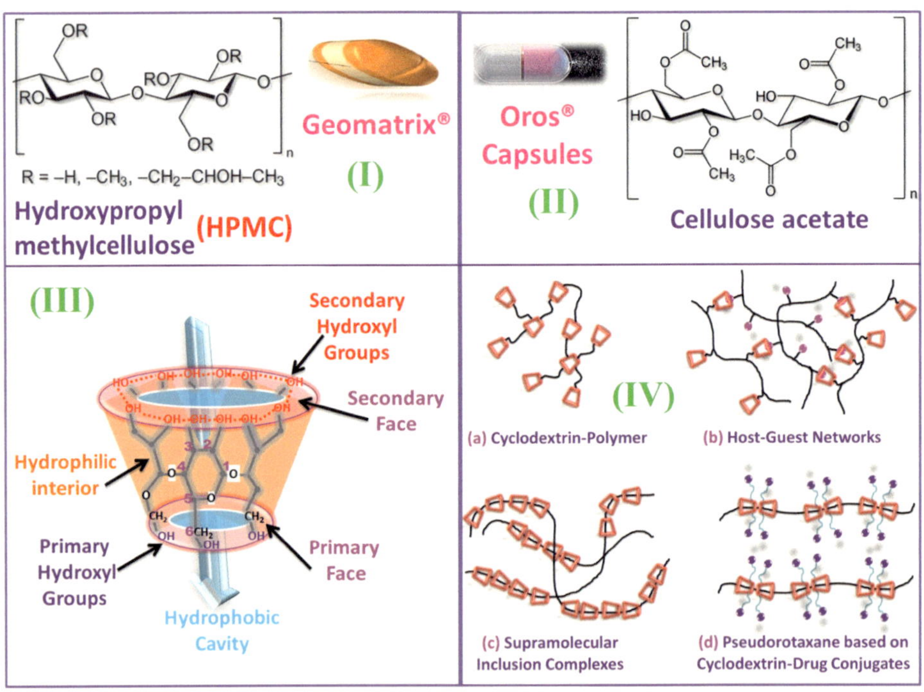

Figure 13.
(I) And (II) represent the chemical structures and examples of macroscale-based DDSs using HPMC, and cellulose acetate; reproduced with permission from ref. [94]. (III) schematic illustration of (a) structure of cyclodextrin polymer; diversity of using cyclodextrins for drug delivery systems via (b) host-guest interactions; (c) formation of supramolecular inclusion complexes (e.g. with PEG); and (d) cyclodextrin-drug conjugates; (IV) conventional representation for native cyclodextrins (CDs) as a truncated cone with "hydrophobic" cavity (blue color) that can accommodate hydrophobic drugs; reproduced with permissions from ref. [103].

α-(1 → 4) linked D-glucose units with occasional α-1,6-glycosidic bonds, which are responsible for the branching. The helical structure of amylopectin is disrupted by the available branched side chains which yield less intense reddish-brown color for the formed amylopectin-iodine complex instead of intense blue-violet color. Another class of polysaccharides nanocarriers is cyclodextrins (CDs) which are crystalline cyclic oligosaccharides consisting of α-1,4-glycosidic bonded D-glycopyranose units with glucose units arranged in a donut shape ring [103]. CDs are produced by enzymatic degradation of starch. CDs are classified as cage molecules with hydrophilic exterior and hydrophobic inner cavity which enables the formation of inclusion complexes with a variety of hydrophobic drug molecules [103], **Figure 13** (III). CDs are categorized based on the number of glucose residues in their structure, for example, CD with the glucose hexamer is named as α-CD, the heptamer as β-CD and the octomer as γ-CD [104]. The designs of supramolecular systems with CD are very diverse; since CDs can be used alone, grafted to other molecules or linked to each other [105], **Figure 13** (IV).

Chitin is the second most abundant natural polysaccharide which can be described as cellulose with one hydroxyl group on each monomer replaced by acetyl amine group. Chitin is abundant in invertebrates, mollusks, the cell walls of fungi, and the exoskeletons of arthropods. Like cellulose, chitin is a hydrophobic and water-insoluble biopolymer with limited application for fabricating DDSs. Chitosan, which is prepared by alkaline or enzymatic hydrolysis of chitin, is considered as the most important derivative of chitin due to its biocompatibility, biodegradability and non-toxic nature [106]. Unlike most anionic polysaccharides, chitosan is classified as a cationic polymer due to the presence of amine group which can be protonated upon dissolving chitosan in dilute acidic solutions such as acetic acid or hydrochloric acid. This unique character allowed chitosan to be used for fabricating various DDSs, such as micro/nanoparticles and hydrogels, *via* formation of polyelectrolyte complexes with various anionic polysaccharides [107, 108]. Another naturally occurring linear polysaccharide is hyaluronic acid (HA) (also called hyaluronan) which is composed of D-glucuronic acid and N-acetyl-D-glucosamine disaccharide. HA acts as an anionic polyelectrolyte at neutral pH, as the pKa of the carboxylic acid groups is ≈ 3–4, which makes HA highly hydrophilic and superabsorbent for water, with ability to expand up to 1000 times its solid volume, leading to loose, hydrated network [97]. Dextran is a water-soluble branched polysaccharide with varied chain lengths and molecular weight in the range of 30,000 – 2,000,000 g/mole [106]. In 1861, Louis Pasteur isolated dextran from wine as a microbial product [109]. Dextran has been applied in nanomedicine, a novel discipline that applies submicron particles for therapeutic and diagnostic purposes. Dextran has been applied in nanomedicine as encapsulating matrix for therapeutic and diagnostic purposes [94], and as an alternative to PEGylation to avoid nanoparticles (NPs) [95] and opsonin interactions [110]. Dextran has been employed for preparing pH-sensitive NPs by polyelectrolyte complexation between dextran sulfates and chitosan [108, 111].

5.2 Proteins

The term protein *was coined in 1838 by the* Swedish chemist Jöns Jacob Berzelius, which was derived from the Greek *prōteios*, meaning "holding first place" [112]. Proteins are versatile biomacromolecules with large and diverse functions in living organisms such as transcription, translation, transport and metabolism [113]. Proteins are key class of biopolymers that have been extensively used as nanocarriers for therapeutic and diagnostic drug delivery applications [114]. Proteins can be classified based on their origin as plant-based proteins and animal-based proteins, **Figure 14**. Detailed description and characteristic for each protein type is provided in the next chapter on proteins. This section provides brief idea about animal-based proteins including gelatin, casein, and albumin.

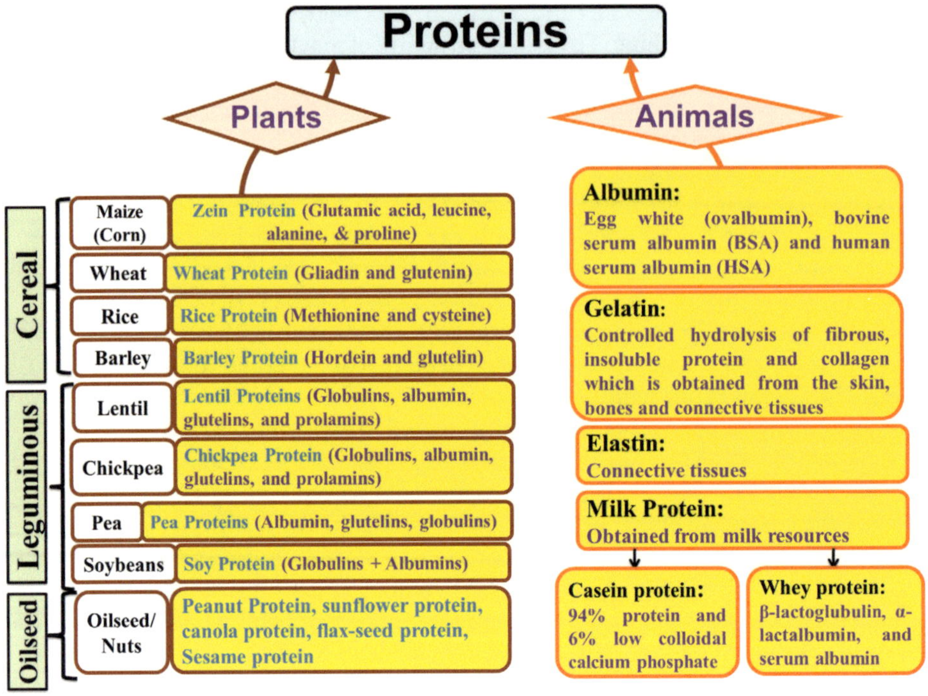

Figure 14.
Classification of proteins based on their origin with the list of the main components.

Collagen is the most abundant protein in mammals which forms 30% of all vertebrate body protein with a majority in bone and skin. Gelatin is a denatured collagen which is obtained by either acid hydrolysis (gelatin type A with isoelectric point ≈ 7–9), or alkaline hydrolysis (gelatin type B with isoelectric point ≈ 4.8–5) [115]. Gelatin is biocompatible and biodegradable with high physiological tolerance and low immunogenicity. Gelatin is classified as "Generally Recognized as Safe" (GRAS) by the US Food and Drug Administration (FDA). Therefore, gelatin have been used for vitamin preparation, drug capsules, scaffolding materials to promote cell migration, wound healing, tissue regeneration and as a nanocarrier for drug and gene delivery [106, 115]. Casein and whey proteins are important protein sources for human nutrition. Casein is one of the oldest natural polymers, used for adhesives, dating back to thousands of years [116]. In contrast to whey proteins, caseins are water-insoluble and account for 80% of total bovine milk proteins. Casein protein is found in milk which serves biologically to transfer nutrients from mother to her offspring. Hence, it can be used as a carrier depot for delivery of drugs. Casein has four constituent phosphate-rich sub-units, which are amphiphilic and self-assemble into a micellar structure in the size range 50–300 nm, held together by calcium phosphate nanoclusters acting as bridges connecting these subunits [117]. Although the word "albumin" is usually associated to serum albumin, it is also employed to describe a family of proteins characterized by their solubility in water [114]. Human serum albumin (HSA) and lactalbumin (known as whey protein) are the most popular albumin proteins employed for drug delivery applications [114]. Besides that, albumins can be found in foods, particularly in seeds and nuts. Serum albumin is the major protein constituent in the blood plasma of all vertebrates. The two main exponents are human (HSA) and bovine serum albumin (BSA). Albumin has diverse physiological functions such as maintaining the pH and colloidal osmotic pressure of plasma, its antioxidant effect by trapping free radicals, and its reversible binding ability to variety of important exogenous and endogenous [118, 119]. Albumin has the ability to bind with positively and negatively charged hydrophobic organic anions such as bilirubin and long-chain fatty acids and divalent cations such as calcium and magnesium [119]. Albumin can bind to different types of compounds including drugs, bile acids, copper, zinc, and even compounds with specific serum binders such as vitamin D and thyroxin [119]. The binding feature of albumin reduces the free concentration of compounds, and hence, limiting their biologic activity, distribution, and rate of clearance [119]. Therefore, HSA is considered an ideal protein for the production of parenteral medications, which has been employed as nanocarrier for drugs, vaccines and genes delivery [120–123].

In 1972, the first protein-based nanoparticle (human serium albumin (HSA) microspheres) was prepared [124]. In January 2005, the first nanotechnology-based drug product, called as Abraxane®, was approved for treatment of metastatic breast cancer [125]. The anticancer and water-insoluble paclitaxel chemotherapeutic agent was easily encapsulated in a shell of protein albumin, where the cancer cells are tricked by the albumin coating into taking the nanospheres embedded with the active cancer-fighting paclitaxel molecules [125]. The encapsulation of paclitaxel drug inside the albumin protein biopolymer provided a harmless way for drug administration as compared to the use of toxic solvents like polyhydroxylated castor oil (Cremophor EL or CrEL), which requires patients to receive premedication for elimination of the allergic reactions and solvent-related hypersensitivity side effects [126]. The FDA approved use of Abraxane® was extended for treatment of non-small-cell lung carcinoma (NSCLC) in 2012, followed by the FDA approval in 2013 for use in treating advanced pancreatic cancer as less toxic alternative to FOLFIRINOX [94]. Gas microbubbles have been encapsulated in the elastic shell of HSA which served as ultrasound contrast agents (e.g. Albunex™ and Optison™ products) for diagnostic applications [127].

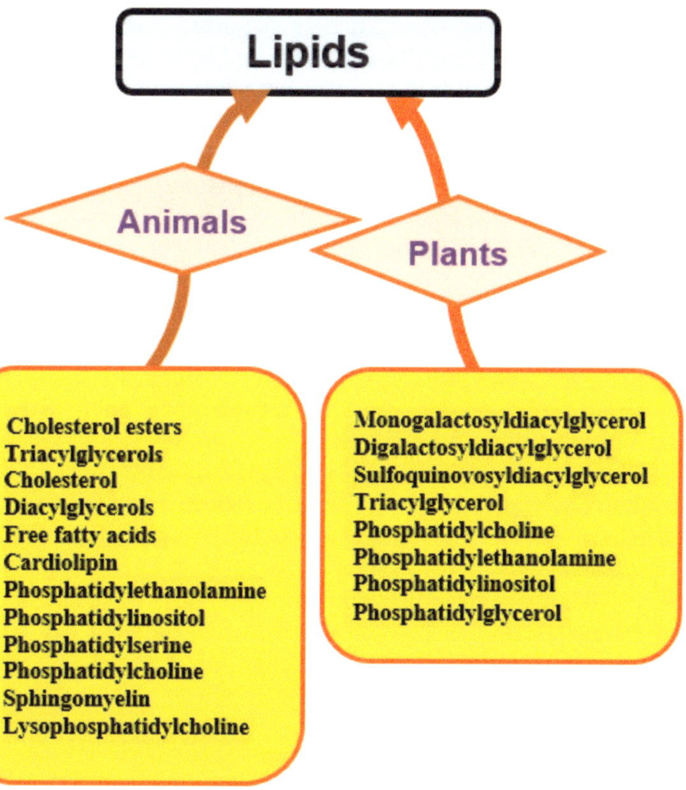

Figure 15.
Classification of lipids based on their origin.

5.3 Lipids

Lipids are heterogenous polymers of fatty acids and in nature occur as fats if solid at ambient temperature, oils if liquids at ambient temperature, fatty acid derivatives, and sterols. A major division among lipids irrespective of their categorization but pertinent for their role in encapsulation and based on polarity divides lipids into polar and non-polar lipids with all types occurring in nature. Polar lipids form aqueous phases with water and occur in nature as constituents of the cell membrane where they form a barrier between the cell and the external water environment. Except for cholesterol, polar lipids have a polar head and a long non-polar tail that aligns itself in a bilayer and include lipids such as glycerophospholipids, sphingolipids and monoglycerides. On the other hand, non-polar lipids such as triglycerides, waxes, are used as energy store and form a solvent for many lyophilic compounds during formulation. Lipids are classified based on origin as shown in **Figure 15**.

6. Lipid-based encapsulation

Lipids are a group of hydrocarbons based organic macromolecules that are rather soluble in non-polar and organic solvents instead of water. Though like carbohydrates in terms of elemental constituents of carbon, hydrogen and oxygen, they differ in containing considerably lower levels of oxygen often attached as part of a single carboxylic acid group at the end of a long hydrocarbon chain. Non-saponifiable lipids such as triglycerides, waxes and phospholipids cannot be hydrolyzed by acid or bases but lipids such as steroids, prostaglandins and terpenes are easily hydrolyzed due to the presence of ester groups. Lipid based encapsulates include liposomes, nanoliposomes, proliposomes, self-assembled micelles, nanostructured lipid carriers, Solid lipid nanoparticles, solid lipid microparticles, liquid lipid nano and micro particles, nanoemulsion, microemulsions, emulsions, nanosuspensions, lipid nanotubes, lipid-polysaccharide complexes and hybrids (**Figure 16**). Some other lipid-based drug delivery systems such as the self-emulsifying microemulsions are not included here because often, they are only encapsulated after ingestion.

A wide range of architectures can be realized depending on the nature and composition of lipids, encapsulation technique, among others. Tuning of process parameters such as pH, temperature, nature and composition of lipid, presence of other constituents such as electrolytes, buffers and sugars will usually determine the size and morphology of the resulting capsules or vesicles. The morphology could be micelles, vesicles, or bilayer sheets. Specific applications will demand specific manipulation of charge, size, pegylation, functionalization, phase transition temperature and drug loading mechanism.

Size: For applications targeting the delivery of macromolecules and tissue penetration, the required size should be below 100 nm but above 5 nm to prevent filtration through the kidney. Multilamellar vesicles are particularly good for depot and sustained release injections while small unilamellar vesicles are good for systemic injections.

Charge: Neutral vesicles usually result in long circulation time and minimal effect of the reticuloenthothelial system. Cationic vesicles however undergo aggregation due to interaction with body protein while anionic vesicles are easily taken up by the liver and spleen.

6.1 Lipids in micro- and nanoencapsulation

Encapsulation processes employed in the use of lipids for formation of micro and nano capsules are similar in principle for both nanocapsules and microcapsules.

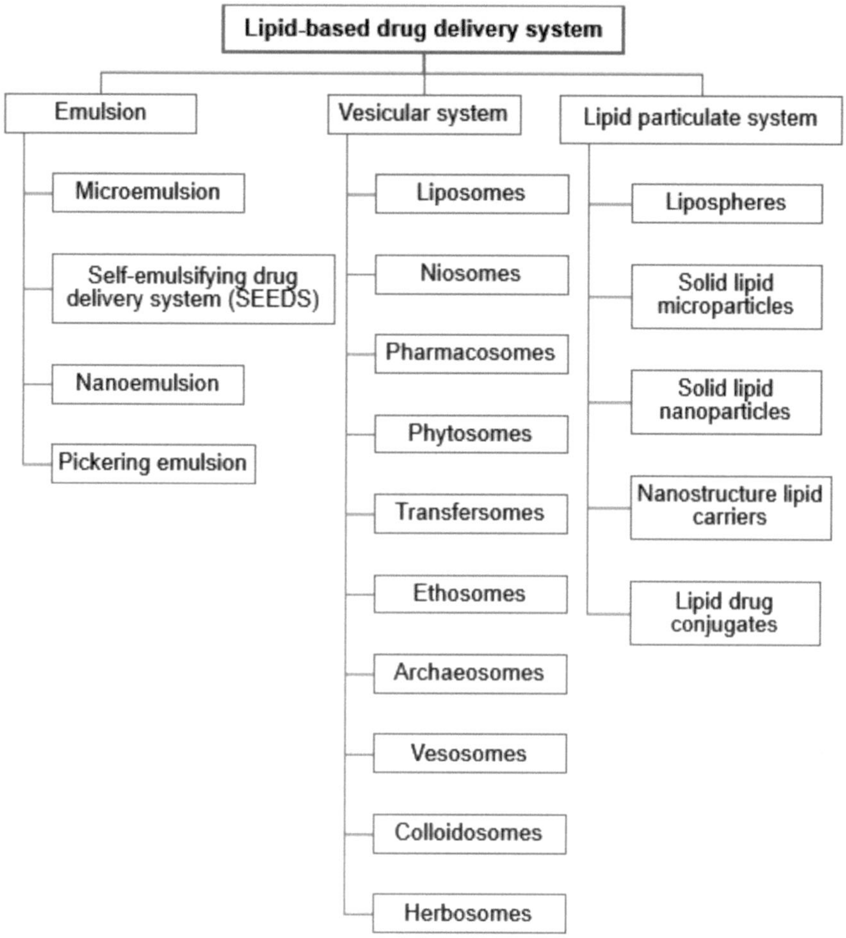

Figure 16.
Classes of lipid-based drug delivery system. Adapted from [128].

Lipids of diverse characteristics and functionalities have in contemporary times remained the focus of hope for the delivery of over 90% new chemical entities in development pipeline that may encounter bioavailability challenges due to their lipophilicity [129]. Likewise, drug delivery systems based on lipids have almost taken center stage in many pharmaceutical companies due to potential profit, both financial and otherwise, accruable to lipid-based reformulation of existing medicines.

Lipids play a major role in many encapsulation processes as either membrane/shell components, core/carrier component, water-insoluble or water-soluble surfactant or as a hydrophilic cosolvent. The type of lipid used for an encapsulation process may depend on several factors that include the target application, size range required for the application, physicochemical properties of the material to be encapsulated. Lipids involved in encapsulation vary widely depending on specific application. There are also a variety of classification system available.

Homolipids: These are also known as simple lipids and are formed by an esterification action of an alcohol with fatty acids which can be short chain (less than 6 carbon atoms), medium chain (6–12 carbons) or long chain (14–24 carbon atoms). Their elemental composition is just carbon, hydrogen, and oxygen. The constituent fatty acid chain may contain a double bond which always occurs in the cis configuration. Examples are naturally occurring glycerides such as fats and oil (coconut oil), cerides such as waxes (beeswax and carnauba wax), and sterides such as esters of fatty acids and cholesterol.

Heterolipids or compound lipids: These contain an additional nitrogen atom or phosphorus atom. They include phospholipids, sulfolipids, and glycolipids (when conjugated with a sugar moiety). Two classes of phospholipids occur in abundance naturally and include sphingolipids such as ceramide and phosphoglycerides. They abound in nature as structural components of membranes.

Complex lipids: These include overly complex lipids such as lipoprotein (when conjugated with protein and are responsible for the transport of cholesterol and other molecules) and chylomicrons.

6.2 Merits and demerits in therapeutic delivery

Challenges abound in the drug delivery terrain particularly for new chemical entities in development pipeline majority of whom are poorly soluble molecules. In addition, better understanding of the molecular basis of diseases is yielding treatment options such as large proteins that pose challenges for delivery. For instance, proteins are easily degraded when administered even parenterally necessitating frequent administrations that contribute to patient cost, side effects and compliance issues. Moreover, often they are large molecules. At the nanosized level, most nanoparticles are easily removed from the circulation by the endoplasmic reticulum. Encapsulation in lipids can solve a great number of these issues. **Figure 17** captures

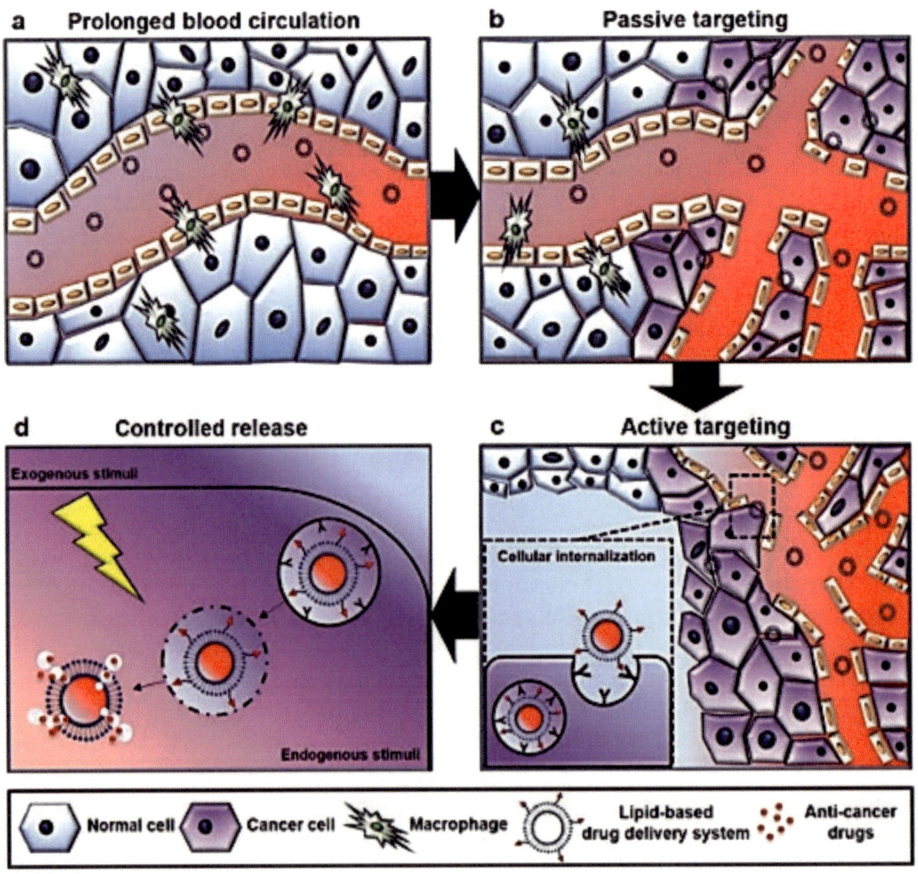

Figure 17.
Some factors contributing to efficiency of lipid encapsulation to therapeutic drug delivery [130].

some of the benefits of lipid encapsulation to drug delivery. The merits of a lipid-based system for drug delivery may vary slightly depending on the type of lipid system and the route of administration.

Modulation of bioavailability: Irrespective of the route of administration or lipid system involved, lipid-based systems have been employed to modulate rate and extent of absorption of active ingredient. They bring about an increase in surface area available for dissolution thereby increasing absorption. In oral delivery, lipid systems have predominantly been used to improve solubilization of poorly soluble solids thereby increasing bioavailability. Solubilization in lipid systems also greatly diminishes intra and inter subject variability enabling caregivers to better adjust dosing to individual needs. Lipid based delivery also reduces the hepatic first pass metabolism for susceptible drugs. The overall improvement may lead to a reduction in the required dose and a proportional decrease in the accompanying side effects and toxicities which may translate to better compliance. An example is the formulation of amphotericin B initially as fungizone with high toxicity as compared to the lipid particle formulation, Abelcet [131]. In addition, existence of areas of opposite polarity within the same systems opens the possibility of delivering 2 physically different compounds through one system.

Lipid based systems in the form of micro and nano particulate systems modulate biodistribution [132]. They are usually used to sustain drug release and target drugs to specific sites. Lipids have been used to deliver large protein macromolecules to specific sites through lipid-drug conjugates. Encapsulation in lipid bilayer membrane spares the drug the attack of the reticuloendothelial system or shield a drug from detection by the immune cells since they have similar membrane. Lipid systems improve or maintain the chemical and physical stability of the included API. They also effectively mask taste, and odor. Formulation efforts are also targeted towards stabilizing the API both during storage and from endogenous enzymes and chemicals until it arrives its site of action. Physicochemical properties of vesicles such as size, charge or surface functionalization with specific ligands can be modulated for specific tasks.

Most lipids used for encapsulation are relatively cheap, biocompatible, biodegradable and exhibit low toxicity and allergenicity. The use of organic solvents is limited in their preparation. Ease of formulation, ease of characterization, sterilization and scale up, and amenability to delivery by various routes all contribute to their versatility.

In spite of the plethora of advantages, lipid-based system has a few challenges.

Digestibility of lipids and drug leakage: Most lipids used for encapsulation and other lipid-based delivery systems are natural. Lipids therefore have a natural propensity to be digested and degraded in the body by enzymes [133]. Digestion of one or more components will break up the membrane or shell which may result in supersaturation, precipitation or dilution depending on the route of administration and may result in toxicity or loss of efficacy.

Drug loading: Passive drug loading may lead to low efficiency, but active drug loading ensures high efficiency depending on the API and the other excipients.

Uncontrolled precipitation and aggregation: many of the lipid systems are prone to physical destabilization of their membranes requiring extra effort to stabilize them. The nanocapsules are prone to aggregation which may lead to non-uniformity of doses.

6.3 Case studies/applications

6.3.1 Encapsulation of small molecules

Small molecules are low molecular weight compounds that include drugs, xenobiotics, lipids, metabolites, metal ions, monosaccharides, second messenger, etcetera. Encapsulation of small molecules using lipids predominantly aims to solubilize poorly soluble molecules, target or control release of the medicament. Lipids being major constituents of the cell membranes can ferry included cargo through the tightly controlled formidable barrier and through various ports of entry such as the stratum corneum, the ocular cornea, parenteral or oral route.

Cantón and colleagues [134] recently reported the preparation of SN-38-β-cyclodextrin complex in solid lipid nanoparticles. The aim was to develop a delivery system that will deliver, stabilize, and protect the FDA approved drug for colorectal cancer. This was necessary since SN-38 is highly insoluble and unstable at physiological pH and easily converts to the carboxylate form that has higher binding affinity to serum and is more stable at the basic pH of the GIT. Initial attempt to include SN-38 -cyclodextrin inclusion complex to a liposome lead to the disassembly of the liposome and the formation of solid lipid nanoparticles. The lipids used were hydrogenated L-α-phosphatidylcholine, 1,2-distearoyl-*sn*-glycero-3- phosphoethanolamine-N-[biotinyl(polyethylene glycol)-2000] (DSPE-PEG-biotin), 1,2-distearoyl-*sn*-glycero-3-phosphoethanolamine-N- [folate(polyethylene glycol)-5000] (DSPE-PEG-folate) 1,2-dihexadecanoyl-*sn*-glycero-3-phosphoethanolamine (DHPE-TR). Evaluation of the stability by determining the presence of the inactive form was undertaken using the size exclusion chromatography. Ultimately, stable, solid lipid particles containing the SN-38 cyclodextrin complex was prepared even though the concentration of the encapsulated drug was narrow.

Photodynamic therapy (PDT) is a treatment modality for cancers that involve the use of reactive oxygen species, photosensitizers, and light for destruction of cancer cells. However, PDT is limited by the inability of high energy light used in PDT to penetrate tissues, and the ability of the body to disperse used photosensitizers systemically [135]. Unfortunately, too, the internal tumor environment is hypoxic, the low oxygen content limiting the efficacy of PDT and being responsible for angiogenesis and subsequent metastasis within cancer cells. Therefore, to improve the outcomes of PDT, particularly for solid tumors, there is a need for the presence of oxygen generator within the tumor cells and the presence of the photosensitizer near the targeted tumor cell. Liu and colleagues [136] developed a calcium peroxide/methylene blue-loaded liposome as an oxygen generating species which targets a photosensitizer, methylene blue in PDT therapy. Many of the oxygen generated previously studied were encapsulated in hydrophobic polymers that had limited capacity for hydrophilic cargo and delayed the generation of oxygen. The use of liposomes provided a hydrophobic shell that served to carry the photosensitizer and a means to penetrate the cell membrane while carrying a hydrophilic cargo in its core. On irradiation, the phospholipid bilayer is easily disrupted causing the release of calcium peroxide which reacts with water rapidly to generate oxygen. On subsequent irradiation, the generated oxygen potentiates the effect of PDT on tumor hypoxia. The first step involved the preparation of calcium peroxide nanoparticles and further encapsulation of the nanoparticles in a pegylated liposome. Composed of DSPE-PEG, DPPC-egg lecithin, and cholesterol. In-vivo tests in a mouse model of mammary cell carcinoma demonstrated the efficacy of the system to limit hypoxia in treated animals when compared to untreated animals.

Kenechukwu and colleagues [137] prepared a lipid matrix made up of sun seed oil: Softisan® in the ratio 1:9 and PEG 4000 by a melt homogenization process for the intravaginal delivery of a poorly soluble drug, Miconazole. The concentration of PEG was varied giving rise to different formulations. The PEG content consequently affected the particle sizes, the encapsulation efficiency, and the loading capacity. The optimum concentration of PEG 4000 according to their study was 40% w/w.

Stella and colleagues [138] investigated the possibility of delivering a doxorubicin pro-drug, squalenoyl-derivative through entrapment in solid lipid nanoparticles. The highly reduced cardiotoxicity of liposomal doxorubicin catapulted the search for other lipid-based carrier systems that will also help in mitigating the resistance to doxorubicin. Squalenoyl derivative is highly lipophilic derivative that has shown capacity to form very stable self-assembles in water. Their absorption in the body had been shown to be mediated by endogenous low-density lipoproteins. Therefore, the researchers initially prepared squalenoyl derivative self-assembly in water using the nanoprecipitation technique. The solid lipid particles were prepared by complex coacervation using fatty acids that were precipitated by acidification and stabilized with poly vinyl alcohol.

Targeting cytotoxic drugs to the tumor environment has always been both desirable and a challenge due to severe side effects to normal cells and the peculiarities of the tumor microenvironment. For instance, multi drug resistance to drugs like doxorubicin has been associated to the hypoxia encountered in tumors. In this study, Xie and colleagues [139] aimed to use methotrexate conjugated with a polymer-lipid hybrid through an imine linkage, as both a targeting moiety and as the drug targeted to the cancer cells, through the nanoplatform of self-assembled lipid micelles also incorporating curcumin. In addition, pH responsiveness and prodrug status were built into the platform using an imine crosslinker. The intent was that at a particular pH unique to the tumor environment, the acid responsive imine aldehyde linkage will be disrupted leading to the release of the active methotrexate. The methotrexate with its strong resemblance to folate will be used as a target to the folate receptors on the tumor. Curcumin, a well-known naturally occurring polyphenol with strong anti-inflammatory and antiproliferative properties was assembled into the hydrophobic core of the resulting lipid-polymer hybrid micelles to forestall drug resistance. In their study, lipid-polymers such as DSPE-PEG and DSPE-Mpeg were used. The first step was the formation of the prodrug complex, DSPE-MPEG-imine- methotrexate, by the conjugation of methotrexate to DSPE-PEG through a Schiff base reaction between the aldehyde group of the polymer and the aromatic group of methotrexate. The resulting prodrug complex was later self-assembled in the presence of the poorly soluble and unstable curcumin. One pot ultra-sonification with solvent evaporation was the method of micelle formation for both drug-loaded and unloaded micelles. The animal studies carried out on HeLA tumor bearing BALB/c nude mice demonstrated the workability of the concept and confirmed the ability of the lipid carrier system to effectively transport the curcumin and methotrexate to the tumor site.

6.3.2 Encapsulation of biologics

Biologics are large high molecular weight proteins, nucleic acids, monoclonal antibodies, vaccines, and enzymes. The delivery of macromolecular proteins is particularly challenging.

Synthetic small interfering RNA, siRNA are nucleic acid fragments that can modify the activities of mRNA when they enter the cell. Many diseases are due to certain abnormality or malefaction at the genetic level and hence the silencing of the specific mRNA can translate to cure. The problem of delivering such proteins are multiple and varied. One of such is the rapid clearance of such protein on systemic administration due to nuclease activity and renal filtration and the induction of immunogenic reactions. In addition, siRNA, and its like are rarely able to diffuse into the cell, hence requiring the complex generation of multiply functionalized systems. Patisiran is the first FDA approved siRNA formulation prepared using lipid nanoparticulate platform for delivery to hepatocytes [140]. It is a double stranded siRNA which degrades 3'untranslated region of the wild type transthyretin by RNA interference [141]. Hereditary transthyretin mediated amyloidosis is a disorder resulting from deposition of abnormal form of the protein produced in liver cells. The entrapment of nucleic acids in lipid nanoparticles require the presence of a cationic lipid to trap the negatively charged nucleic acid. Secondly, the pKa of the lipid should be such that at physiological pH, there is a net neutral charge. The lipid should also display a positive charge when in the endosome environment and finally, it must display the hexagon shape. For proteins, there must be rational design to take into cognizance; linkers, acyl chains and the ionizable groups required.

Vascular endothelial growth factor, VEGF, has been implicated in tumor progression and metastasis. It has been shown that in cancer and some other diseases such as age-related macular degeneration, the expression for VEGF is usually upregulated to promote angiogenesis. The possibility of using RNA interference to silence genes through the interference of siRNA will be a welcome option in the battle against tumors. Important barriers to the use of siRNA is the availability of vectors, low transfection efficiency and stability. Polymeric lipids have been in the lead as a choice for siRNA delivery material. Cationic lipids are of importance due to the need for a positive charge to stabilize the negatively charged nucleic acid and for internalization. Cationic lipids however pose a problem of toxicity and may offer no protection to the nucleic acid. In Chen and co-workers' study [142], polyethyleneimine (PEI) was used for protonation of the polycation liposome while 1,2-dioleoyl-*sn*-glycero-3-phosphoethanolamine (DOPE), was used as a destabilizer to promote the escape of siRNA into the cytosol. siRNA was conjugated to calcium phosphate nanoparticles which has shown low toxicity, biocompatibility and biodegradability in previous studies involving the delivery of DNA and siRNA. siRNA-calcium phosphate nanoparticles were first prepared and introduced as an aqueous solution into a polycation liposome prepared by the film dispersion method using equimolar concentration of DOPE and PEI-Cholesterol. The in vitro gene silencing assay was performed using human breast adenocarcinoma cell lines while animal studies were done in tumor infected BALB/C-nu female mice. The results obtained showed the superior silencing effect of the siRNA delivered through the core-shell polycationic liposome.

Antibodies can be generated as inhibitory agents to many diseases causing proteins in the cytosol. Unfortunately, this has not been effectively utilized in treatment modalities due to inability of the large antibody proteins to transverse the cytosol. Wang and coworkers [143] developed a lipid carrier for immunoglobulin G, IgG, by first conjugating it with anionic polypeptides and subsequently complexed them (through electrostatic interactions) with cationic lipids previously used for the delivery of nucleic acids. They initially fused the polypeptide to a photoreactive antibody binding domain and subsequently to a chain of IgG without disturbing the IgG binding site and enabling the easy exchange of cargo functionalization of of-the-shelf IgG. The functionalized IgG was subsequently complexed with diverse types of cationic lipids and evaluated comparatively with cell penetrating peptides for cytosolic delivery of about 500 nM of IgG. The lipid complexed IgG was functional and also capable of inhibiting the drug efflux pump MRP I (responsible for multi drug resistance) and the transcription factor NFκB. Results also showed the supremacy of this method over traditional cell penetrating peptide method (delivering small proteins) in terms of delivering very large proteins.

Kose and coworkers [144] developed a lipid nanoparticle encapsulated mRNA encoding the antibody against chikungunya virus. The lipid nanoparticle system was prepared by the ethanol drop nanoprecipitation using ionizable lipid, lipid-polymer hybrid, cholesterol and DSPC in a microfluidic mixer. The lipid nanoparticle system provided approximately 90% encapsulation with particle sizes in the range of 80–100 nm. The protective ability of the developed system was tested in AG129 mice. The study showed that treatment lipid encapsulated mRNA protected the mice in a dose dependent manner.

6.3.3 Encapsulation of diagnostics

Certain factors can trigger responses in lipid particles of vesicles and include pH, reactive oxygen species, redox agents' presence of biomolecules, as well as certain environmental stimuli such as temperature, and light. Biosensors constitute a receptor that will interact with the stimuli to be detected and a transducer that will translate the analyte/stimuli -receptor information to measurable signal. Treatment and survival for many terminal and chronic diseases depend on early detection and diagnosis. Fortunately, many biosensing and bioimaging materials are being developed for possible use in diagnosis and treatment. There is a need to transport these nanoplatforms to the targeted site in a non-invasive and hidden manner to avoid destruction by the bodyguards of the body. One way this has been mitigated is by enclosure into vesicles that have a close resemblance to the body's own cells, the liposomes. Encapsulation based on lipid systems is driving the development of bioimaging and biosensing devices towards picogram detection thereby aiding both treatment such as fluorescence guided surgeries and survival. Some of the challenges being mitigated by lipid based or encapsulated devices include targeting, sustained release, and circulation.

Photoacoustic tomography (PAT) that makes use of light and sound has been considered a viable alternative to overcoming some of the limitations of conventional imaging systems such as computed tomography (CT) and magnetic resonance imaging (MRI), in early detection of atypical liver cancers that are less than 10 mm diameter. In addition, surgical resection remains about the most viable treatment option. Gold nanorods, due to their easy effusion into solid tumors, biocompatibility, and low toxicity [135] is usually considered good for PAT. It is also possible to move its absorption peak from red to near infrared (NIR) due to its anisotropic shape and enhancing its photoacoustic signal with large absorption cross section. Exploiting these factors, Guan and coworkers [145] developed dual PAT-NIR probe to aid early liver cancer detection and for guided surgical resection. They tapped a sort of synergistic effect of both gold nano rods and indocyanine green, an FDA approved photoacoustic NIR fluorescent dye that has dominated clinical practice for a while, and played down on some limitations of indocyanine green such as aggregation, rapid clearance, low energy conversion efficiency as a dual photoacoustic and fluorescence dye, and fluorescence quenching. In a relatively facile process, indocyanine green liposomes were prepared with phosphatidylcholine and cholesterol using the thin film hydration method. Pegylated gold nanorods were subsequently encapsulated with the indocyanine green liposomes by ultrasonication overnight. The dual system was used for resection surgery in tumor infected laboratory animals and proved successful.

Nucleolin is a nuclear and cytoplasmic protein also expressed on the cell surface and partly responsible for angiogenesis and by extension metastasis and tumor progression. Unlike other markers of tumor progression, that become less prominent as the tumor size increases, nucleolin is detected even in big tumors. It could therefore be mapped as a means of tracking metastasis. In current practice, Nucleolin is tracked using biopsy which is invasive and cannot indicate the full extent of metastasis or spread. Zhang and colleagues [146] developed a nucleolin targeted ultrasound contrast agent for detecting the presence of nucleolin in cells. The contrast agent is microbubble which is an encapsulated air commonly generated by sonicating a polymer solution in the presence of air or by compressing air into a polymer solution and then releasing it through specialized nozzles. In this study, Zhang and colleagues [146] synthesized an F3 peptide that has been shown to target nucleolin and conjugated it to the surface of generated microbubbles. Subsequently, they evaluated the ability of the F3 conjugated nucleolin targeting microbubble to detect the presence of nucleolin non-invasively. They initially synthesized the F3 peptides, lipo-peg peptides. Subsequently the microbubble which was encapsulated in a liposomal shell was synthesized using disteroylphosphatidylcholine (DSPC), 1,2-distearoyl-*sn*-glycero-3-phosphoethanolamine-N-[methoxy(polyethylene glycol)-2000] (ammonium salt) (DSPE-PEG2K), and lipo-peg-peptide earlier synthesized. The liposomal shell was prepared using the thin film hydration method and the microbubble generated by shaking the liposomal solution in air and used within 2 hours of purification. Two batches were made, one batch without the targeting peptide contained just the lipids DSPC: DSPE-PEG2K in the ratio of 90:10 while the targeted batch had I % of the lipo-peg-peptide replacing part of the DSPE-PEG2K. Evaluation of the contrast media in tumor infected female FVB mice in vivo and nucleolin expressing breast cancer cell line in vitro demonstrated that the accumulation of the contrast media facilitated the detection of murine breast tumors.

Deng and colleagues [147] recently developed a multicomponent system for diagnosis and treatment of cancers. They combined near infrared luminescence of quantum dots and thermo-sensitivity of magnetic liposomes to encapsulate and control drug localization and release. They prepared thermosensitive liposomes that were eventually loaded with drug, paclitaxel, magnetic nanoparticles and NIR luminescent quantum dots. The liposomes were prepared by the thin film hydration method using dipalmitoylphophatidylcholine, DPPC, 1,2-diaccyl-sn-glycero-3-phosphoethanolamine-N-(methoxy [polyethylene glycol]-2000 (DSPE–MPEG-2000), 1,2-diaccyl-sn-glycero-3-phosphoglycerol sodium (DSPG-Na). Effect of the developed systems were studied on cancer cell MCF-7 and SKOV-3 cell lines and uptake of the drug followed in real time by confocal scanning microscope. **Tables 2** and **3**

Micro-encapsulating materials	Active compounds	Micro-encapsulation technique	Diagnostic applications	EE %	Ref.
DPPC, DSPE–MPEG-2000 and DSPG-Na.	Paclitaxel	Liposomes	NIR imaging	86.46 ± 1.43%.	[147]
DPPC, CHOLESTEROL, DSPE-PEG-MALEIMIDE, DSPE-PEG-PDP.	Indocyanine green liposomes/ Perfluorobutane	Microbubble/ liposomes	Fluorescence and ultrasound imaging	—	[148]
DSPC, DSPE-PEG2K	Gas	microbubble	Ultrasound imaging	Not applicable	[146]
Lipids	perfluoropropane	microbubble	Ultrasound imaging	Not applicable	[149]
DSPC, PEG40 stearate, DSPE-PEG3400-maleimide	Perfluorocarbon	Emulsion/ microbubble decorated with antibody	Tumor cell isolation	—	[150]
DMPA, DPPC, DPPA, Cholesterol	Perfluoropentane	Emulsion containing perfluoropentane loaded liposome	Ultrasound guided tumor destruction.	—	[151]
DSPC	Perfluorobutane	Gene loaded microbubble	Ultrasound guided tumor destruction	—	[152]
Cholesterol, DDSPC, DSPE-PEG and DOPC	Magnetic iron oxide nanoparticles	Liposome	Magnetic resonance imaging contrast agent	—	[153]

Note: 1,2-dimyristoyl-sn-glycero-3-phosphatidic acid: DMPA, 1,2 Distearoyl-sn-glycero-3-phosphocholine: DSPC, Distearoyl-sn-glycero-3-phosphoethanolamine-N-[methoxy(polyethylene glycol)-2000: DSPE-MPEG2000, 1,2 dipalmitoyl-sn-glycero-3-phosphate: DPPA, 1,2-dipalmitoyl-sn-glycero-3-phospho-ethanolamine: DPPE, 1,2-distearoyl-sn-glycero-3-phosphoethanolamine-N-[carboxy(polyethylene glycol)-2000]): DSPE-PEG-COOH, 1,2-distearoyl-sn-glycero-3-phosphoethanolamine-N-[PDP(polyethylene glycol)-2000]: DSPE-PEG-PDP, 1,2-dioleoyl-sn-glycero-3-phosphatidylcholine: DOPC; EE: Encapsulation Efficiency.

Table 2.
Plant and animal lipid-based microencapsulating carriers for diagnostic applications.

Nano-encapsulating materials	Active compounds	Nano-encapsulation technique	Diagnostic applications	EE %	Ref.
DPPC, Stearic acid	Sulfur hexafluoride	Nanobubble	Ultrasound imaging	Not Applicable	[154]
Lipoid S75–3	oil	Phase inversion	O_2 sensor for MRI	—	[155]
DPPC, DSPC, DSPE-PEG 2000	Topotecan	liposomes	MRI guided focused ultrasound	—	[156]
DSPE-PEG2000-amine, DPPC	perfluoro-15-crown-5-ether	Pressure extrusion	MRI	—	[157]
DSPC, DSPE-PEG	camptothecin-floxuridine	Nanoprecipitation/ microbubble	Focused ultrasound	56.7 ± 2.3	[158]
DSPC, DSPE-PEG3400-maleimide, DSPE-PEG-1000	Perfluorohexane (antibody ligated)	Emulsion	Isolation of Circulating Tumor Cells.	—	[159]
Phosphatidylcholine, cholesterol.	Indocyanine green and gold nanorods	Liposomes	Photoacoustic and fluorescence imaging	97% (implied)	[145]
DPPC, DPPA, DPPE, DSPE-PEG-COOH	Pentafluoroctane	Antibody conjugated nanobubble	Contrast agent for ultrasound imaging for ovarian cancer diagnosis	Not applicable	[160]
DPPC, DSPE-MPEG, DPPA, DPPE	pentafluoroctane	Nanobubble	Contrast agent for ultrasound imaging	Not applicable	[161]
DSPC, DPPE, DSPE-PEG2000-Biotin.	octafluoropropane	Nanobubble	Ultrasound imaging for cancer detection	Not applicable	[162]

Note: 1,2-dimyristoyl-sn-glycero-3-phosphatidic acid: DMPA, 1,2 Distearoyl-sn-glycero-3-phosphocholine: DSPC, Distearoyl-sn-glycero-3-phosphoethanolamine-N-[methoxy(polyethylene glycol)-2000: DSPE-MPEG2000, 1,2 dipalmitoyl-sn-glycero-3-phosphate: DPPA, 1,2-dipalmitoyl-sn-glycero-3-phosphoethanolamine: DPPE, 1,2-distearoyl-sn-glycero-3-phosphoethanolamine-N-[carboxy(polyethylene glycol)-2000]): DSPE-PEG-COOH, 1,2-distearoyl-sn-glycero-3-phosphoethanolamine-N-[PDP(polyethylene glycol)-2000]: DSPE-PEG-PDP, 1,2-dioleoyl-sn-glycero-3-phosphatidylcholine: DOPC; EE: Encapsulation Efficiency.

Table 3.
Plant and animal lipids-based nano-encapsulating carriers for diagnostic applications.

indicate diagnostic applications based on micro- and nano-encapsulation utilizing animal/plant lipids as encapsulating materials.

7. Conclusions and future trends

Application of natural polymers and their semi-synthetic polymer derivatives provide the basis for many commercially available DDSs that range from the traditional macroscale DDSs to microscale, nanoscale, targeted, and stimuli- responsive DDSs. The effective encapsulation technique and the achieved encapsulation efficiency depend on the physical and chemical properties of the selected natural polymer (e.g. polysaccharides, proteins, lipids) such as solubility, thermal stability, and its ability to form stable colloidal particles in a specific system. Therefore, various encapsulation methods including chemical, physical, physicochemical, mechanical and thermal encapsulation were discussed in details, **Table 1**.

Lipid vesicles nanocarriers have been discovered in 1960s, and later became known as "liposomes". In 1995, the first nano-drug based on Pegylated liposomal doxorubicin "DOXIL" was approved by FDA for cancer treatment. Polymer-drug conjugates and liposomes represent most of the marketed NP therapeutics and continue to be investigated extensively. Nanoencapsulation using lipid nanoparticles offers a practical approach to increase the solubility of water-insoluble drugs or poorly water soluble agents. Lipids have shown to be effective natural material for micro- and nanoencapsulation of bioactive small molecules and biologics for therapeutic and diagnostic drug delivery applications. Compared to other encapsulating materials, lipid-based encapsulation systems offer advantages such as low-cost and easy to scale-up and sterilize high biocompatibility, higher encapsulation efficiency, higher drug loading, and feasibility of carrying both hydrophilic and hydrophobic drugs.

Author details

Ndidi C. Ngwuluka[1*], Nedal Y. Abu-Thabit[2*], Onyinye J. Uwaezuoke[3], Joan O. Erebor[4], Margaret O. Ilomuanya[5], Riham R. Mohamed[6], Soliman M.A. Soliman[6], Mahmoud H. Abu Elella[6] and Noura A.A. Ebrahim[7]

1 Department of Pharmaceutics, Faculty of Pharmaceutical Sciences, University of Jos, Jos, Nigeria

2 Department of Chemical and Process Engineering Technology, Jubail Industrial College, Jubail Industrial City, 31961, Saudi Arabia

3 Department of Pharmaceutics and Pharmaceutical Technology, Faculty of Pharmacy, Olabisi Onabanjo University, Ago-Iwoye, Ogun State, Nigeria

4 Department of Pharmacy Practice, College of Pharmacy and Pharmaceutical Sciences, University of Toledo, Toledo, Ohio, USA

5 Center for Biomedical Research, Population Council, New York, 10065, USA

6 Chemistry Department, Faculty of Science, Cairo University, Giza, Egypt

7 Pathology Department, National Cancer Institute, Cairo University, Giza, Egypt

*Address all correspondences to: ndidi.ngwuluka@biodrudel.com and abuthabit_nidal@yahoo.com

IntechOpen

© 2020 The Author(s). Licensee IntechOpen. This chapter is distributed under the terms of the Creative Commons Attribution License (http://creativecommons.org/licenses/by/3.0), which permits unrestricted use, distribution, and reproduction in any medium, provided the original work is properly cited.

References

[1] Devi N, Sarmah M, Khatun B, Maji TK. Encapsulation of active ingredients in polysaccharide–protein complex coacervates. Advances in Colloid and Interface Science. 2017;**239**:136-145

[2] Ngwuluka NC, Ochekpe NA, Aruoma OI. Naturapolyceutics: The science of utilizing natural polymers for drug delivery. Polymers. 2014;**6**(5):1312-1332

[3] Ngwuluka NC, Ochekpe N. Natural Polymers: Drug Delivery. In: Mishra M, (ed). Encyclopedia of Biomedical Polymers and Polymeric Biomaterials, 11 Volume Set: CRC Press; 2015. p. 5603-5618.

[4] Čalija B, Cekić N, Milić J. Influence of Polycation functional properties on Polyanion micro/nanoparticles for NSAIDs reinforced via polyelectrolyte complexation: Alginate–chitosan case study. Microsized and Nanosized Carriers for Nonsteroidal Anti-Inflammatory Drugs: Elsevier; 2017. p. 133-160.

[5] Sinha N, Kulshreshtha NM, Dixit M, Jadhav I, Shrivastava D, Bisen PS. Nanodentistry: Novel approaches. Nanostructures for Oral Medicine: Elsevier; 2017. p. 751-776.

[6] Hrkach J, Langer R. From micro to nano: Evolution and impact of drug delivery in treating disease. Drug Delivery and Translational Research. 2020:1-4

[7] Fu F, Lin L, Xu E. Functional pretreatments of natural raw materials. Advanced High Strength Natural Fibre Composites in Construction: Elsevier; 2017. p. 87-114.

[8] Lengyel M, Kállai-Szabó N, Antal V, Laki AJ, Antal I. Microparticles, microspheres, and microcapsules for advanced drug delivery. Scientia Pharmaceutica. 2019;**87**(3):20

[9] Bochenek MA, Veiseh O, Vegas AJ, McGarrigle JJ, Qi M, Marchese E, et al. Alginate encapsulation as long-term immune protection of allogeneic pancreatic islet cells transplanted into the omental bursa of macaques. Nature Biomedical Engineering. 2018;**2**(11):810-821

[10] Arhewoh, Matthew., Okhamafe, Augustine., Auriemma, Finizia., Claudio, De., Di Girolamo, Rocco. Microencapsulated *Garcinia kola* and *Hunteria umbellata* seeds aqueous extracts – Part 1: Effect of microencapsulation process. International Journal of Phytopharmacy. 2016;6(1):1-9.

[11] Bremer-Hoffmann S, Halamoda-Kenzaoui B, Borgos SE. Identification of regulatory needs for nanomedicines. Journal of Interdisciplinary Nanomedicine. 2018;**3**(1):4-15

[12] Bayraktar O, Erdoğan İ, Köse MD, Kalmaz G. Nanocarriers for plant-derived natural compounds. In Ficai A., editors. Nanostructures for Antimicrobial Therapy: Elsevier. 2017:395-412

[13] Montalbán MG, Coburn JM, Lozano-Pérez AA, Cenis JL, Víllora G, Kaplan DL. Production of curcumin-loaded silk fibroin nanoparticles for cancer therapy. Nanomaterials. 2018;**8**(2):126

[14] Tammaro O, di Polidoro AC, Romano E, Netti PA, Torino E. A microfluidic platform to design multimodal PEG-crosslinked hyaluronic acid nanoparticles (PEG-cHANPs) for diagnostic applications. Scientific Reports. 2020;**10**(1):1-11

[15] Barenholz YC. Doxil®—The first FDA-approved nano-drug: Lessons

learned. Journal of Controlled Release. 2012;**160**(2):117-134

[16] George A, Shah PA, Shrivastav PS. Natural biodegradable polymers based nano-formulations for drug delivery: A review. International Journal of Pharmaceutics. 2019;**561**:244-264

[17] Moncada-Basualto M, Matsuhiro B, Mansilla A, Lapier M, Maya J, Olea-Azar C. Supramolecular hydrogels of β-cyclodextrin linked to calcium homopoly-l-guluronate for release of coumarins with trypanocidal activity. Carbohydrate Polymers. 2019;**204**:170-181

[18] Narayanaswamy R, Torchilin VP. Hydrogels and their applications in targeted drug delivery. Molecules. 2019;**24**(3):603

[19] Boffito M, Tonda-Turo C, Ciardelli G. Design of electrospun fibrous patches for myocardium regeneration. In: Guarino V, Ambrosio L, editors. Electrofluidodynamic Technologies (EFDTs) for Biomaterials and Medical Devices: Elsevier. 2018:221-250

[20] Biswas S, Sharmeen S, Islam MM, Rahman MM, Haque P, Mallik AK. Pharmaceutical Applications of Okra Gum. In: Nayak A, Hasnain M, Pal D, (eds). Natural Polymers for Pharmaceutical Applications. CRC Press; 2019. p. 183-202.

[21] Trojanowska A, Nogalska A, Valls RG, Giamberini M, Tylkowski B. Technological solutions for encapsulation. Physical Sciences Reviews. 2017;**2**(9):20170020

[22] Bazylińska U, Wawrzyńczyk D, Kulbacka J, Frąckowiak R, Cichy B, Bednarkiewicz A, et al. Polymeric nanocapsules with up-converting nanocrystals cargo make ideal fluorescent bioprobes. Scientific Reports. 2016;**6**(1):29746

[23] Zhang Z, Li L, Sun D, Wang M, Shi J, Yang D, et al. Preparation and properties of chitosan-based microspheres by spray drying. Food Science & Nutrition. 2020;**8**(4):1933-1941

[24] Mishra MK. Microencapsulation. In: Kirk-Othmer Encyclopedia of Chemical Technology. 3rd Edition, John Wiley & Sons; 2019. p. 1-35

[25] Sosnik A, Seremeta KP. Advantages and challenges of the spray-drying technology for the production of pure drug particles and drug-loaded polymeric carriers. Advances in Colloid and Interface Science. 2015;**223**:40-54

[26] Zhang S, Chen J, Yin X, Wang X, Qiu B, Zhu L, et al. Microencapsulation of tea tree oil by spray-drying with methyl cellulose as the emulsifier and wall material together with chitosan/alginate. Journal of Applied Polymer Science. 2017;**134**(13):44662

[27] Wei Y, Huang Y, Cheng K, Song Y. Investigations of the influences of processing conditions on the properties of spray dried chitosan-tripolyphosphate particles loaded with theophylline. Scientific Reports. 2020;**10**(1):1155

[28] Coulomb D. Refrigeration. In: Cachon R, Girardon P, Voilley A, (eds). Gases in Agro-Food Processes. 1st Edition. Academic Press; 2019. p. 223-318.

[29] Oxley J. Chapter 4 - Overview of Microencapsulation Process Technologies. In: Microencapsulation in the food industry. Academic Press; 2014. pp. 35-46

[30] Russo P, Morello S, Pinto A, Del Gaudio P, Auriemma G, Aquino RP. Zinc and calcium cations combination in the production of floating alginate beads as prednisolone delivery systems. Molecules. 2020;**25**(5):1140

[31] Singh MN, Hemant KSY, Ram M, Shivakumar HG. Microencapsulation: A promising technique for controlled drug delivery. Research in Pharmaceutical Sciences. 2010;**5**(2):65-77

[32] Frey CR. Encapsulation via Pan-Coating. In: Mishra M, (ed). Handbook of Encapsulation and Controlled Release: CRC Press; 2015. p. 147.

[33] Amaral PHRd, Andrade PL, Conto LCd. Microencapsulation and its uses in food science and technology: A review. In: Salaün F, (ed). Microencapsulation - Processes, Technologies and Industrial Applications: IntechOpen; 2019.

[34] de Souza L. Franquelin Gomes, Nitz M. Taranto OP. Film Coating of Nifedipine Extended Release Pellets in a Fluid Bed Coater with a Wurster Insert. BioMed Research International. 2014;**2014**:e520758

[35] Patil H, Tiwari RV, Repka MA. Hot-melt extrusion: From theory to application in pharmaceutical formulation. AAPS PharmSciTech. 2015;**17**(1):20-42

[36] Muley S, Nandgude T, Poddar S. Extrusion–spheronization a promising pelletization technique: In-depth review. Asian Journal of Pharmaceutical Sciences. 2016;**11**(6):684-699

[37] Kallakunta VR, Sarabu S, Bandari S, Tiwari R, Patil H, Repka MA. An update on the contribution of hot-melt extrusion technology to novel drug delivery in the twenty-first century: Part I. Expert Opinion on Drug Delivery. 2019;**16**(5):539-550

[38] Azad MOK, Kang WS, Lim JD, Park CH. Bio- fortification of Angelica gigas Nakai Nano-powder using bio-polymer by hot melt extrusion to enhance the bioaccessibility and functionality of nutraceutical compounds. Pharmaceuticals. 2020;**13**(1):3

[39] Gately NM, Kennedy JE. The development of a melt-extruded shellac carrier for the targeted delivery of probiotics to the colon. Pharmaceutics. 2017;**9**(4):38

[40] Castro N, Durrieu V, Raynaud C, Rouilly A, Rigal L, Quellet C. Melt extrusion encapsulation of flavors: A review. Polymer Reviews. 2016;**56**(1):137-186

[41] Chang D, Hayat K, Abbas S, Zhang X, Chang D, Hayat K, et al. Ascorbic acid encapsulation in a glassy carbohydrate matrix via hot melt extrusion: Preparation and characterization. Food Science and Technology. 2019;**39**(3):660-666

[42] Khor CM, Ng WK, Kanaujia P, Chan KP, Dong Y. Hot-melt extrusion microencapsulation of quercetin for taste-masking. Journal of Microencapsulation. 2017;**34**(1):29-37

[43] Shinde T, Sun-Waterhouse D, Brooks J. Co-extrusion encapsulation of probiotic lactobacillus acidophilus alone or together with apple skin polyphenols: An aqueous and value-added delivery system using alginate. Food and Bioprocess Technology. 2014;**7**(6):1581-1596

[44] Silva MP, Tulini FL, Martins E, Penning M, Fávaro-Trindade CS, Poncelet D. Comparison of extrusion and co-extrusion encapsulation techniques to protect lactobacillus acidophilus LA3 in simulated gastrointestinal fluids. LWT. 2018;**89**:392-399

[45] Demont A, Marison IW. Microencapsulation by dripping and jet break-up. In: Mishra M, editor. Handbook of. Encapsulation and Controlled Release: CRC Press; 2015

[46] Martin-Banderas L, Ganan-Calvo M, Fernandez-Arevalo A. Making drops in microencapsulation

processes. Letters in Drug Design & Discovery. 2010;**7**(4):300-309

[47] Dorati R, Genta I, Modena T, Conti B. Microencapsulation of a hydrophilic model molecule through vibration nozzle and emulsion phase inversion technologies. Journal of Microencapsulation. 2013;**30**(6):559-570

[48] Bidoret A, Martins E, De Smet BP, Poncelet D. Cell microencapsulation: Dripping methods. Methods in Molecular Biology. 2017;**1479**:43-55

[49] Carneiro J, Campos JBLM, Miranda JM. High viscosity polymeric fluid droplet formation in a flow focusing microfluidic device - experimental and numerical study. Chemical Engineering Science. 2019;**195**:442-454

[50] Nooranidoost M, Haghshenas M, Muradoglu M, Kumar R. Cell encapsulation modes in a flow-focusing microchannel: Effects of shell fluid viscosity. Microfluidics and Nanofluidics. 2019;**23**(3):31

[51] Ciriza J, Saenz del Burgo L, Hernández RM, Orive G, Pedraz JL. Use of Flow Focusing Technique for Microencapsulation of Myoblasts. In: Opara EC, (ed). Cell Microencapsulation: Methods and Protocols New York, NY: Springer; 2017. p. 207-216.

[52] Li W, Zhang L, Ge X, Xu B, Zhang W, Qu L, et al. Microfluidic fabrication of microparticles for biomedical applications. Chemical Society Reviews. 2018;**47**(15):5646-5683

[53] Cam ME, Zhang Y, Edirisinghe M. Electrosprayed microparticles: A novel drug delivery method. Expert Opinion on Drug Delivery. 2019;**16**(9):895-901

[54] Guan B, Cole RB. The background to electrospray. In: Gross ML, Caprioli RM, editors. The Encyclopedia of Mass Spectrometry. Boston: Elsevier; 2016. pp. 132-140

[55] Parhizkar M, Reardon PJT, Knowles JC, Browning RJ, Stride E, Pedley RB, et al. Performance of novel high throughput multi electrospray systems for forming of polymeric micro/nanoparticles. Materials and Design. 2017;**126**:73-84

[56] Wang J, Jansen JA, Yang F. Electrospraying: Possibilities and challenges of engineering carriers for biomedical applications - A mini review. Frontiers in Chemistry. 2019;**7**:258

[57] Xie J, Jiang J, Davoodi P, Srinivasan MP, Wang C. Electrohydrodynamic atomization: A two-decade effort to produce and process micro−/nanoparticulate materials. Chemical Engineering Science. 2015;**125**:32-57

[58] ShamsT, IllangakoonUE, ParhizkarM, Harker AH, Edirisinghe S, Orlu M, et al. Electrosprayed microparticles for intestinal delivery of prednisolone. Journal of the Royal Society Interface. 2018;**15**(145):20180491

[59] Yuan S, Lei F, Liu Z, Tong Q, Si T, Xu RX. Coaxial electrospray of curcumin-loaded microparticles for sustained drug release. PLoS One. 2015;**10**(7):e0132609

[60] Gómez-Mascaraque LG, Ambrosio-Martín J, Perez-Masiá R. Lopez-Rubio A. Impact of Acetic Acid on the Survival of *L. plantarum* upon Microencapsulation by Coaxial Electrospraying. Journal of Healthcare Engineering. 2017;**2017**:4698079

[61] Lee H, An S, Kim S, Jeon B, Kim M, Kim IS. Readily Functionalizable and stabilizable polymeric particles with controlled size and morphology by electrospray. Scientific Reports. 2018;**8**(1):15725

[62] Paulo BB, Ramos FM, Prata AS. An investigation of operational parameters of jet cutting method on the size of Ca-alginate beads. Journal of Food Process Engineering. 2017;**40**(6):e12591

[63] Ammendola M, Rodrigo Gomez R, Garcia VR. Perfume encapsulation via vapor induced phase separation. PRO. 2019;7(12):865

[64] Song Y, Fan J, Wang S. Recent progress in interfacial polymerization. Materials Chemistry Frontiers. 2017;**1**(6):1028-1040

[65] Perrier E, Hart J. Smart vectorization: Enzymatically activated encapsulation technologies. In: Rosen M, editor. Delivery System Handbook for Personal Care and Cosmetic Products Norwich. NY: William Andrew Publishing; 2005. pp. 797-816

[66] Kanellopoulos A, Giannaros P, Palmer D, Kerr A, Al-Tabbaa A. Polymeric microcapsules with switchable mechanical properties for self-healing concrete: Synthesis, characterisation and proof of concept. Smart Materials and Structures. 2017;**26**(4):045025

[67] Ishizuka F, Stenzel MH, Zetterlund PB. Microcapsule synthesis via RAFT photopolymerization in vegetable oil as a green solvent. Journal of Polymer Science Part A: Polymer Chemistry. 2018;**56**(8):831-839

[68] Nguon O, Lagugné-Labarthet F, Brandys FA, Li J, Gillies ER. Microencapsulation by in situ polymerization of amino resins. Polymer Reviews. 2018;**58**(2):326-375

[69] Jiang T, Mo R, Bellotti A, Zhou J, Gu Z. Gel - liposome-mediated Co-delivery of anticancer membrane-associated proteins and small-molecule drugs for enhanced therapeutic efficacy. Advanced Functional Materials. 2014;**24**(16):2295-2304

[70] Racoti A, Rusen E, Dinescu A, Ion VA, Calinescu I, Mocanu A, et al. Ginger essential oil encapsulation in PMMA microcapsules–part II. University Politehnica Of Bucharest Scientific Bulletin Series B-Chemistry and Materials Science. 2016;**78**(3):87-96

[71] Iqbal M, Zafar N, Fessi H, Elaissari A. Double emulsion solvent evaporation techniques used for drug encapsulation. International Journal of Pharmaceutics. 2015;**496**(2):173-190

[72] Urbaniak T, Musial W. Influence of solvent evaporation technique parameters on diameter of submicron lamivudine-poly-Îµ-caprolactone conjugate particles. Nanomaterials. 2019;**9**(9):1240

[73] Hoa LTM, Chi NT, Nguyen LH, Chien DM. Preparation and characterisation of nanoparticles containing ketoprofen and acrylic polymers prepared by emulsion solvent evaporation method. Journal of Experimental Nanoscience. 2012;**7**(2):189-197

[74] Jiang J, Ao J, He C, Xiong J, Zhao J, Liu J, et al. Preparation and characterisation of ginkgolide nanoparticles via the emulsion solvent evaporation method. Micro Nano Letters. 2018;**13**(5):636-640

[75] Martínez Rivas CJ, Tarhini M, Badri W, Miladi K, Greige-Gerges H, Nazari QA, et al. Nanoprecipitation process: From encapsulation to drug delivery. International Journal of Pharmaceutics. 2017;**532**(1):66-81

[76] Yesenia Hernández-Giottonini K, Josefina Rodríguez-Córdova R, Alejandra Gutiérrez-Valenzuela C, Peñuñuri-Miranda O, Zavala-Rivera P, Guerrero-Germán P, et al. PLGA nanoparticlepreparationsbyemulsification

and nanoprecipitation techniques: Effects of formulation parameters. RSC Advances. 2020;**10**(8):4218-4231

[77] Corrêa-Filho LC, Moldão-Martins M, Alves VD. Advances in the application of microcapsules as carriers of functional compounds for food products. Applied Sciences. 2019;**9**(3):571

[78] Capelezzo AP, Mohr LC, Dalcanton F, Mello JMM de, Fiori MA. β-Cyclodextrins as Encapsulating Agents of Essential Oils. In: Arora P, Dhingra N. (eds). Cyclodextrin - A Versatile Ingredient: IntechOpen. 2018. P. 169-200.

[79] Brito de Souza V, Thomazini M, Chaves IE, Ferro-Furtado R, Favaro-Trindade C. Microencapsulation by complex coacervation as a tool to protect bioactive compounds and to reduce astringency and strong flavor of vegetable extracts. Food Hydrocolloids 2020;98:105244.

[80] Lemos YP, Marfil PHM, Nicoletti V. Particle size characteristics of Buriti oil microcapsules produced by gelatin-sodium alginate complex coacervation: Effect of stirring speed. International Journal of Food Properties. 2017;**20**:1438-1447

[81] Ariga K, Ahn E, Park M, Kim B. Layer-by-layer assembly: Recent Progress from layered assemblies to layered Nanoarchitectonics. Chemistry - An Asian Journal. 2019;**14**(15): 2553-2566

[82] Bah MG, Bilal HM, Wang J. Fabrication and application of complex microcapsules: A review. Soft Matter. 2020;**16**(3):570-590

[83] Piccinino D, Capecchi E, Botta L, Bizzarri BM, Bollella P, Antiochia R, et al. Layer-by-layer preparation of microcapsules and nanocapsules of mixed polyphenols with high antioxidant and UV-shielding properties. Biomacromolecules. 2018;**19**(9):3883-3893

[84] Rochín-Wong S, Rosas-Durazo A, Zavala-Rivera P, Maldonado A, Martínez-Barbosa ME, Vélaz I, et al. Drug release properties of Diflunisal from layer-by-layer self-assembled Î°-carrageenan/chitosan nanocapsules: Effect of deposited layers. Polymers. 2018;**10**(7):760

[85] Paşcalău V, Tertis M, Pall E, Suciu M, Marinca T, Pustan M, et al. Bovine serum albumin gel/polyelectrolyte complex of hyaluronic acid and chitosan based microcarriers for Sorafenib targeted delivery. J Appl Polym Sci 2020;N/A:49002.

[86] Soh SH, Lee LY. Microencapsulation and nanoencapsulation using supercritical fluid (SCF) techniques. Pharmaceutics. 2019;**11**(1):21

[87] Zhu L, Lan H, He B, Hong W, Li J. Encapsulation of menthol in beeswax by a supercritical fluid technique. International Journal of Chemical Engineering. 2010;**2010**:e608680

[88] Karim FT, Ghafoor K, Ferdosh S, Al-Juhaimi F, Ali E, Yunus KB, et al. Microencapsulation of fish oil using supercritical antisolvent process. Journal of Food and Drug Analysis. 2017;**25**(3):654-666

[89] Leon M. Si-based inorganic microencapsulation. Physical Sciences Reviews. 2016;**1**(3):20150008

[90] Ashraf MA, Khan AM, Sarfraz M, Ahmad M. Effectiveness of silica based sol-gel microencapsulation method for odorants and flavors leading to sustainable environment. Frontiers in Chemistry. 2015;**3**:42

[91] Gonzalez Gomez A, Syed S, Marshall K, Hosseinidoust Z. Liposomal Nanovesicles for efficient encapsulation

of staphylococcal antibiotics. ACS Omega. 2019;**4**(6):10866-10876

[92] Rahman A, Uahengo V, Likius D, Rahman A, Uahengo V, Likius D. Mini review on emerging methods of preparation of liposome and its application as liposome drug delivery systems. Open Journal of Pharmacology and Pharmacotherapeutics. 2018;**3**(1):005-021

[93] Cheirsilp B, Rakmai J. Inclusion complex formation of cyclodextrin with its guest and their applications. Biology, Engineering and Medicine 2017;2(1).

[94] Abu-Thabit N, Makhlouf ASH. Historical development of drug delivery systems: From conventional macroscale to controlled, targeted, and responsive nanoscale systems. Stimuli Responsive Polymeric Nanocarriers for Drug Delivery Applications, Volume 1: Elsevier; 2018. p. 3-41.

[95] Makhlouf ASH, Abu-Thabit N. Stimuli Responsive Polymeric Nanocarriers for Drug Delivery Applications: Volume 1: Types and Triggers: Woodhead Publishing; 2018.

[96] Makhlouf ASH, Abu-Thabit N. Stimuli Responsive Polymeric Nanocarriers for Drug Delivery Applications: Volume 2: Advanced Nanocarriers for Therapeutics: Woodhead Publishing; 2019.

[97] Kamaly N, Yameen B, Wu J, Farokhzad OC. Degradable controlled-release polymers and polymeric nanoparticles: Mechanisms of controlling drug release. Chemical Reviews. 2016;**116**(4):2602-2663

[98] Nicolas J, Mura S, Brambilla D, Mackiewicz N, Couvreur P. Design, functionalization strategies and biomedical applications of targeted biodegradable/biocompatible polymer-based nanocarriers for drug delivery. Chemical Society Reviews. 2013;**42**(3):1147-1235

[99] ASPINALL GO. Classification of polysaccharides. The polysaccharides: Elsevier; 1983. p. 1-9

[100] Ngwuluka NC. Responsive polysaccharides and polysaccharides-based nanoparticles for drug delivery. In: Makhlouf ASH, Abu-Thabit N. (eds). Stimuli Responsive Polymeric Nanocarriers for Drug Delivery Applications: Volume 1: Types and triggers: Elsevier; 2018. p. 531-554

[101] Abu-Thabit N, Judeh AA, Umar Y, Ahmad A, Hakeem AS, Ul-Hamid A. Isolation and characterization of microcrystalline cellulose from date seeds (Phoenix dactylifera L.). International Journal of Biological Macromolecules. 2020;**155**:730-739

[102] Rodriguez CF, Bruneau N, Barra J, Alfonso D. Hydrophilic cellulose derivatives as drug delivery carriers: Influence of substitution type on the properties. Handbook of pharmaceutical controlled release technology. 2000;**1**

[103] Parmar V, Patel G, Abu-Thabit N. Responsive cyclodextrins as polymeric carriers for drug delivery applications. In: Makhlouf ASH, Abu-Thabit N. (eds). Stimuli Responsive Polymeric Nanocarriers for Drug Delivery Applications, Volume 1: Elsevier; 2018. p. 555-580.

[104] Wang J, Qiu Z, Wang Y, Li L, Guo X, Pham D, et al. Supramolecular polymer assembly in aqueous solution arising from cyclodextrin host-guest complexation. Beilstein Journal of Organic Chemistry. 2016;**12**(1):50-72

[105] Simoes SMN, Rey-Rico A, Concheiro A, Alvarez-Lorenzo C. Supramolecular cyclodextrin-based

drug nanocarriers. Chemical Communications. 2015;**51**(29):6275-6289

[106] Efthimiadou EK, Theodosiou M, Toniolo G, Abu-Thabit N. Stimuli-responsive biopolymer nanocarriers for drug delivery applications. In: Makhlouf ASH, Abu-Thabit N. (eds). Stimuli Responsive Polymeric Nanocarriers for Drug Delivery Applications, Volume 1: Elsevier; 2018. p. 405-432.

[107] Emmanuel BD, Abu-Thabit N, Ngwuluka NC. Responsive poly-electrolyte complexes based on natural polysaccharides for drug delivery applications. In: Makhlouf ASH, Abu-Thabit N. (eds). Stimuli Responsive Polymeric Nanocarriers for Drug Delivery Applications, Volume 1: Elsevier; 2018. p. 267-287.

[108] Wu D, Zhu L, Li Y, Zhang X, Xu S, Yang G, et al. Chitosan-based colloidal polyelectrolyte complexes for drug delivery: A review. Carbohydrate Polymers. 2020;**116126**

[109] Pasteur L. Sur la fermentation visquese et la fermentation butyrique. Bull. Soc. Chim. Paris. 1861;**11**:30-31

[110] Wasiak I, Kulikowska A, Janczewska M, Michalak M, Cymerman IA, Nagalski A, et al. Dextran nanoparticle synthesis and properties. PLoS One. 2016;**11**(1):e0146237

[111] Delair T. Colloidal polyelectrolyte complexes of chitosan and dextran sulfate towards versatile nanocarriers of bioactive molecules. European Journal of Pharmaceutics and Biopharmaceutics. 2011;**78**(1):10-18

[112] Koshland DE, Haurowitz F. Protein Biochemistry. 2020; Available at: https://www.britannica.com/science/protein. Accessed 27th May 2020.

[113] Pieters BJGE, Van Eldijk MB, Nolte RJM, Mecinović J. Natural supramolecular protein assemblies. Chemical Society Reviews. 2016;**45**(1):24-39

[114] Gabrani R, Ghildiyal R, Pratap N, Sharma G, Dang S. Applications of Protein Nanoparticles as Drug Delivery Vehicle. Smart Healthcare Systems: Chapman and Hall/CRC; 2019. pp. 199-215

[115] Elzoghby AO. Gelatin-based nanoparticles as drug and gene delivery systems: Reviewing three decades of research. Journal of Controlled Release. 2013;**172**(3):1075-1091

[116] Guo M, Wang G. Milk protein polymer and its application in environmentally safe adhesives. Polymers. 2016;**8**(9):324

[117] Gandhi S, Roy I. Doxorubicin-loaded casein nanoparticles for drug delivery: Preparation, characterization and in vitro evaluation. International Journal of Biological Macromolecules. 2019;**121**:6-12

[118] Iwao Y, Ishima Y, Yamada J, Noguchi T, Kragh-Hansen U, Mera K, et al. Quantitative evaluation of the role of cysteine and methionine residues in the antioxidant activity of human serum albumin using recombinant mutants. IUBMB Life. 2012;**64**(5):450-454

[119] Levitt DG, Levitt MD. Human serum albumin homeostasis: A new look at the roles of synthesis, catabolism, renal and gastrointestinal excretion, and the clinical value of serum albumin measurements. International journal of general medicine. 2016;**9**:229-255

[120] Kunda NK, Alfagih IM, Dennison SR, Tawfeek HM, Somavarapu S, Hutcheon GA, et al. Bovine serum albumin adsorbed PGA-co-PDL nanocarriers for

vaccine delivery via dry powder inhalation. Pharmaceutical Research. 2015;**32**(4):1341-1353

[121] Guan G, Song B, Zhang J, Chen K, Hu H, Wang M, et al. An effective cationic human serum albumin-based gene-delivery carrier containing the nuclear localization signal. Pharmaceutics. 2019;**11**(11):608

[122] Jin Q, Qiao C, Li J, Li J, Xiao X. An engineered serum albumin-binding AAV9 capsid achieves improved liver transduction after intravenous delivery in mice. Gene Therapy. 2019;**27**:237-244

[123] Lomis N, Westfall S, Farahdel L, Malhotra M, Shum-Tim D, Prakash S. Human serum albumin nanoparticles for use in cancer drug delivery: Process optimization and in vitro characterization. Nanomaterials. 2016;**6**(6):116

[124] Scheffel U, Rhodes BA, Natarajan TK, Wagner HN. Albumin microspheres for study of the reticuloendothelial system. Journal of Nuclear Medicine. 1972;**13**(7):498-503

[125] Criswell B. Connecting acids and bases with encapsulation... and chemistry with nanotechnology. Journal of Chemical Education 2007;84(7):1136.

[126] Damascelli B, Cantu G, Mattavelli F, Tamplenizza P, Bidoli P, Leo E, et al. Intraarterial chemotherapy with polyoxyethylated castor oil free paclitaxel, incorporated in albumin nanoparticles (ABI-007). Cancer. 2001;**92**(10):2592-2602

[127] Solbiati L, Martegani A, Leen E. Contrast-Enhanced Ultrasound of Liver Diseases: Springer Science & Business Media; 2003.

[128] Shrestha H, Bala R, Arora S. Lipid-Based Drug Delivery Systems. Journal of pharmaceutics 2014;2014:801820).

[129] Kalepu S, Nekkanti V. Insoluble drug delivery strategies: Review of recent advances and business prospects. Acta Pharmaceutica Sinica B. 2015;**5**(5):442-453

[130] Kim MW, Kwon S, Choi JH, Lee A. A promising biocompatible platform: Lipid-based and bio-inspired smart drug delivery systems for cancer therapy. International Journal of Molecular Sciences. 2018; **19**(12):3859

[131] Savla R, Browne J, Plassat V, Wasan KM, Wasan EK. Review and analysis of FDA approved drugs using lipid-based formulations. Drug Development and Industrial Pharmacy. 2017;**43**(11):1743-1758

[132] Krstić M, Medarević Đ, Đuriš J, Ibrić S. Chapter 12 - Self-nanoemulsifying drug delivery systems (SNEDDS) and self-microemulsifying drug delivery systems (SMEDDS) as lipid nanocarriers for improving dissolution rate and bioavailability of poorly soluble drugs. In: Grumezescu AM, editors. Lipid Nanocarriers for Drug Targeting: William Andrew Publishing. 2018:473-508

[133] Sassene PJ, Michaelsen MH, Mosgaard MD, Jensen MK, Van Den Broek E, Wasan KM, et al. In vivo precipitation of poorly soluble drugs from lipid-based drug delivery systems. Molecular Pharmaceutics. 2016;**13**(10):3417-3426

[134] Cantón AS, Broek N van den, Danelon C. Development of a lipid-based delivery system for the chemotherapeutic compound SN-38. bioRxiv 2019.

[135] Conde J, Rosa J, Lima JC, Baptista PV. Nanophotonics for molecular diagnostics and therapy applications. International Journal of Photoenergy. 2011;**2012**:e619530

[136] Liu L, Zhang Y, Qiu W, Zhang L, Gao F, Li B, et al. Dual-stage light amplified photodynamic therapy against hypoxic tumor based on an O2 self-sufficient Nanoplatform. Small. 2017;**13**(37):1701621

[137] Kenechukwu FC, Attama AA, Ibezim EC, Nweke LI, Ahiabuike JE. Physicochemical and safety characteristics of novel microstructured lipid-based drug delivery system encapsulating miconazole nitrate. Journal of Pharmaceutical and Allied Sciences. 2017;**14**(4):2646-2658

[138] Stella B, Peira E, Dianzani C, Gallarate M, Battaglia L, Gigliotti CL, et al. Development and characterization of solid lipid nanoparticles loaded with a highly active doxorubicin derivative. Nanomaterials. 2018;**8**(2):110

[139] Xie J, Fan Z, Li Y, Zhang Y, Yu F, Su G, et al. Design of pH-sensitive methotrexate prodrug-targeted curcumin nanoparticles for efficient dual-drug delivery and combination cancer therapy. International Journal of Nanomedicine. 2018;**13**:1381-1398

[140] Hoy SM. Patisiran: First global approval. Drugs. 2018;**78**(15):1625-1631

[141] Zhang X, Goel V, Robbie GJ. Pharmacokinetics of patisiran, the first approved RNA interference therapy in patients with hereditary transthyretin-mediated amyloidosis. The Journal of Clinical Pharmacology. 2020;**60**(5):573-585

[142] Chen J, Sun X, Shao R, Xu Y, Gao J, Liang W. VEGF siRNA delivered by polycation liposome-encapsulated calcium phosphate nanoparticles for tumor angiogenesis inhibition in breast cancer. International Journal of Nanomedicine. 2017;**12**:6075-6088

[143] Wang HH, Tsourkas A. Cytosolic delivery of inhibitory antibodies with cationic lipids. Proceedings of the National Academy of Sciences. 2019;**116**(44):22132-22139

[144] Kose N, Fox JM, Sapparapu G, Bombardi R, Tennekoon RN, de Silva AD, et al. A lipid-encapsulated mRNA encoding a potently neutralizing human monoclonal antibody protects against chikungunya infection. Sci Immunol 2019;4(35):eaaw6647.

[145] Guan T, Shang W, Li H, Yang X, Fang C, Tian J, et al. From detection to resection: Photoacoustic tomography and surgery guidance with indocyanine green loaded gold nanorod@liposome Core-Shell nanoparticles in liver cancer. Bioconjugate Chemistry. 2017;**28**(4):1221-1228

[146] Zhang H, Ingham ES, Gagnon MK, Mahakian LM, Liu J, Foiret JL, et al. In vitro characterization and in vivo ultrasound molecular imaging of nucleolin-targeted microbubbles. Biomaterials. 2017;**118**:63-73

[147] Deng Y, Huang H, Chen M, Chen G, Zou W, Zhao Y, et al. Comprehensive effects of near-infrared multifunctional liposomes on cancer cells. Molecules. 2020;**25**(5):1098

[148] Cool SK, Geers B, Roels S, Stremersch S, Vanderperren K, Saunders JH, et al. **Coupling of drug containing liposomes to microbubbles improves ultrasound triggered drug delivery in mice**. **Journal of Controlled Release**. **2013;172(3):885-893**

[149] Wang D, Yang K, Gao Y, Tan K, Liu Z. Preparation and characterization of a nanoscale ultrasound contrast agent. Clinical Imaging. 2010;**34**(4):288-292

[150] Shi G, Cui W, Benchimol M, Liu Y, Mattrey RF, Mukthavaram R, et al. Isolation of rare tumor cells from blood cells with buoyant immuno-microbubbles. PLoS One. 2013;**8**(3):e58017

[151] Ninomiya K, Yamashita T, Tanabe Y, Imai M, Takahashi K, Shimizu N. Targeted and ultrasound-triggered cancer cell injury using perfluorocarbon emulsion-loaded liposomes endowed with cancer cell-targeting and fusogenic capabilities. Ultrasonics Sonochemistry. 2016;**28**:54-61

[152] Carson AR, McTiernan CF, Lavery L, Hodnick A, Grata M, Leng X, et al. Gene therapy of carcinoma using ultrasound-targeted microbubble destruction. Ultrasound in Medicine & Biology. 2011;**37**(3):393-402

[153] Kostevšek N, Cheung CC, Serša I, Kreft ME, Monaco I, Comes Franchini M, et al. Magneto-liposomes as MRI contrast agents: A systematic study of different liposomal formulations. Nanomaterials. 2020;**10**(5):889

[154] Prabhakar A, Banerjee R. Nanobubble liposome complexes for diagnostic imaging and ultrasound-triggered drug delivery in cancers: A theranostic approach. ACS Omega. 2019;**4**(13):15567-15580

[155] Nel J, Franconi F, Joudiou N, Saulnier P, Gallez B, Lemaire L. Lipid nanocapsules as in vivo oxygen sensors using magnetic resonance imaging. Materials Science and Engineering: C. 2019;**101**:396-403

[156] Centelles MN, Wright M, So P, Amrahli M, Xu XY, Stebbing J, et al. Image-guided thermosensitive liposomes for focused ultrasound drug delivery: Using NIRF-labelled lipids and topotecan to visualise the effects of hyperthermia in tumours. Journal of Controlled Release. 2018;**280**:87-98

[157] Gambino G, Gambino T, Angelovski G. Combination of bioresponsive chelates and perfluorinated lipid nanoparticles enables in vivo MRI probe quantification. Chemical Communications. 2020;**56**(66):9433-9436

[158] Liang X, Xu Y, Gao C, Zhou Y, Zhang N, Dai Z. Ultrasound contrast agent microbubbles with ultrahigh loading capacity of camptothecin and floxuridine for enhancing tumor accumulation and combined chemotherapeutic efficacy. NPG Asia Materials. 2018;**10**(8):761-774

[159] Wang G, Benasutti H, Jones JF, Shi G, Benchimol M, Pingle S, et al. Isolation of breast cancer CTCs with multitargeted buoyant immunomicrobubbles. Colloids and Surfaces B: Biointerfaces. 2018;**161**:200-209

[160] Gao Y, Hernandez C, Yuan H, Lilly J, Kota P, Zhou H, et al. Ultrasound molecular imaging of ovarian cancer with CA-125 targeted nanobubble contrast agents. Nanomedicine: Nanotechnology, Biology and Medicine. 2017;**13**(7):2159-2168

[161] Wu H, Abenojar EC, Perera R, An T, Exner AA. Time-intensity-curve analysis and tumor extravasation of nanobubble ultrasound contrast agents. Ultrasound in Medicine & Biology. 2019;**45**(9):2502-2514

[162] Jiang Q, Zeng Y, Xu Y, Xiao X, Liu H, Zhou B, et al. Ultrasound molecular imaging as a potential non-invasive diagnosis to detect the margin of hepatocarcinoma via CSF-1R targeting. Frontiers in Bioengineering and Biotechnology. 2020;**8**:783

Chapter 2

Natural Polymers in Micro- and Nanoencapsulation for Therapeutic and Diagnostic Applications: Part II - Polysaccharides and Proteins

Ndidi C. Ngwuluka, Nedal Y. Abu-Thabit, Onyinye J. Uwaezuoke, Joan O. Erebor, Margaret O. Ilomuanya, Riham R. Mohamed, Soliman M.A. Soliman, Mahmoud H. Abu Elella and Noura A.A. Ebrahim

Abstract

Encapsulation remains a fundamental and consistent approach of fabrication of drug and diagnostic delivery systems in the health space and natural polymers such as polysaccharides and proteins continue to play significant roles. Micro- or nanoencapsulation is employed for the conventional pharmaceuticals, biopharmaceuticals, or biologics, bioactives from natural sources and diagnostics such as biomarkers. The outcome of any encapsulation depends on the technique employed and the encapsulating material. The encapsulating materials employed influence the physical and chemical attributes of the fabricated micro- and nanocapsules. The encapsulating materials could be natural or synthetic, however, natural polymers are preferred because they are human and environmentally friendly. Polysaccharides and proteins are abundant in nature, biogenic, biocompatible, biodegradable and possess biological functions making them materials of choice for encapsulation of drugs and diagnostics. This chapter reviews the recent and advanced applications of polysaccharides and proteins as nanocarrier materials for micro- and nanoencapsulation of therapeutics and diagnostics.

Keywords: natural polymers, biopolymers, drug delivery, nanoencapsulation, microencapsulation, polysaccharides, proteins, therapeutic, diagnostic

1. Introduction

Encapsulation remains a fundamental and consistent approach of fabrication of drug and diagnostic delivery systems in the health space and natural polymers such as polysaccharides and proteins continue to play significant roles. Natural polymers (polysaccharides, proteins, and lipids), the macromolecules found in nature are integral in the existence of living organisms especially polysaccharides and proteins. Natural polymers constitute a huge portion of the earth's organic matter because they are synthesized by living organisms such as plants, animals, bacteria, and fungi during their entire life cycle. Polysaccharides also referred to as glycans are the most abundant organic compounds on earth. Polysaccharides are involved in many vital functions in nature such as provision of support and stability for cells and tissues, facilitation of cell communications, storage of energy, protection, lubrication, and cell recognition. Proteins are regarded as the 'workhorses' of cells being involved in many processes necessary for life including being the expressions of genetic information.

Polysaccharides, proteins, and lipids interact in nature to enhance day to day functions in living organisms. Polysaccharides bind with protein and lipids to form glycoproteins and glycolipids respectively which can be used for cell communications. Other processes modulated by glycoconjugates (glycoproteins and glycolipids) include molecular targeting, cell migration, cell–cell interactions, immune responses, and blood clotting. Polysaccharides influence how proteins function and how cells respond to stimuli. The behavior of a protein is affected by which glycan is attached to it. Glycoproteins are abundant in the cells where they can serve as regulatory switches.

Since natural polymers are biogenic, when used for therapeutic applications, the body would usually identify with them and not treat as foreign bodies thereby bypassing the body's defense mechanisms leading to long circulation of the delivery system and possible targeting to the site of action. The biological properties of polysaccharides and proteins such as cell recognition and interactions, enzymatic degradability, semblance to extracellular matrix and their chemical flexibility [1] make them materials of choice for encapsulation of drugs and diagnostics. In addition, they are preferred to synthetic polymers because they are less toxic, eco-friendly, biodegradable, biocompatible and renewable. Polysaccharides and proteins are used for micro- and nanoencapsulation because they exhibit good process efficiency, are modifiable and can be tailored to target the desired site of action, have good rheological and emulsification/emulsion stabilizing properties, gelling and film forming [2, 3]. In addition, use of polysaccharides and proteins align with the interest and advocacy for 'green' production of drugs and diagnostics. This chapter reviews the applications of polysaccharides and proteins as preferred encapsulating materials in micro- and nanoencapsulation of therapeutics and diagnostics.

2. Polysaccharide-based encapsulation

Carbohydrate monosaccharide molecules that are cohesively bound together by glycosidic chains are termed polysaccharides [4]. The nature, sequence, and glycosidic monosaccharide chains inherent in polysaccharides influence the molecular and structural properties of polysaccharides. Water retention ability, digestibility, gelation, and solubility properties of polysaccharides are dependent on the composition of their glycosidic monosaccharide chains [5–7]. Polysaccharides are usually obtained through low cost production techniques with raw materials obtained from natural sources. These polymers possess essential properties critical for drug delivery systems [8–11]. Polysaccharides are macromolecules structured in a linear or branched pattern extensively used in both conventional and advanced drug delivery systems as carriers, building blocks, bioactive materials and excipients. Due to their flexibility, they can be derivatized and tailored to achieve certain functionalities that can enhance targeting and delivery properties. Some of the derivatives of polysaccharides called semi-synthetic polysaccharides include carboxymethylcellulose, starch acetate, methylcellulose, ethylpullulan, and chitosan sulfate. Polysaccharides and their derivatives enhance delivery and diagnostic properties such as mechanical strength, stability, protection, solubility, targeting, stimuli responsiveness, controlled release, self-regulation, adhesion, bioimaging, labeling, site-specificity and multifuntionality which equip them to respond to stimuli, diagnose, image, target and treat as single devices [12]. These potentials of polysaccharides make them convenient materials for encapsulation conferring on the encapsulated product the various benefits of encapsulation.

2.1 Polysaccharides in micro- and nanoencapsulation

Drug delivery systems make use of a wide range of polysaccharide-based delivery systems from plant (khaya gum, starch and cellulose) [13, 14], animal (chitosan) [15], algae (alginate and carrageenan) and microbial (dextran and xanthan gum) sources [16, 17] and cyclodextrins [18]. These polysaccharides delivery systems can interact with bioactive compounds ensuring that they act as innate drug carriers which bind and encapsulate hydrophilic and hydrophobic functional compounds [19]. The size, shape, and internal structure of these polysaccharide delivery systems differ depending on several factors including the method of formulation and the polysaccharide used in formulation [9]. Size is an integral component of drug delivery systems since it affects their physicochemical stability, encapsulation and release characteristics, and biological activity [9]. Encapsulation of bioactive drug compounds can be achieved via a single or a combination of polysaccharides.

Polysaccharides used for micro- or nanoencapsulation include varied types of polysaccharides and utilization of specific polysaccharides for encapsulation is dependent on its chemical non reactivity with active pharmaceutical ingredient, chemical compatibility as well as stability target-selected delivery [20]. Micro and nanoencapsulation are achieved majorly via chemical (emulsification, polymerization, and liposomes) or physical (freeze-drying/lyophilization, spray drying, co-crystallization, fluidized-bed coating encapsulation processes). Drugs with low solubility and high permeability i.e. BCS class 2 drugs are usually formulated via encapsulation to optimize bioavailability, stability, and controlled release of drugs [20].

2.2 Merits and demerits in therapeutic delivery

Despite the many advances of encapsulation process, relatively few of these products have been made commercially available due to many reasons which include degradation of highly temperature sensitive compounds, difficulty in controlling the particle size especially as the size of the yield is usually small [21]. Long processing times, expensive costs of production and storage of these dosage forms are also of concern. **Table 1** shows varying polysaccharides utilized on the encapsulation process stating the merits and demerits of each application.

2.3 Case studies/applications

2.3.1 Encapsulation of small molecules

Mankala *et al.*, [19] incorporated aceclofenac, a nonsteroidal anti-inflammatory drug (NSAID) with biological half-life of 4.3 h and a BCS class 2 drug into

	Polysaccharide	Encapsulation type	API	Significance of the study	Demerits of the encapsulation process/study set back	Reference
1.	Chitosan	Microencapsulation	Isoniazid and rifabutin	Spray-dried chitosan microparticles inhibited bacterial growth by 96%, demonstrating that microencapsulation preserved drug antibacterial activity *in vitro*. Overall, the obtained data suggest the potential of chitosan microparticles for inhalable lung tuberculosis therapy.	Microparticles were sensitive to high temperatures and the yield was extremely small. Control of the particle size during the production process was difficult.	[22]
		Nanoencapsulation	Tamoxifen	Compared to tamoxifen citrate suspension, the amount of the drug permeated using the nano formulation was increased from 1.5 to 90 times, in absence or in presence of pancreatin or lipase. The encapsulation of tamoxifen in lecithin/chitosan nanoparticles improved the non-metabolized drug passing through the rat intestinal tissue via paracellular transport.	The effect of enzymes on intestinal permeation of tamoxifen was shown only when tamoxifen-loaded nanoparticles were in intimate contact with the mucosal surface. The nanoparticle yield was extremely small.	[23]
		Nanoencapsulation	Gallic acid	Gallic acid (GA) loaded chitosan nanoparticles (GANP) treated mice, reversed the scopolamine induced amnesia in mice which may be attributed to its antioxidant properties and improved cholinergic functions. These effects were significantly increased by the administration of GANP compared with pure GA administration, but no significant change was observed for GANP.	The nanoparticles required coating with Tween 80 to enhance the stability of the product. The yield of the nanoparticles was extremely small.	[24, 25]
2.	Alginate	Microencapsulation	Gallic acid	Electro-spraying microencapsulation of Gallic acid calcium alginate for use in management of dementia provided alginate beads with a size of 200 μm - 1.3 mm. Loading capacity acid varied from 7 to 12 g/100 g. There was a faster release profile in simulated intestinal fluid than in gastric fluid.	Difficulty in controlling particle size, moderate yields for small batches was experienced. The need for special handling and storage conditions was required.	[26, 27]
		Nanoencapsulation	IgY	Controlled delivery of therapeutic agents by alginate nanoparticles became an attractive issue in the gastric organ. Some therapeutic agents such as proteins could not tolerate severe conditions in the gastrointestinal tract. Concentrations of a specific IgY as a prophylactic	The yield was small, and the formulation was not stable at high temperatures. Degradation of highly temperature- sensitive compounds was also experienced because of the nanoencapsulation process.	[28]

	Polysaccharide	Encapsulation type	API	Significance of the study	Demerits of the encapsulation process/study set back	Reference
				agent against *E. coli* O157: H7 was entrapped in 0.2% $^{w}/_{v}$ sodium alginate nanoparticles by ionic gelation method. Alg NPs prepared from 0.2%$^{w}/_{v}$ stock solution could be appropriate candidates for efficient and safe delivery of IgY through the gastrointestinal tract.		
		Microencapsulation	Paclitaxel	Alginate microparticles were fabricated by an emulsification technique and characterized. The *in vitro* cytotoxicity activity of paclitaxel loaded microparticles was assessed using human non-small cell lung cancer cell lines (A549 and Calu-6). Results showed that exposure of cells to pure paclitaxel and paclitaxel loaded microparticles effectively inhibited the growth of A549 and Calu-6 cells similarly in a concentration- and time-dependent manner thus its use in management of primary or metastatic lung cancer.	The yield was small, and the formulation was not stable at high temperatures. Clearance of the microparticles by macrophages is expected to be high. This will alter its overall bioavailability.	[29]
3.	Hyaluronate	Nanoencapsulation	Recombinant neuroglobin	The formulation of sodium hyaluronate nanoparticles loaded with neuroglobin, showed that the formulation is highly compatible for pharmaceutical use and may act as a delivery system to transport neuroglobin within the blood. After a stroke, the sodium hyaluronate nanoparticles loaded with neuroglobin injected intravenously at the onset of the reperfusion period, can cross the BBB. They quickly reached the damaged nerve cells, being detected inside cytoplasm. This delivery system successfully carried the neuroprotective oxygen-sensing protein NGB to the damaged ischemic brain after 2 hr. and was retained after 24 hr. of reperfusion.	The nano particles must be preserved at low temperatures.	[30]
		Microencapsulation	—	Sodium hyaluronate was evaluated as a material for inhalation due to its therapeutic potential, utility as a formulation excipient or drug carrier, and ability to target lung inflammation and cancer.	The microparticles was fabricated over long processing time and incurred expensive process costs.	[31]

	Polysaccharide	Encapsulation type	API	Significance of the study	Demerits of the encapsulation process/study set back	Reference
4.	Cellulose derivatives	Nanoencapsulation	—	Tempo-oxidized bacterial cellulose (TOBC) and sodium alginate (SA) composites were prepared to improve the properties of hydrogel for cell encapsulation. The compression strength and chemical stability of the TOBC/SA composites were increased compared with the SA hydrogel, which indicated that TOBC performed an important function in enhancing the structural, mechanical and chemical stability of the composites.	Nanocellulose-alginate hydrogel for cell encapsulation are not easily adapted for encapsulation of biologics. The encapsulation process is time consuming.	[32]
		Nanoencapsulation	Celecoxib	Amorphous drug/polymer nanoparticles containing celecoxib were prepared using ethyl cellulose. Nanoparticles released celecoxib rapidly and provided higher dissolved-drug concentrations than micronized crystalline drug. Nanoparticle suspensions were stable for several days and can be spray-dried to form dry powders resuspendable in water. Drug/polymer nanoparticles are well suited for providing rapid oral absorption and increased bioavailability of BCS Class II drugs.	Absorption profile must be monitored as the formulation showed enhanced bioavailability of the API to avoid dose dumping.	[33]
		Microencapsulation	Probiotic bacteria	Novel carboxymethyl cellulose-chitosan hybrid microparticles were prepared in aqueous media for delivery of probiotic bacteria. The model probiotic bacteria (*Lactobacillus rhamnosus*) was successfully encapsulated in carboxymethyl cellulose based particles with acceptable viability count for its potential delivery in the intestinal tract with the purpose of modulating gut microbiota and improving human health.	The microparticles produced must be protected from environmental stresses i.e. heat	[34]

Table 1.
Polysaccharides used in encapsulation of various active pharmaceutical ingredients showing the merits and demerits in therapeutic delivery.

polymeric microcapsules. Aceclofenac-loaded microcapsules was formulated using ionic gelation technique employing sodium alginate as the coat material in combination with some mucoadhesive polysaccharide derivatives such as hydroxypropyl methyl cellulose (HPMC), sodium carboxymethyl cellulose (SCMC) and methylcellulose. The microcapsules were spherical (**Figure 1**) with microencapsulation efficiency of 83.25–99.94%, good mucoadhesive property to enhance bioavailability and ensured over 15 hr. sustained release of aceclofenac via zero order kinetic super case 2 transport [19]. The formulation composition of drug:sodium alginate:HPMC in the ratio of 2:4:1 displayed a sustained release of up to 24 hr. In another study using aceclofenac, Dharmendra *et al.*, [20] developed a LbL self-assembly which was utilized to make aceclofenac single bilayer microcapsules produced by sequential adsorption of positively charged chitosan and negatively charged pectin, a polysaccharide on the external surface of negatively charged aceclofenac microcrystals. This enabled targeted release of aceclofenac in the colon.

Glipizide an antidiabetic agent with short biological half-life was microencapsulated using polysaccharide coat comprising alginate alone or in combination with chitosan via ionotropic gelation process [35]. Abdelbary *et al.*, [35] showed that the microencapsulated glipizide enhanced drug bioavailability causing significant hypoglycaemic activity compared to innovator product. Microencapsulation provides a physical barrier against digestive enzymes, whilst offering protection against the acidic gastric environment. Cholesterol-lowering efficacy of yoghurt formulation containing microencapsulated bile salt hydrolase (BSH)-active *Lactobacillus reuteri* for management of hypercholesterolaemia adults was evaluated by Martoni *et al.* [36]. Microencapsulation of bile salt hydrolase-active *Lactobacillus reuteri* using sodium alginate showed superiority over traditional probiotic therapy and may be an exceptional choice as a cholesterol-lowering agent to be administered alone or in combination with other cholesterol-lowering agents [36].

Karan *et al.*, [37] developed novel polymeric microspheres of 5-fluorouracil (5-FU) using natural polysaccharide gum katira via microencapsulation to obtain an optimal therapeutic response at the colon. This controlled release delivery system of 5FU released the chemotherapeutic agent at a controlled rate whilst retarding gastric degradation of the drug. Utilization of natural polysaccharides in microencapsulation of 5FU via optimized katira gum microsphere ensured that a micro-carrier for efficient colon drug targeting was developed.

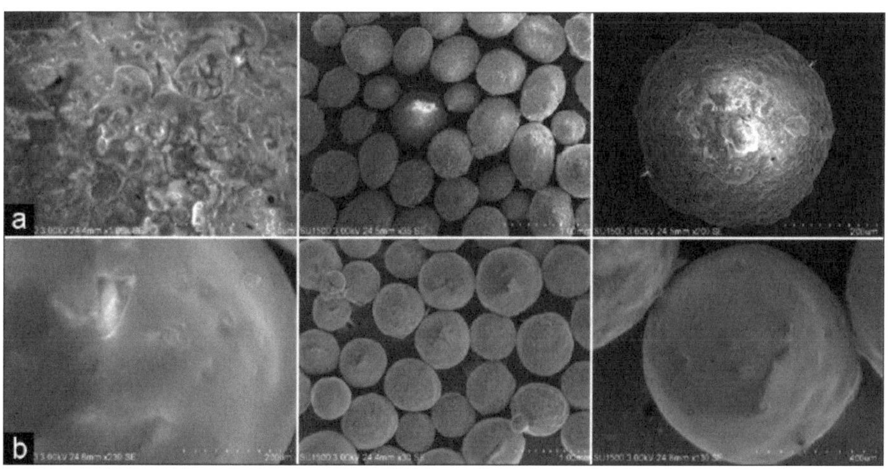

Figure 1.
(a) SEM images of aceclofenac mucoadhesive microcapsules formulated with HPMC; (b) SEM images of aceclofenac mucoadhesive microcapsules formulated with SCMC [19].

The use of polysaccharides for microencapsulation of bicalutamide was utilized by Tekade *et al.*, [38] to develop bicalutamide microspheres using guar gum as a polymer via oil-in-water emulsion solvent diffusion method. The microencapsulated dosage forms containing 2.5% of guar gum, 0.25% span 80 as dispersing agent showed the optimum drug release of 94.22% within 24 hrs, devoid of drug excipient interactions. The potential to enhance bicalutamide bioavailability and sustained release especially due to the polymorphic nature of the drug could be further optimized using nanoencapsulation. This will create a channel for precision targeting of the non-steroidal antiandrogen to a greater extent than microencapsulation [39] especially where these microencapsulated solid dosage forms have not met the pharmacological need of the patient.

Molecular Envelope Technology (MET) nanoparticles fabricated from complex polysaccharide chains of N-palmitoyl-N monomethyl- N, N-dimethyl-N,N,N-trimethyl-6-O-glycol chitosan, a self-assembling polymer amphiphile has been utilized in delivery of formulations to target sites of action across the blood brain barrier [40]. Fisusi *et al.*, [40] developed drug loaded MET formulations containing Lomustine for management of Glioblastoma multiforme. The MET envelope utilizing the complex polysaccharide for nanoencapsulation optimized biodistribution and pharmacodynamics whilst reducing the toxic effects of the active drug, lomustine thereby providing better outcomes for patients managed for brain cancer. As the active pharmaceutical ingredient is protected from degradation, the MET envelope ensures targeted drug delivery due to PEGylation of the polysaccharide to facilitate extended circulation time within the body [40, 41]. Lekshmi *et al.*, [42] prepared and characterized repaglinide loaded ethylcellulose nanoparticles by the solvent evaporation method for the management of type 2 diabetes. The polysaccharide encapsulated nanoparticles showed high encapsulation efficiency suggesting that nanoencapsulation of repaglinide in biodegradable, biocompatible polymer was able to improve its pharmacological activity via modification of surface function and charge to promote cell entry.

Di Martino and co-workers fabricated polysaccharide-based polyelectrolyte nanocomplexes which exhibited the several benefits of encapsulation [43]. Polyelectrolyte nanocomplexes were formed between chitosan (CS) and alginic acid (ALG) and then chitosan and polygalacturonic acid (PGA). Solutions of the polycation (CS in acidic medium) and the polyanions (ALG and PGA in alkaline medium separately) were prepared. The drugs, temozolomide (TMZ) and fluorouracil (5-FU) were dissolved in aqueous solution and added to the separate solutions of the polyanions. The drug(s)-polyanions solutions were added dropwise into increasing concentrations of CS. Characterization of the encapsulated product revealed spherical nanoparticles with diameters within 100–200 nm, increased encapsulation efficiency with increasing concentration of CS, controlled release of drugs, pH sensitivity making it a possible system for colon delivery, stability of drugs especially TMZ. A setback is the burst release which may be due to several factors such as drying method (freeze drying), and degree of complexation. This setback can be modulated by adjusting the ratio of CS:ALG or CS:PGA, harvesting of the nanoparticles early from the fabrication medium. Spray drying may be an alternative to freeze drying to reduce migration of the drugs to the surface during drying. In addition, derivatization of the polysaccharides without loss of their polyelectrolytic nature may increase their mechanical strength, reduce pores within and enhance entrapment.

Gastrointestinal intolerance of metformin HCl may be reduced by encapsulation which provides controlled release of the drug ensuring therapeutic efficacy and minimizing adverse effects. Extended release formulation became necessary to improve patient adherence and reduce gastrointestinal intolerance (GI) experienced by the patients when on immediate release formulation [44, 45]. It is envisaged the metformin HCl-loaded tamarind seed polysaccharide-alginate encapsulated beads fabricated by Nayak and co-workers [46] will control the release of metformin HCl, improve GI tolerability and more. The drug release was pH sensitive as less than 20% of metformin released in two hours while in acidic medium. Most of the drug was released in pH 7.4, suggesting the maximal absorption may occur in the duodenum and jejunum and possibly increasing the bioavailability of metformin. The release of metformin followed a zero-order pattern which suggests that metformin will be released at a constant rate thereby maximizing its therapeutic efficacy and minimizing adverse effects.

2.3.2 Encapsulation of biologics

In a study undertaken by Sari and colleagues [47], chitosan was used as adjuvant and encapsulating material for the formulation of an anti-botulism single shot vaccine. The toxoids type C and D were encapsulated in chitosan by coacervation method using sodium sulfate as the precipitating agent. The toxoids-loaded chitosan microspheres were compared with the conventional method of mixing the toxoids with aluminum hydroxide which served as an adjuvant. The protein encapsulation efficiency obtained was 41.03% for toxoid C and 32.3% for toxoid D. It is envisaged that modulation of parameters such as protein and chitosan concentration may enhance the encapsulation efficiency. The comparative vaccination in guinea pigs and the neutralization bioassay indicated that the animals were able to develop titers of 10 and 2 IU/mL against *C. botulinum* type C and D respectively for both toxoid-loaded chitosan microspheres and the conventional method of delivery. However, aluminum hydroxide is fraught with adverse reactions such as local pain, swelling, irritation at the injection site, erythema, subcutaneous nodules, contact hypersensitivity and granuloma and allergic reactions [48, 49] making chitosan as an adjuvant a better alternative. Chitosan enables humoral and cellular immune responses and so it is efficient and safe compared to aluminum hydroxide [47].

Sodium alginate was used as an encapsulating material for the encapsulation of mesenchymal stem cells (MSCs), a promising cell-based therapeutic agent for the treatment of cancers, tissue injury, immune disorders, cardiovascular and neurological diseases [50]. MSCs were mixed with alginate solution and cell-encapsulated alginate beads were fabricated by ionotropic gelation with calcium chloride as the crosslinking agent. The cell-encapsulated beads were characterized to assess the ability of the cells to execute their functions despite encapsulation. MSCs were able to proliferate within the alginate beads at different times. Expression of genes proceeded unhindered. In comparison to 2D cultured cells, the 3D (three-dimensional microenvironment provided by the alginate microbeads) cells showed a significant increase in expression of pro-angiogenic genes hypoxia-inducible factor-1 (HIF-1 – 80.4%) and VEGF (74%). Seven paracrine signaling factors such as VEGF, TGF-β, TNF-α, IFN-γ, IL-10, IL-6, and IL-1β were secreted. There was an indication that the 3D microenvironment could enhance pluripotency of MSCs. The alginate beads facilitated proper growth and viability of MSCs contributing to the higher therapeutic efficiency of MSCs in vivo. Encapsulated MSCs exhibited anti-cancer activity against breast cancer stem cells, suppressed cancer-associated genes, inhibited migration and angiogenesis of breast CSCs among other activities making encapsulated MSCs a promising cell-based therapy for targeting cancer cells and reducing the burden of cancer.

Insulin-loaded arabinoxylan microspheres were fabricated by crosslinking of arabinoxylan employing enzymatic reaction and characterized [51]. Insulin solution was prepared in 0.25 mM HCl and thereafter, glutamic acid was added, and pH adjusted to 4. The insulin solution was added to a solution of arabinoxylan in 0.1 M acetate buffer and then agitated. The enzyme, laccase was added as the crosslinking agent and dropwise extrusion into a hydrophobic liquid, and the microspheres were formed and harvested after 6 hr. The insulin-loaded arabinoxylan microspheres were characterized extensively in vitro and in vivo in diabetic induced Wistar rats. Average size of the spherical shaped and smooth surfaced microspheres was 322 μm having irregular pore sizes and geometries. Insulin aggregates in the microspheres were stabilized by presence of glutamic acid yielding a homogenously distribution of insulin. However, at higher insulin/arabinoxylan mass ratio, micro-phase separation occurred. Arabinoxylan microspheres minimized release of insulin in the gastric and small intestine facilitating delivery of insulin to the colon and limiting degradation by the digestive enzymes. Controlled release of insulin over 10 hr. was observed in vitro. For in vivo studies, insulin was first labeled with RITC before encapsulation. It was observed that the insulin-RITC-loaded arabinoxylan microspheres were relatively intact in the upper GIT releasing about 13–21% of the total RITC load. Maximum amount of RITC was found in the colon, about 78.8% after 8 hr. possibly due to the degradation of arabinoxylan microspheres by the colonic microflora. The blood glucose in the diabetic induced rats decreased by 70% between 9 and 12 hr. after three treatments orally while hyperglycemia was sustained in the control groups. Arabinoxylan microspheres protected insulin from enzymatic degradation, retained a high percentage of insulin for delivery and release in the colon exerting significant hypoglycemic effect.

Microneedle technology, an encapsulation technology used for biologics and small molecules as an alternative to hypodermic injection and implantation was used to encapsulate etanercept, for transdermal delivery for rheumatoid arthritis [52]. Microneedles fabricated are microscopic needles of lengths 50–900 μm (**Figure 2**) which pierces the stratum corneum barrier generating transient microchannels for delivery of encapsulated biologic or small molecule without triggering the nerves and injuring the blood vessels. Etanercept is a human dimeric fusion protein which is fully soluble and is a tumor necrosis factor (TNF) inhibitor as it binds to TNF preventing the activation of the inflammatory cascade. It is a fusion protein of recombinant human TNF-receptor p75 fused with the Fc domain of human Immunoglobulin G1 (IgG1).

Acrylate modified-hyaluronic acid was used to fabricate the microneedles and on application to the skin released etanercept which was absorbed by the blood capillary and etanercept was transported to the arthritic tissue where it exerted therapeutic effect by binding to TNF (**Figure 3**). The etanercept-loaded microneedles were fabricated by micromoulding method. Thereafter, the microneedles were detached from the mold and crosslinked by exposing to UV light to enhance mechanical strength. Drug loading and in vitro bioactivity were evaluated. Skin penetration, microneedle dissolution and skin recovery, therapeutic

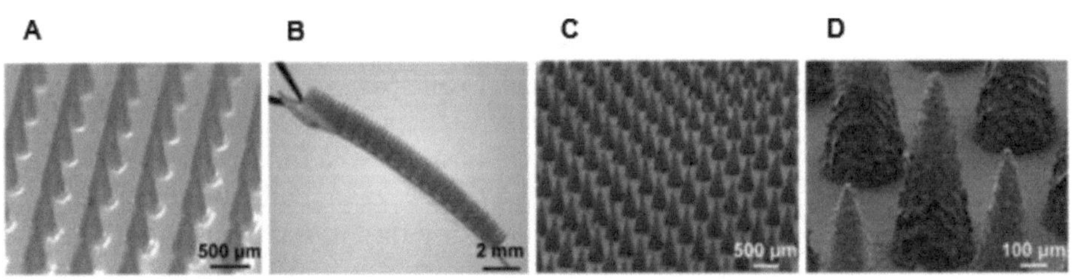

Figure 2.
Images of microneedles: (A) microscopic image – 500 μm, (B) microscopic image – 2 mm, (C) scanning electron microscopic (SEM) image – 500 μm, and (D) SEM image – 100 μm [52].

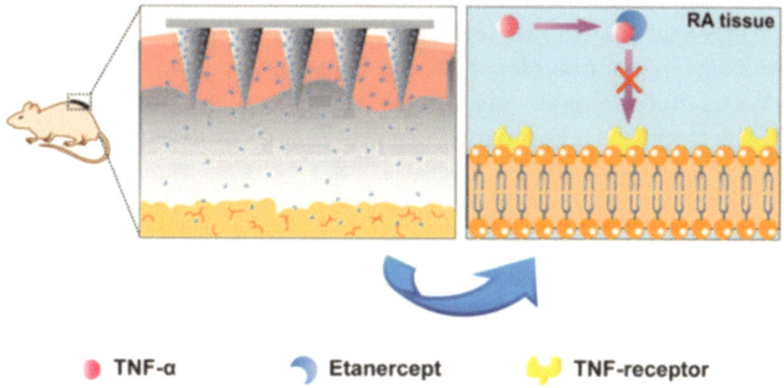

Figure 3.
Schematic illustration of microneedle-assisted transdermal delivery of etanercept from application on the dorsal skin of the mouse to binding of etanercept to TNF [52].

effect were determined with mice. Average etanercept per microneedle was 42.72 ± 5.81 μg which was sufficient for in vivo evaluation. The microneedles exhibited sufficient mechanical strength, complete dissolution of microneedles in the skin after 90 min, quick recovery of skin after 120 min, good biocompatibility, little interference with bioactivity of etanercept and high anti-inflammatory efficacy. There was evidence of reduction of TNF-α and IL-6 in serum, protection of the joint from erosion and microneedle system showed good bioequivalence to the classical subcutaneous route.

Hydrogel encapsulation systems compare better than use of autologous chondrocytes and the marrow stimulating technique for cartilage repair because hydrogel encapsulation systems do not just encapsulate chondrocytes but also maintain both cell viability and phenotype and support neocartiliage formation [53]. Fenbo and co-workers [54] fabricated chondrocytes-loaded alginate-chondroitin sulfate hydrogel beads by mixing solutions of sodium alginate and chondroitin sulfate and chondrocytes was added to the mixture which was transferred dropwise into a solution of strontium chloride with a syringe. The beads were harvested, rinsed to remove excess strontium chloride, and then cultured. Characterization of the chondrocytes-loaded hydrogel beads showed that low molecular weight alginate-chondroitin sulfate hydrogel promoted high cell viability and up-regulated the expression of collagen II and B cell leukemia 2 (Bcl-2). The study suggests that low molecular weight alginate-chondroitin sulfate hydrogel beads promotes cartilage formation and decreases inflammation and may be a promising system for cartilage tissue repair. The study observed that molecular weight of encapsulating materials is an important parameter in tissue engineering.

2.3.3 Encapsulation of diagnostics

Encapsulation of biomarkers such as microRNAs (miRNAs or miRs) confer stability on them. MiRNAs are a class of small endogenous non-coding RNAs comprising 18–22 nucleotides regulating various biological processes by preventing expression of target genes [55, 56]. MiRNAs have been suggested and explored as therapeutics and biomarkers for various diseases such as cancer, diabetes, cardiovascular diseases, and other diseases whose etiology is related to atypical gene expression [57]. MiRNAs can be employed in disease environment for diagnosis, treatment, and reoccurrence prediction. Moraes and colleagues [57] modified pullulan by linking quaternized ammonium groups to its backbone. The pullulan derivative interacted with miRNA to form stable polyplexes which were characterized for physicochemical properties and cellular uptake. Elemental analysis, SEC-MALLS analysis, and IR and NMR spectra confirmed the modification of pullulan. Average size of polyplexes was 130 ± 30 nm, zeta potential was −12 ± 5 mV and morphology study showed homogenous spherical particles. Agarose gel electrophoresis confirmed the presence of miRNA within the polyplexes and loading efficiency was 80%. There was no indication of degradation or fragmentation of miRNA suggesting that cationic quarternized pullulan could protect miRNA. The polyplexes were found to be stable, cytocompatible, and the complexation of miRNA with quartenized pullalan facilitated the uptake of miRNA into the cells.

Cellulose nanofibers are appealing cargo carriers due the unique barrier, chemical, interfacial, mechanical, and optical properties of nanocellulose [58]. Cellulose nanofibers-based microcapsules were fabricated as a diagnostic device with glucose oxidase encapsulated within for glucose monitoring [58]. Cellulose nanofibers (CNF), apple pectin (AP) and xyloglucan-amyloid (XyG) were used to fabricate the microcapsules using layer by layer ((LbL - CNF/XyG/CNF/AP)2CNF) technique on top of fluorescein isothiocyanate (FITC) – labeled glucose oxidase-loaded calcium carbonate particles to build the capsule wall. The FITC-glucose oxidase-$CaCO_3$ particles were crosslinked with glutaraldehyde forming the templates on which LbL microcapsules were fabricated. After LbL fabrication, calcium carbonate was removed with 100 mM EDTA in water. The microcapsules collapsed on drying after removal of the $CaCO_3$ core. The glucose oxidase-loaded microcapsules fabricated were porous, spherical, uniform and structurally stable, and the encapsulation efficiency of glucose oxidase was 68 ± 2%. The microcapsules were used to monitor/measure glucose. An interaction of glucose oxidase and glucose produced hydrogen peroxide which was transported through channels to an external flow-cell where hydrogen peroxide was oxidized electrically producing current that was recorded and used to determine the concentration of glucose. The microcapsules immobilized the enzymes as well as provided a favorable microenvironment for the sustained biocatalytic activity of glucose oxidase. The nanocellulose microcapsules show promise as a device for in vivo monitoring of analytes.

A glucose biosensor fabricated based on gum tragacanth was tested on actual blood samples. Cadmium Telluride Quantum Dots (CdTe QDs) and glucose oxidase were encapsulated in tragacanth gum for glucose detection [59]. Tragacanth gum nanohydrogels were prepared by adjustment of pH, sonication followed by precipitation. Modified tragacanth gum was prepared by radial graft copolymerization of acrylic acid (AA: 0–5 mL), using N,N′-methylenebisacrylamide (MBA: 0.1–0.3 g) as a crosslinker in potassium persulfate solution (initiator) followed by precipitation after agitation for 4 hr. at 70°C. The nanohydrogels were characterized and the composition with the desired mechanical strength and highest swelling ratio was used in fabrication of superabsorbent biosensor nanohydrogels. The biosensor nanohydrogels were tested for leakage of CdTe QDs and glucose oxidase, encapsulation efficiency and glucose detection. The QDs leakage was about 1.48% for 2 hr. There was insignificant change in fluorescence intensity of QDs after 45 days at 4°C and 17% decrease in fluorescence intensity at ambient temperature after 45 days. Enzyme was stable at 4°C and unstable with time at ambient temperature. Fluorescence intensity decreased significantly with increase in hydrogen peroxide concentration indicating the encapsulated glucose oxidase was able to catalyze the oxidation of glucose to hydrogen peroxide and gluconic acid.

Enzymatic reaction, base stacking (aptamers) and antigen–antibody linkers are possible approaches to cholesterol detection; however, they are fraught with some limitations and foreign interference [60]. Chebi and co-workers [60] fabricated a nano-sensor for cholesterol sensing without enzymatic reaction using curcumin

(CUR) as a fluorescence probe, polyelectrolyte, chitosan oligosaccharide lactate (COL) as the encapsulating material and silica nanoparticles as the core (**Figure 4**). The nanohybrid particles were fabricated by precipitation technique. Solutions of COL and curcumin were mixed under agitation and a dispersion of silica nanoparticles was added dropwise and agitated overnight. The nanocapsules formed were harvested and characterized. When not aggregated, the sizes of the spherical particles were 25–35 nm. In the presence of cholesterol, a large blue shift $>$ 100 nm was observed in the fluorescence intensity of nanohybrid particles. The fluorescence intensity of the nanohybrid particles were not affected by interfering substances such as ascorbic acid, uric acid and glucose indicating specificity, selectivity and sensitivity of cholesterol determination using the fabricated nano-sensor.

Urea is a waste product of metabolism and is eliminated from the body through the kidney. Evaluation of urea content is used to assess kidney function and other possible implications. Increased level of urea in the urine and blood indicates the presence of some acute and chronic diseases such as kidney failure, and myocardial infarction, or dehydration, gastrointestinal hemorrhage, high protein diet, aging and catabolic states such as trauma, severe infection, starvation and drugs. Decreased urea content is indicative of pregnancy, low protein diet, overhydration, advanced liver disease and reduced urea synthesis. While there are several techniques for determining urea content, there is a growing need for easy to fabricate, easy to use and cheap diagnostic tools. Khattab and co-workers [61] fabricated crosslinked calcium alginate microcapsules containing urease and tricyanofuran hydrazone fixed on cotton fibers to create a colorimetric cotton strip as a sensor for determining urea content. Solutions of sodium alginate, urease and tricyanofuran hydrazone was mixed and overlaid on cotton fiber strips and dried. Thereafter the dried cotton fiber strips were immersed in a solution of calcium choride for the crosslinking process. The microcapsules were characterized, and the sensor was used to determine urea content. The urea content assay using the sensor fabricated, displayed a visual color change from light yellow to purple indicating the presence

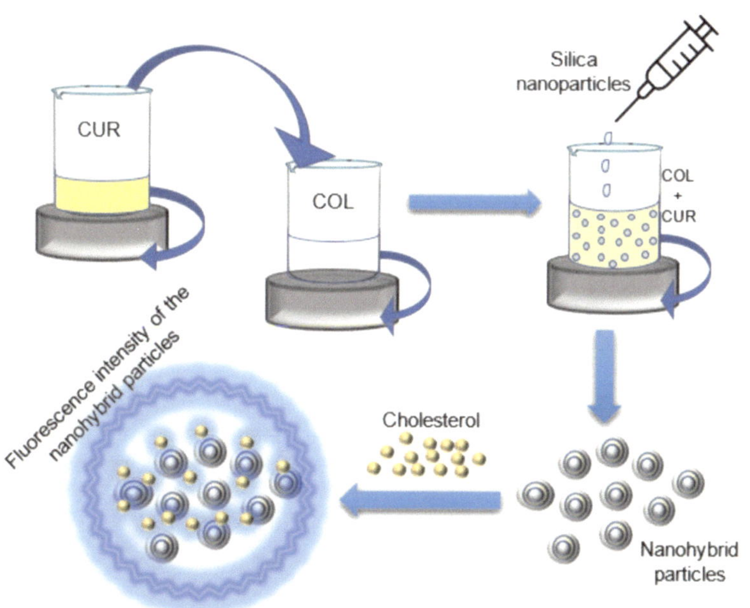

Figure 4.
Schematic illustration of the fabrication of nanohybrid particles and the fluorescence intensity in the presence of cholesterol.

Micro-encapsulating materials		Active compounds	Micro-encapsulation technique	Application	EE %	Ref.
Polysaccharide	**Other materials**					
Gum katira		5-fluorouracil	Emulsion solvent evaporation	Treatment of colon cancer	59.45 ± 3.18–79.25 ± 4.25	[37]
Guar gum		Bicalutamide	Emulsion solvent diffusion	Treatment of prostate cancer	69.43 ± 1.06–74 ± 1.07	[38]
Tamarind seed polysaccharide/alginate		Metformin HCl	Ionotropic gelation	Diabetes	94.86 ± 3.92	[46]
Arabinoxylan		Insulin	Enzymatic crosslinking	Diabetes	—	[51]
Hyaluronic acid	Methacrylic anhydride	Etanercept	Micromoulding	Rheumatoid arthritis	—	[52]
Alginate	Eudragit E100 Eudragit L30D-55	Indomethacin	Ultrasonic atomization/ polyelectrolyte complexation	Inflammation, pain	74 ± 1	[62]
Gellan gum		Methotrexate	Emulsion solvent diffusion method	Cancers and auto-immune diseases	50.78–84.8	[63]
Esterified Agave Fructans		Ibuprofen	Coacervation	Inflammation, pain	0.8–21.5	[64]
Chitosan		Astragalus Polysaccharide	Spray-drying	Allergic rhinitis		[65]
Galactomannan *(**Delonix regia**)*	pluronic® F127	Riboflavin	Spray-drying	Energy conversion, growth of cells and health of eyes and skin	87.14–88.53	[66]
β-glucan		Anthocyanins	Spray-drying	Antioxidant/therapeutic	45	[67]
psyllium husk mucilage		Curcumin	Precipitation	Antioxidant, antifungal and antibacterial	56	[68]
Cyanobacterial polysaccharide		Vitamin B12	Spray drying	Cell metabolism, blood cell production		[69]
Pectin-Alginate		Vitamin E	Emulsification-ionic gelation	Antioxidant	52.91	[70]
β-cyclodextrin		Caffeine	Freeze drying	Psychostimulant	74	[71]
Sodium alginate		Urease/tricyanofuran hydrazone	Ionotropic gelation	Urea detection	38.5–55.5	[61]

Table 2.
Polysaccharide-based micro-encapsulating carriers for delivery of bioactive compounds.

Nano-encapsulating materials		Active compounds	Micro-encapsulation techniques	Applications	EE %	Ref.
Polysaccharide	**Other materials**					
Chitosan derivative		Lomustine	Molecular Envelope Technology/ Probe sonication	Treatment of Glioblastoma multiforme		[40]
Ethyl cellulose		Repaglinde	Solvent evaporation	Diabetes Mellitus	58.8 ± 0.724–86.4 ± 0.31	[42]
Chitosan/alginic acid		Temozolomide/fluorouracil	Polyelectrolyte complexation	Cancer	43 ± 3–76 ± 8	[43]
Pullulan derivative		miRNA	Polyelectrolyte complexation	Gene delivery/biomarker	80	[57]
Cellulose/pectin/xyloglucan		Glucose oxidase	Layer by layer	Glucose detection	68 ± 2	[58]
Tragacanth gum	Acrylic acid	Glucose oxidase/cadmium telluride quantum dots	Copolymerization-precipitation	Glucose detection		[59]
Chitosan oligosaccharide lactate	Silica	Curcumin	Precipitation	Cholesterol detection		[60]
Auricularia auricular polysaccharide/chitosan		Doxorubicin HCl	Polyelectrolyte complexation	CANCER	74.1 ± 2.2	[72]
Pectin-chitosan		Nisin	Polyelectrolyte complexation	Antimicrobial	42.3 ± 3.7–65.9 ± 6.1	[73]
Depolymerized holothurian glycosaminoglycan		Doxorubicin	Polyelectrolyte complexation	Cancers	55–64.2	[74]
Mango gum		Donezepil	Emulsion crosslinking	CNS - dementia	85 ± 2.14	[75]
Azivash gum	Polyvinyl alcohol	Catechin	Electrospinning	Antioxidant	87.4–99	[76]
Cashew gum	N-isopropylacrylamide	Epirubicin	Self-assembly	Cancer	63.67 ± 1.4%	[77]
Chitosan-fucoidan		Red ginseng extract	Nanoprecipitation/ionic gelation	Thrombosis	22.63 40.13	[78]
Cactus mucilage (*Opuntia monacantha*)		Zeaxanthin	Nano emulsification	Antioxidant	96.57	[79]

Table 3.
Polysaccharide-based nano-encapsulating carriers for delivery of bioactive compounds.

of urea. The detection ability of the sensor was determined by the color strength and the International Commission on Illumination – CIE L*, a*' and b* color coordinates. The dye and enzyme-loaded crosslinked alginate microparticles coated cotton sensor strips were effectively employed to determine unknown concentrations of urea. The spectroscopic parameters indicated the microencapsulated sensor displayed a detection range of 0.1 ppm to 250 ppm. **Tables 2** and **3** indicate applications based on micro- and nano-encapsulation utilizing natural polysaccharides as encapsulating materials.

3. Protein-based encapsulation

3.1 Proteins in micro- and nanoencapsulation

Protein-based delivery systems can be synthesized via different kinds of animal and plant proteins using a range of different production methods. A fabricator should pick the most fitting protein for a certain application, after making sure of all safety requirements. The main elements influencing the selection of the protein and encapsulation methods are:

a. Nanocarrier chemical or physical compatibility with food components.

b. Nanocarrier stability under processing, storage, or during its application.

c. Possible release mechanism(s) and conditions affecting the rate of release.

d. Biodegradability of the protein-based nanocarrier in the body.

e. Cost-effectiveness of nanocarriers when synthesized on a large scale for real applications.

Figure 5 is a schematic illustration of polymeric encapsulation of bioactive agents.

3.1.1 Applications and clinical usage

Protein-based nanoparticles (PBNs), recently reported, are of great interest due to their various advantages. They confirmed their high activity in both clinical and medicinal fields. Several formulations have been developed and suggested as potential future therapeutic products [80]. Besides, some PBNs have been officially accepted by US food and drug administration [81]. In addition, protein-based nanoparticles functional groups (e.g. carboxylic and amino groups) facilitate the particles surface modification, which makes them suitable for tumor targeting strategies. On the other hand, protein-based nanoparticles (PBNs) surface can be modified by attachment of targeting ligands such as peptides, antibodies, vitamins, hormones, and enzymes. These surface modifications allow specific targeting and accumulation of the particles at the desired site such as a tumor. Each protein tends to encapsulate either hydrophobic or hydrophilic molecules. Gelatin, silk, gliadin, and legumin have higher encapsulation efficiency for hydrophilic drugs. While collagen, casein, and zein proteins have higher encapsulation efficiency for hydrophobic drugs. Albumin, however, can bioconjugate with hydrophilic drugs and interact with highly hydrophobic drugs. Besides, each protein has some characteristics that enhance its selectivity to be a better carrier for a certain drug. Albumin,

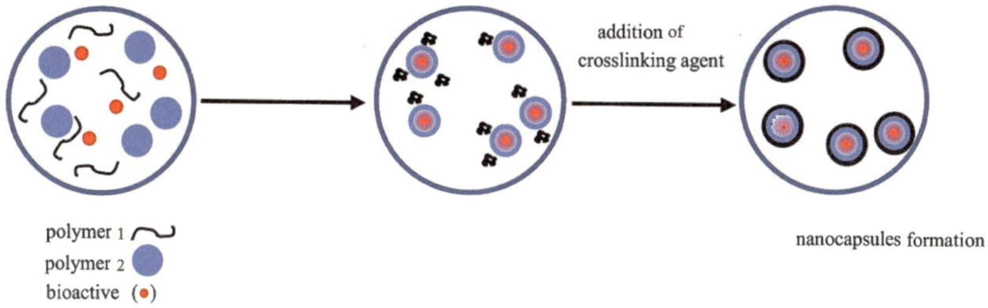

Figure 5.
Schematic illustration of encapsulation of bioactive agents.

for example, is the most abundant plasma protein, which makes it non-toxic, biodegradable, and non-immunogenic. It has also good connectivity to many drugs and it is extremely robust to various conditions. Gelatin and collagen possess many carboxyl groups with possible crosslinking functions. These parameters are important for selecting the nanoparticles synthesis method. The protein selection depends on drug properties, and on the target of the nanoparticles to be prepared. The selected protein properties such as functionality, molecular weight, and hydrophobicity can affect particle size, drug loading and loading efficiency, and dissolution or release profile of the drug to the surrounding environment of the nanoparticles. The proteins have the chance to target a specific place in vivo and secure the encapsulated active molecules from biodegradation and undesirable metabolism - **Figure 6**. Protein nanoparticles, however, have unique properties when compared to other nanoparticles since they are extracted from natural origins that exist in nature, easy to handle, and most importantly they are non-toxic as they do not leave undesirable biodegradation products.

3.1.2 Physicochemical properties of proteins

The physicochemical properties of proteins such as isoelectric point (pI), chemical compositions, denaturation thermal temperature (Tm), and solubility are necessary for the fabrication of the protein-based micro- and nanoencapsulation delivery systems (**Table 4**) [82–90]. Some micro- and nanoencapsulation processes use protein as a wall material to act as a barrier which is used to protect bioactive agents against the surrounded environmental conditions including pH, temperature, moisture, and oxygen and form stable capsules (they are in a range size between few micrometers and millimeters in microencapsulation methods and from 10 nanometers to one micrometer in nanoencapsulation methods) with high encapsulation efficiency (EE) due to their excellent gel, film and emulsifying formation properties, and promising improvements such as water solubility, stability, and bioavailability [91, 92]. Besides,

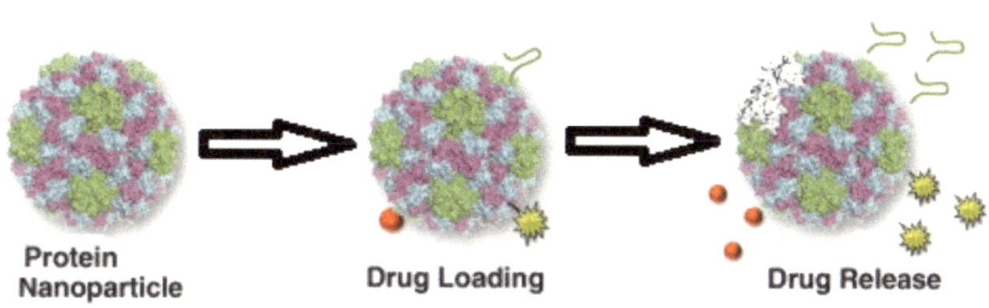

Figure 6.
Drug loading and release from protein-based nanoparticles.

their functional groups possess the ability to protect, reverse binding, and interact with numerous bioactive compounds. Nowadays, two sources of proteins; plant proteins such as soy, pulses, and cereals proteins and animal proteins such as bovine serum albumin, casein and whey proteins are widely used as encapsulating agents in micro- and nanoencapsulation techniques. Proteins are employed to encapsulate solids and liquids including oils. Their ability to encapsulate oils depends on their capacity to adsorb at the interface and form stable emulsions. The following factors affect their emulsifying properties [93]:

- The molecular size of proteins
- Hydrophobicity of the protein surface
- The flexibility of protein compounds
- Protein solubility

Protein	Source	Main composition	Properties	pI	Tm (°C)
1.1. Soy protein	Soybean	Albumins and globulins	Globular and water soluble	4.5	67–87
1.2. Cereal proteins 1.2.1. Zein protein	Maize (corn)	Glutamic acid, leucine, alanine, and proline	Soluble in aqueous alcohol	6–7	75–95
1.2.2. Wheat protein	Wheat	Gliadin and glutenin	Soluble in aqueous alcohol	5–8	90
1.2.3. Barley protein	Barley	Hordein and glutelin	Soluble in alkali	5	115
1.3. Pulse proteins					
1.3.1. Pea protein	Pea	Albumins,glutelins and globulins	Water soluble	4.3–4.5	85–90
1.3.2. Chickpea	Chickpea	Glutein, albumin, prolamine, and globulin	Water soluble	4.5	90
1.3.3. Lentil	Lentil	Globulins, albumin, glutelins, and prolamins	Water soluble	4.5	90
2.1. Whey protein	Cheese or casein	β-lactoglubulin, α-lactalbumin, and serum albumin	Globular and water soluble	4.4–5.5	60–90
2.2. Casein protein	Milk	94% protein and 6% low Mwt colloidal calcium phosphate	Rheomorphic, poorly water soluble, and highly stable	4.6–4.8	125–140
2.3. Bovine serum albumin	Bovine serum or milk	583 amino acids and contains three domains: I, II, and III	Globular, water soluble, and antioxidant	4.7	70–90
2.4. Gelatin	Collagen	Acid (Type-A) gelatin and basic (Type-B) gelatin	Linear, soluble in hot water, and highly stable	4.8	40

pI: Isoelectric point and Tm: denaturation thermal temperature.

Table 4.
Physicochemical properties of plant and animal proteins used for the delivery of bioactive ingredients.

- Preparation methods of protein compounds
- Environmental conditions include pH of solvent and ionic strength

Protein ingredients have been vastly used as good encapsulating agents alone or in combination with either another protein or polysaccharides which occurs through different possible interactions (such as covalent, electrostatic, H-bonding, hydrophobic, van der Waals, and disulfide interactions) for delivery of various bioactive compounds (**Figure 7**) [94]. Different polysaccharides can be used to fabricate bilayer on the oil droplets surface with protein compounds to increase the physical stability of both emulsion and the interfacial modifying properties [95].

3.1.3 Plant proteins

Plant proteins have different types such as soy proteins, cereals proteins (e.g., zein, wheat, and barley proteins), and pulses proteins (e.g., pea, chickpea, and lentil proteins).

3.1.3.1 Soy proteins

Soy proteins are globular proteins and are considered as one of the most important food proteins that are applied significantly in human diets because they have good nutritional values, health-benefiting effects, and high functionalities. They are mainly composed of albumins and globulins which represent around 50–90% of total seed proteins. They are divided according to their sedimentation coefficients into four fractions: 2S, 7S, 11S, and 15S fractions. The 2S fraction corresponds to albumins, while the globulins are present in 7S, 11S, and 15S fractions. Also, glycinin (named as 11S or SG, and Mwt 350 kDa) and β-conglycinin (named as 7S or SC, and Mwt of about 70 kDa are two globulin forms). Soy protein isolate (SPI) is considered as an essential product of soy proteins and contains protein range from 85 to 90% as a dry basis [96, 97]. Due to the good properties of soy proteins such as water solubility, fat and water absorption, gel, film, and foaming-formation and emulsion stabilization properties, they have been used as wall materials for micro- and nanoencapsulation of different bioactive ingredients alone or in combination with either proteins or polysaccharides [98].

3.1.3.2 Cereal proteins

Cereal grains are grown worldwide and they comprise three main biopolymers which are roughly classified into three groups - protein, starch, and non-starch polysaccharides [99]. Cereal micro- and nanotechnology for biomedical, food, and pharmaceutical applications focus on fabricating highly functional micro- and nanostructures from cereal biopolymers. Cereal proteins (e.g., zein, barley, and wheat proteins) are considered a vital protein source in the diet. Cereal proteins have excellent properties such as low cost, widely available, and versatile molecules which are valuable compounds for nano- and microtechnology applications. They are classified into four classes according to the solubility of fractionations: (a) albumins; proteins soluble in water, (b) globulins; proteins soluble in the diluted salt solution, (c) prolamins; proteins soluble in the aqueous alcohol, and (d) glutelins; proteins soluble in the diluted acid or alkali [100, 101].

3.1.3.3 Maize (Zein) protein

Zein protein is classified as a storage prolamine protein that makes up 35–60% of total protein in corn (maize). Pure zein protein is one of the important plant

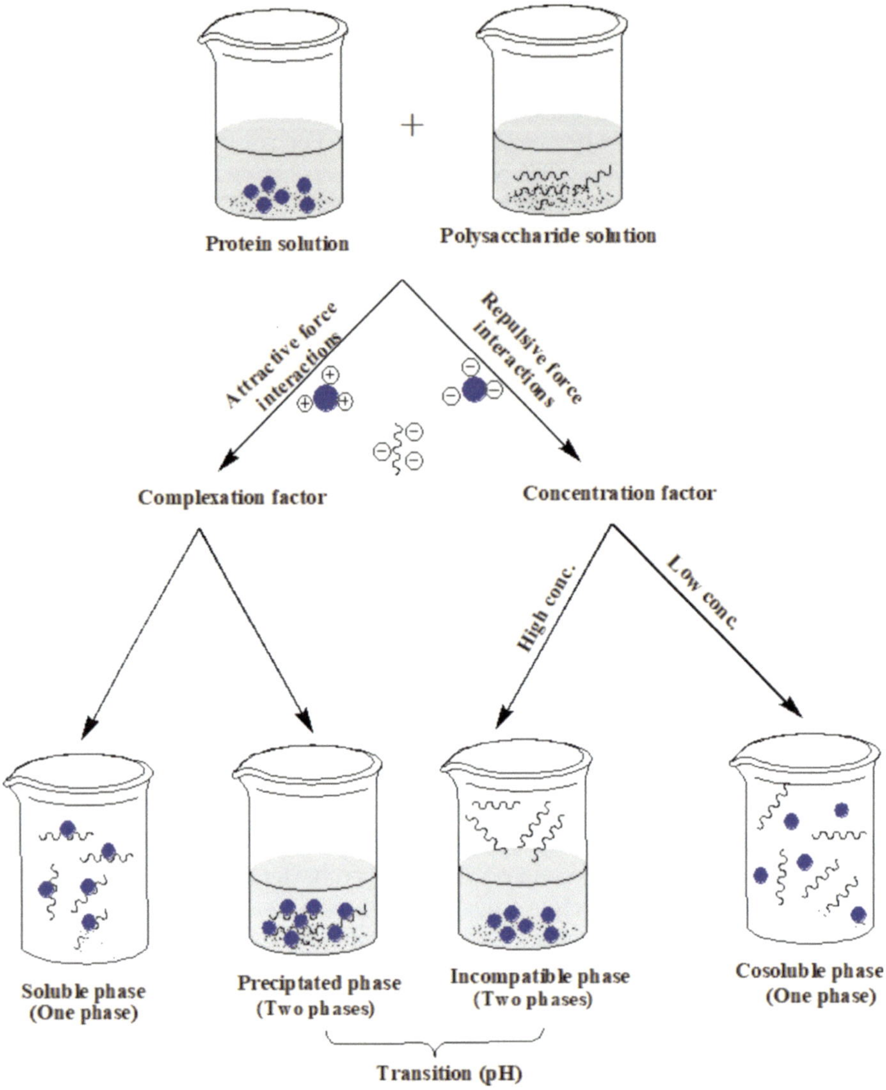

Figure 7.
Suggested interactions in two biopolymers components (e.g., protein and polysaccharide) system.

proteins due to its properties such as clear, tasteless, odorless, and edible properties, making it widely used a protein in different industrial applications [102]. The main composition of zein proteins is amino acids such as glutamic acid, leucine, alanine, and proline that are combined via disulfide bonds. It has four fractions: α, β, and γ as major fractions (accounts for 80% of the total zein protein), while the last one named δ-zein is a minor fraction. α-Zein protein is the main zein type commercially available in the market. It is water-insoluble because of the presence of non-polar amino acids which are previously mentioned but is soluble in the aqueous alcohol (50–95%). Its poor solubility in water due to the absence of essential amino acids including tryptophan and lysine decreased its usage in food products for human consumption, so zein protein nanocarriers have been applied to encapsulate core materials to enhance their distribution in water environment [103, 104]. Prolamine protein as zein protein is a valuable compound used to prepare micro-and nanoscale systems that are stable in water because these systems do not need a post-production hardening step that stables the integrity of prepared particles, as the constituting protein does not require to re-dissolve in water [105].

3.1.3.4 Wheat proteins

Wheat proteins are obtained during the isolation of starch polysaccharide from wheat flour as a byproduct and account for 80% of total wheat seed proteins; it is also used as an essential food source for both humans and animals [106]. Wheat flour is a complex material which composes of small polysaccharide fraction as starch and protein. The latter composes of two main components as gliadin and glutenin. The constitution of gliadin is single chain polypeptides (average molecular weight, Mwt, ranged from 25 KDa to 100 KDa) which are linked by intramolecular disulfide bonds and soluble in the aqueous alcohol (70% ethanol), while glutenin is a soluble fraction and is similar to gliadin composition but they are linked via intermolecular disulfide bonds with Mwt higher than 105 KDa [106, 107]. Wheat proteins have different interesting physicochemical properties such as gel- and film-forming properties due to its low water solubility and viscoelasticity [108].

3.1.3.5 Barley protein

Barley crop is a very adaptable crop. It is cultivated for both animal feed and brewing industry, in which, the by-product becomes livestock feed. Barley crops and by-products are rich and affordable protein sources which include 8–13% and 20–30%, respectively [109]. Barley proteins composed of two major protein fractions: hordein and glutelin (about 35–55% and 35–40%, respectively). Hordein fraction (alcohol extracted fraction) is divided into five groups - B hordein, C hordein, γ-hordein, D hordein, and A hordein - based on their amino acid compositions and electrophoretic mobility. On the other hand, glutelin is an alkali-soluble protein after hordein extraction, so it is not possible to extract glutelin fraction free from hordein fraction contamination. Barley proteins are highly hydrophobic and they exhibit excellent foaming, emulsifying and film-forming properties indicating that the emulsifying-stabilization process can prepare micro- and nanocapsules from barley protein [110–112].

3.1.3.6 Pulse proteins

Pulse crops are invaluable agricultural commodities that are grown in cool seasons annually. They are grown in many regions around the world such as North America (particularly Canada), Asia, and the Middle East (particularly India and Egypt). They are considered an important source of dietary protein, fiber, essential vitamins, minerals, and carbohydrates. So, they have a health value that relates to decrease of HDL cholesterol, heart disease, and type-2 diabetes. The pulse proteins including lentil, pea, and chickpea proteins which show an attractive alternative to soy proteins because they have a low risk for allergen and non-genetically modified status [113, 114]. Pulse proteins are classified according to their solubility into glutelins (dilute acid and alkaline-soluble and makes up 10–20% of the total pulse protein), globulins (soluble in water-salt solution and accounts for 70% of the total pulse protein), and albumin (water-soluble and represents about 10–20% of the total pulse protein) [113].

3.1.3.7 Pea protein

Pea protein is extracted from pea seeds which represents 18–30% fraction. It is mainly composed of globulins (65–80%) that include three various proteins: legumin, convicilin, and vicilin [115]. Also, it contains albumins and glutelins as two minority fractions. Pea legumin protein (denoted 11S globulin) has molecular weight ranged 350–400 KDa while convicilin and vicilin (denoted 7S globulin) have a molecular weight of about 150 KDa [98]. Pea proteins have interesting emulsifying and gel-forming properties, so they are used alone or in combination with either proteins or polysaccharides. This interaction creates a stable emulsion that improves the efficiency of a micro/nanoencapsulation technique as it gives good particle size distribution. Also, encapsulation occurs without chemical or enzymatic modification, due to the surfactant, foaming, and solubility properties. Besides, they are cheap and highly nutritious [116, 117].

3.1.3.8 Chickpea protein

Chickpea protein possesses many excellent advantages such as low cost, biodegradable, biocompatible, and non-toxic, hence, its use in the encapsulation field. Moreover, it is generally safe for use in the food industry because of little or no toxicity and side reactions [118–120]. Chickpea protein contains glutein, albumin, prolamine, and globulin with different percentage contents as the main composition: 3.12–6.89%, 8.39–12.31%, 19.38–24.40%, and 53.44–60.29%, respectively, and represents about 28.6% of total chickpea crops [121, 122]. It is a low-cost wall material and possesses high encapsulating ability, emulsifying properties, nutritional value, and beneficial health effects. Additionally, it can form thick viscoelastic films around oil droplets thus enhancing their stability through processing. The chickpea protein is widely used in different culinary applications because it has sustained nutritional benefits, and it is used in stews, soups, and salads [84, 93, 123, 124].

3.1.3.9 Lentil protein

Lentil crops are implanted in over 48 countries around the world and they contain soluble and dietary fiber more than in both pea and chickpea crops, besides, they are rich in protein sources which ranged from 20.6–31.4% of the total lentil plant. Lentil protein comprises globulins (Mwt 320–380 KDa), albumin (Mwt20 KDa), glutelins (Mwt 17–46 KDa), and prolamins (Mwt 16–64 kDa) with different percentages: 70%, 16%, 11%, and 3%, respectively [125–127]. It has good properties such as good solubility, drying, and emulsifying properties that lead to being widely used as a wall material to form stable capsules with high EE % [128].

3.1.4 Animal proteins

Animal proteins are amphiphilic compounds because they compose of block copolymers with both hydrophilic and hydrophobic amino acid residues. There are various types of animal proteins such as milk proteins: whey proteins and casein, gelatin, and bovine serum albumin which can be used in micro- and nanoencapsulation processes as wall materials either alone or in combination with other biopolymers: proteins (as soy protein) and polysaccharides (as chitosan) [91, 129]. Also, they possess many advantages more than plant protein as good wall materials as summarized below:

- More soluble than plant proteins over the wide pH range,

- Lower Mwt than plant proteins (e.g., soy protein has Mwt: 350 kDa, while casein protein has Mwt: 20 kDa)

- More flexible.

3.1.4.1 Milk proteins

Milk proteins can be divided into two groups: casein and whey proteins which can bind their hydrophilic and hydrophobic moieties with different substances with various affinities [130]. They are considered a good choice for micro- and nanoencapsulation of bioactive materials as wall materials due to their physico-chemical properties. They are available commercial products, they are flexible materials to encapsulate hydrophilic, hydrophobic and viable bioactive compounds, and they are rich bioactive peptide sources of various physiological effects. Also, they have a variety of characteristics including pH-responsiveness, self-assembly, and gel swelling behavior that lead to their use as good candidates for bioactive delivery systems [91, 131, 132].

3.1.4.2 Whey proteins

Whey proteins are produced from the manufacture of either cheese or casein as the dairy byproduct. They compose of a mixture of β-lactoglubulin, α-lactalbumin, and serum albumin which are water-soluble, so they have a variety of applications [133]. They are considered complete proteins because they have nine essential amino acids, in addition, low in lactose content. The three forms of whey protein are:

- Whey protein concentrate (WPC) which contains low fat and carbohydrate levels. The protein percentage in WPC is ranged between 30% and 90%.
- Whey protein isolate (WPI) which contains zero fat and lactose contents, and it contains high protein level ($\geq$ 90%)
- Whey protein hydrolysate (WPH) which has been subjected to partial hydrolysis process. So, it is a predigested form of whey protein.

Whey proteins are widely used as good wall coating materials in micro- and nanoencapsulation processes for the controlled release of different bioactive materials such as oils/fats, vitamins, and volatile compounds because of the high encapsulation efficiency and stability during storage [134–137].

3.1.4.3 Casein proteins

Casein is a major amphiphilic milk protein (it makes up about 80% of total milk protein) which is an essential part of the global daily diet. It has a variety of interesting physicochemical properties such as its availability, low-cost, non-toxicity, high stability, biocompatibility, biodegradability, binding of small and ions molecules, excellent emulsification, and self-assembly that increase its efficacy in both encapsulation and loading efficiency of the loaded bioactive ingredients [130, 138]. Casein protein's composition is 94% protein and 6% low Mwt colloidal calcium phosphate. There are four different casein fractions: αS1-, αS2-, β, and κ-casein which are amphiphilic structures in proportions of 4:1:4:1 by weight, respectively. Mwt is ranged from 19 kDa to 25 kDa [139–141]. Casein micro- and nanoencapsulation carrier systems have attracted attention in recent years for controlled and sustained release delivery of bioactive compounds because of the following advantages: their cheap price, digestibility, good dispersibility in an aqueous system, good amphiphilicity, the capability to encapsulate a variety of drug and nutrients, and form uniform spherical structures [142–144].

3.1.4.4 Bovine serum albumin

Bovine serum albumin (BSA) is a globular natural albumin protein. Its origin is either bovine serum or milk which is transferred between bovine plasma and milk through the lactating cells [131, 145]. Its structure composes a single chain of 583 amino acids with Mwt of 62.2 kDa and contains three domains: I, II, and III which are divided into two helical subdomains (A and B which bond through 17 disulfide bridges) which is specified to bind lipid, nucleotide, and metal ion [130, 146, 147]. Additionally, BSA is negatively charged at physiological pH (pH 7.4). Moreover, BSA is one of the most common protein plasma that is widely used in many applications such as drug and antigen delivery and food industry because it has good features: biocompatibility, biodegradability, non-toxicity, no immunogenicity, good stability, low cost, abundance, ease of purification and unusual ligand-binding. Consequently, its micro- and nano-capsule carriers have gained traction in recent years [145, 148].

3.1.4.5 Gelatin protein

Gelatin protein is not available in nature, but it is extracted from partially hydrolyzed collagen which is the most abundant protein in the skin and bones of the animal bovine or fish. Also, it is a linear denatured protein which is carrying dual charges: positively charged (when it is extracted with acid hydrolysis of collagen, it is known as type –A gelatin and its pI is ranged 7–9.4) and negatively charged (if it is extracted with alkaline hydrolysis, it is known as type –B gelatin and its pI is ranged 4.8–5.5) and its thermal denaturation temperature is about 40°C [149, 150]. In addition, gelatin protein is a good coating material due to its amphoteric nature, and so it is widely used as coating materials in combination with different polysaccharides such as chitosan, pectin, and alginate to form hard and soft capsules (in range of micro- and nanoscale) in food and pharmaceutical applications [151–154].

3.2 Merits and demerits in therapeutic delivery

The link of a drug with a delivery system is named “controlled drug delivery”. This link can control drug pharmacokinetics. Various delivery systems were aroused. Among them, we can cite nanoparticles, liposomes, surface-modified nanoparticles, and solid-lipid nanoparticles. Among nanoparticles, protein-based nanoparticles (PBNs) have special merits because they are metabolizable, biodegradable, and can be easily controlled as there are different chances for surface improvement for drug fixation [155].

Many proteins have functional merits making them suitable for encapsulation of bioactive agents, such as pharmaceuticals and nutraceuticals. Natural proteins are biological polymers composed of amino acid chains linked together via peptide bonds, which serve in important biological functions, such as enzyme catalysis, signaling, transport, and structure formation [156]. Some of the proteins’ chemical and physical characteristics can be used to construct encapsulation and carrier systems. Proteins used in the nanoparticles field can be classified as animal proteins and plant proteins, and both have advantages and disadvantages.

Low toxicity of the end product using animal proteins gives them an advantage over synthetic polymers. The major drawback of animal proteins is the risk of infection from any pathogenic contamination, although, it is not important as animal proteins can be disinfected. As for plant proteins, their hydrophobic character is the main advantage compared to animal proteins. This could lead to avoiding toxic chemical cross-linkers [157]. Besides, plant proteins are also cheaper than animal proteins.

3.3 Case studies/applications

3.3.1 Encapsulation of small molecules

3.3.1.1 Hydrophobic compounds

It is used with hydrophilic compounds to improve stability and bioavailability of certain compounds such as lipid vitamins (eg: A, D, E, and K). Vitamin A (VA) and VE were also successfully incorporated into biodegradable gelatin nanofibers. Curcumin is a fat-soluble polyphenol that possesses significant antioxidant and anticarcinogenic activities [158]. The release profile showed sustained release behavior of curcumin for over 7 days (around 75%) without significant burst effect when curcumin was encapsulated within amaranth protein isolate (API)/pullulan nanofibers. Dextran and whey protein concentrate (WPC) and chitosan were used as matrix materials to encapsulate lycopene by emulsion electrospinning. WPC afforded the greatest EE (around 75%), and it was also able to protect lycopene against moisture and thermal degradation [158]. Zein nanoparticles were used as delivery nano-system to enhance the oral bioavailability of quercetin (3,3′,4′,5,7-pentahydroxyflavone), which is found in tea, red wine, fruits, and some vegetables. Zein is a protein extracted from corn (with molecular weight usually from 22 to 27 kDa). It has a high content of hydrophobic amino acids, such as proline, glutamine, and asparagine. The encapsulation of quercetin ameliorates its anti-inflammatory effect on endotoxemia was studied in a mouse model [159]. Okagu et al., [160] studied the encapsulation of hydrophobic nutraceuticals (curcumin) by biopolymer nano-complexes based on insect proteins as uncoated or coated with chitosan. The authors explained the interaction between curcumin and insect via hydrophobic forces. They observed under gastrointestinal conditions, over 90% of the nutraceutical was released. Hu et al. [161] formed biopolymer-based nanoparticles through ionic gelation between stearic acid-chitosan conjugate (SA-CS) and sodium caseinate (NaCas) and cross-linked using oxidized dextran (Odex) via Schiff base reaction, as shown in **Figure 8**. The prepared nanoparticles were used to encapsulate Astaxanthin (ASTX) to improve its bioavailability and solubility in an aqueous medium. The authors successfully prepared nanoparticles with a diameter of 120 nm with good dispersity. They estimated the capability of loading ratio of 6% loading ratio and high efficiency of encapsulation.

Xiang et al. [162] formed nanocomplexes composed of ovalbumin (OVA) and methoxy pectin (PEC) to encapsulate Vitamin D3 (VD3). Vitamin D3 is fat-soluble and readily degrades under acidic conditions. The authors observed the efficiency of VD3 encapsulation up to 96.37%. Whey proteins (positive proteins) (4% w/w), and pectin (negatively charged polysaccharides) (1% w/w) were used to form nanocomplexes which were used to encapsulate D-limonene [163]. Resulted nanocomplexes have spherical shaped nanoparticles with an average diameter of 100 nm. The efficiency of D-limonene encapsulation was about 88%.

3.3.1.2 Hydrophilic compounds

Hydrophilic compounds are encapsulated to prevent their interactions with different compounds or to guarantee a certain release pattern. A study was undertaken to assess the release kinetics of prepared nano-encapsulated folic acid using a double W1/O/W2 emulsion [164]. Initially, loaded W1/O nano-emulsions with folic acid were formed and then re-emulsified into an aqueous stage (W2) having a concentrate on a single whey protein (WPC) layer or double-layered complex of WPC-pectin for W1/O/W2 emulsions formation. Single-layer WPC encapsulated

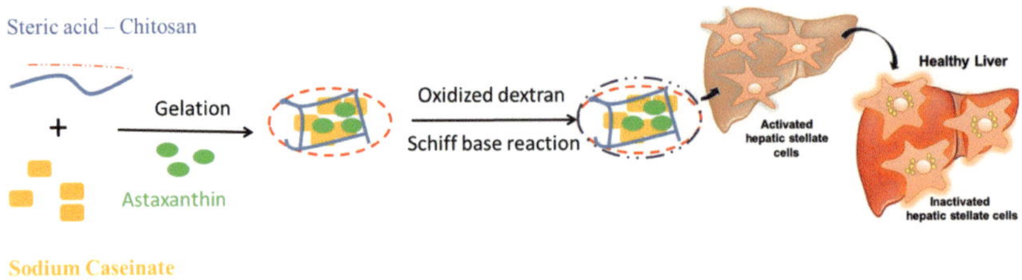

Figure 8.
General mechanism of ASTX loaded SA-CS/NaCas/Odex nanoparticles formulation and its application.

powders was the best model that fits for folic acid release pattern observed with the highest R^2. Enzymes are particularly important in therapeutics because of their catalytic activity and specificity. The challenge in the intracellular delivery of enzymes is that enzymes are unstable and have a huge size. Estrada et al. [165] developed β-Galactosidase delivery nanoparticles based on a protein. β-Galactosidase (β-gal) is an important enzyme, and its deficiency leads to several lysosomal storage disorders. The authors observed that protein-enzyme nanoparticles showed internalization in multiple cell lines in vitro higher than soluble enzyme. Authors based on the result concluded that protein nanoparticles are a biocompatible and display good efficiency for active enzyme therapeutics delivery.

3.3.2 Encapsulation of biologics

Noorani et al. [166] fabricated albumin nanoparticles enhancing anticancer efficiency of albendazole in the xenograft model of ovarian cancer. Nanoparticles based albumin was formulated with the diameter in the range of 7 to 10 nm. Loaded albendazole onto albumin nanoparticles showed the highest killing effect with specificity against ovarian cancer cells studied ex vivo [167].

Trafani de Melo et al. [168] studied the design of whey protein drug delivery system for a photoactive compound, aluminum phthalocyanine chloride for targeting of glioblastoma brain cancer. Nanoparticles were fabricated by spray drying technique with particle size between 100 and 300 nm. Authors based on their results concluded that a combination of hydrophobic drugs and irradiation achieve efficient treatment.

Stein et al. formulated mTHPC-albumin nanoparticles using nab-technology [169]. Nanoparticles showed colloidal stability over a wide range of pH and in physiological NaCl with different concentrations. The authors observed cell culture uptake of mTHPC in a cholangiocarcinoma cell line (TFK-1).

3.3.3 Encapsulation of diagnostics

Nanoscale materials permit nanodevices to enter novel scientific and technological frontiers in different diseases especially cancer diagnosis. Proteinticles are nanoscale protein particles designated by engineering, which are very useful in changing different properties based on surface area and size of various conventional things [170]. Combined detection of two serum biomarkers is also feasible through multiplexed viral detection. The disease detection method is imperative in diseases such as AIDS and hepatitis. Such a protocol is based on lateral flow assay (LFA) for protein nanoparticles. Proteinticles were found to have better biocompatibility and biodegradability with compliance with surface modifications. These nanoparticles are formed by using different proteins like elastin, gliadin, gelatin, zein, legumin, albumin, soy protein, and milk protein. Various methods used for the formulation include emulsification, desolvation, electrospray, and coacervation. Characterization parameters of these nano-formulations involve morphology of particle, size of a particle, their surface charge, entrapment of drug, loading of a drug, structure of the particle, and in vitro drug release. Different methods for the application of route of administration for protein nanoparticles have been studied by renowned researchers [170]. In nature, particular proteins have a self-assembling property inside cells leading to the formation of nanoscale particles (called "proteinticles") with constant surface topology and structure [171]. Unlike chemically synthesized nano-formulations (e.g., various carbon, metal and polymer nanoparticles), a set of effective proteinticles can be easily produced through genetic modulation of the proteinticles surface, i.e., by inserting or adding specified peptides/proteins to the C- or -N-terminus or the internal region of the modified protein. Proteins/peptides were presented that were proven to recognize specific antibodies in certain diseases that were recognized on the outer surface of human ferritin based proteinticles purposed at accurate 3D diagnosis of human infectious and autoimmune diseases. The surface exhibited the extracellular domain of myelin oligodendrocyte glycoprotein (MOG) with native conformation successfully differentiated between autoantibodies to denatured or native MOG, leading to an accurate diagnosis of multiple sclerosis. Different antigenic peptides from the hepatitis C virus (HCV) were displayed simultaneously on the same proteinticles surface with modification of the composition of each peptide. Proteinticles having heterogeneous peptide surfaces were detected with anti-HCV antibodies in patient serum with 100% accuracy. The desired method of proteinticles engineering can be used in general to the specific and sensitive diagnosis of several human diseases [171].

The aptamer is defined as an oligonucleotide-based nano-formulation. Unique characteristics of aptamer exhibit specificity and high-binding affinity with target molecules both intra- and extracellular. It functions as an agonist or antagonist in a biological system [170]. Recently, numerous aptamers were used for the detection of disease, with curative purposes under development for the identification of different molecules of HCC (hepatocellular carcinoma). The aptamer has been proved to improve the effectiveness of conventional chemotherapies and decrease the growth of HCC cells in vitro. Aptamer was proved to elicit antitumor activity and cell death in vivo. The overall data showed that aptamer possessed reduced toxicity levels. Moreover, it may provide a safer base in the field of personalized medicine [170].

Tumor Necrosis Factor-α (TNF-α) by gold protein chip was sensed using a total internal reflection fluorescence microscopy (TIRFM) as a detection method for a nano-based single biomarker for oral cancer diagnosis. Authors observed this method which is an attomolar (aM) concentration level leading to a higher sensitivity of oral cancer detection [172].

Apoferritin Ferritin is a complex of an iron-containing protein having 24 self-assembled polypeptide subunits with external and internal diameters of 12 and 7.6 nm, respectively [173]. These protein-based cage-like networks show three characteristic interfaces, the interior, exterior, and the interface present between the subunits, which exhibit functionalization. When the iron core from the inner cavity is removed, it results in a hollow protein cage-like called the Apoferritin nanocage, which is subjected to assembling and disassembling as a result of the change in the environment surrounding the molecule. Apoferritin nanocage can be utilized to insert inorganic metals inside its cavity purposing at scavenging ROS which are generated during several mechanisms in the cellular environment. This character has been used as a template for the synthesis of an array of nanocomposites for theragnostic applications in cancer treatment. Apoferrtin

Micro-encapsulating materials		Active compounds	Micro-encapsulation techniques	Applications	EE %	Ref.
Protein	Other materials					
Barley protein	—	Fish oil	Spray drying	Reducing the inflammation and improving the hypertriglyceridemia	EE: 92.9%	[174]
Chickpea and lentil proteins	Maltodextrin	Flaxseed oil	Spray drying	Reducing the coronary heart risks	EE:88.0% (Lentil) & EE:86.3% (Chickpea)	[175]
WPI protein	—	Docosahexan-oic acid	Spray drying	Improving the hypertriglyceridemia	EE: 93.2%	[176]
Zein and WPI proteins	—	β-carotene	Spray drying	Inhibiting the DNA damage and enhancing the immune system	EE: 74.0%	[177]
Casein protein	Lactose	Oil/milkfat compounds	Spray drying	Reducing the lipid oxidation problem	EE: 95.2%	[178]
Gelatin	—	Ciprofloxacin	Spray drying	Respiratory tract infection treatment	EE: 80.0%	[179]
	Ethyl cellulose	Curcumin	Spray drying	Bladder cancer treatment	—	[180]
	GPTMS	Vancomycin	Emulsification	Skin and joint infections treatment	—	[181]
WPI	—	Riboflavin	Desolvation and Spray drying	Ariboflavinosis treatment	EE: 96.6%	[182]
BSA protein	Ch and HA	Sorafenib	Complexation	Hepatocellular carcinoma treatment	EE: 45.6%	[183]
	—	Hemoglobin	Co-precipitation	Erythrocytes Shortage treatment	EE: 82.0%	[184]
Pea protein	Polyglycerol polyricinoleate	Riboflavin	Emulsification	Ariboflavinosis treatment	EE: 84.0%	[185]

EE: Encapsulation Efficiency; GPTMS: 3-glycidoxypropyltrimethoxysilane; WPI: Whey protein isolate; BSA: Bovine serum albumin; Ch: Chitosan; HA: hyaluronic acid.

Table 5.
Plant and animal proteins-based micro-encapsulated carriers for delivery of bioactive compounds.

nanoparticles enter the targeted tumor cells via clathrin-mediated endocytosis, receptor-mediated endocytosis, and macropinocytosis processes.

A ferritin-based multifunctional nanomaterial was prepared for MR and fluorescence simultaneous imaging of lung cancer cells. Human H-chain ferritin was engineered with green fluorescent protein aiming at stable fluorescence in the cells. Moreover, arginylglycylaspartic acid peptide was fused on the external surface of the ferritin cage for αvβ3 integrin receptors targeting human tumor cells (human glioblastoma U87MG cells and A549 cells) [173]. Multifunctional nanostructures based on ferritin (RGD-GFP-ferritin [RGF]/Fe_3O_4, rHF/Fe_3O_4,

Nano-encapsulating materials		Active compounds	Nano-encapsulation techniques	Applications	Particle size (nm) and EE %	Ref.
Protein	**Other materials**					
Barley protein	—	β-carotene	Emulsification	Inhibiting the DNA damage and enhancing the immune system	90 nm EE: 93.5%	[186]
Zein protein	—	Doxorubicin	Phase separation	Cancer Treatment	247 nm EE: 90.1%	[187]
WPC protein	Maltodextrin	Vitamin B9	Nano-emulsification	Folate deficiency treatment	100 nm EE: 86.6%	[188]
SPI protein	Folic acid	Doxorubicin	Nano-precipitation	Cancer treatment	200 nm EE: 83.8%	[189]
WPI protein	Ch	Trypsin	Nano-precipitation	Satietogenic and inflammation treatment	109 nm EE: 98.5%	[190]
BSA protein	—	Resveratrol	Coacervation	Inflammation and cancer treatment	175 nm EE: 60%	[191]
	Folic acid	Paclitaxel and CDF	Modified desolvation	Ovarian and cervical Cancer treatment	197.8 nm, EE: 78.4% (CDF) & EE:77.4% (Paclitaxel)	[192]
	Starch and chitosan	Curcumin	Coacervation	Cancer treatment	200 nm EE: 92.1%	[193]
Pea Protein	—	Vitamin D	Nano-emulsification	Deficient Vitamin D treatment	233 nm EE: 96.0%	[194]
	CMCFG	Curcumin	Nano-precipitation	Inflammation treatment	100 nm EE: 99.2%	[195]
Casein protein	—	Celecoxib	Coacervation	Inflammation treatment	216.1 nm EE: 90.7%	[196]
	—	Mequindox	Spray drying	Inhibition of pathogenic bacteria	262.5 nm EE: 72.2%	[197]
Gelatin	Folic acid	Irinotecan	Nano-precipitation	Metastatic colorectal cancer	200 nm EE:11.2%	[198]
	—	17β-estradiol (E2)	Modified desolvation	Ischemic stroke treatment	362.3 nm EE: 95.5%	[199]

EE: Encapsulation Efficiency; SPI: Soy protein isolate; WPC: Whey protein concentrate; WPI: Whey protein isolate; Ch:Chitosan; CDF: di-fluorinated curcumin; CMCFG: carboxymethylated corn fiber gum.

Table 6.
Plant and animal proteins-based nano-encapsulated carriers for delivery of bioactive compounds.

and GFP-rFH/Fe_3O_4) were prepared by synthesizing iron oxide (Fe_3O_4) nanoparticles in the previously engineered ferritin cages. Imaging of these cages with fluorescence targeted to αvβ3 integrin-positive A549 and U87MG cells showed higher-intensity fluorescence with RGF, when compared to GFP-rHF control cells. Furthermore, MRI with RGF showed significant enhancement of the signal to facilitate meticulous diagnosis, when compared to GFP-rHF/Fe_3O_4 or without contrast agent. Therefore, efficient targeting and fluorescence imaging of lung cancer cells utilizing engineered nanocages were proved to be a useful vehicle among the different multifunctional, nanostructured, protein-based tools to be used in fluorescent imaging.

The antioxidant enzymes present normally inside the human body, like catalase, superoxide dismutase (SOD), and peroxidase, fail in the protection of the cells under sudden oxidative damage/stress conditions Thus, further studies have developed artificial antioxidants capable of decreasing oxidative stress during lung cancer treatment [173]. Apoferritin-encapsulated protein nanoparticles have been prepared as artificial antioxidants on account of their peroxidase, catalase, and SOD-mimicking activity. Apoferritin-CeO_2 nano-truffle has been used as an artificial redox enzyme owing to its ability to mimic SOD activity. This character can be utilized to combat ROS-mediated lung cancer by scavenging hydrogen superoxide, peroxide, and other small molecules triggered in sudden oxidative damage. Thus, these systems show potential for hopeful application in lung cancer treatment [173]. **Tables 5** and **6** indicate applications based on micro- and nano-encapsulation utilizing animal/plant proteins as encapsulating materials.

4. Conclusions and future trends

This chapter describes in details the applications of polysaccharides, and proteins, as natural nanocarriers for encapsulation and safe delivery of various therapeutic, diagnostic and theragnostic agents. The chapter provides detailed discussion with recent examples and case studies for using polysaccharides and proteins as biocompatible, biodegradable nanocarriers for encapsulation and delivery of small molecules, biologics, and diagnostics.

Encapsulation will remain a valuable process in the design and development of drug delivery systems and fabrication of diagnostic tools. Advances in naturapolyceutics and encapsulation technologies will continue to drive the applicability of natural polymers and encapsulation in drug delivery and diagnostics. More of polymer blending or interactions; increasing combination of the classes of natural polymers will be observed to achieve the evolving need to improve on the delivery of existing drugs and drugs in the development pipeline. The desire to enhance selectivity, specificity and sensitivity of biosensors will continue to drive the innovations and applications of natural polymers in diagnostic space. Filling the gaps in patient related therapies will place encapsulation as the main stay technology in solving delivery related problems and diagnostic challenges. The quest for maximization, cost effectiveness, reducing patient complications, and optimization of systems and devices will lead to increased assembling of multifunctional all-in-one devices. Theragnostics has come to stay and will precipitate combination of natural polymers and encapsulation technologies to achieve the desired theragnostics that will detect biomarkers, bioimage; and target, deliver and monitor drugs at the site of action. As drug delivery and diagnostics advance, natural polymers will remain materials of focus due to their biogenicity, biodegradability, biocompatibility, good interactions with living cells, suitability for long circulation and targeting, and cell recognition.

Author details

Ndidi C. Ngwuluka[1*], Nedal Y. Abu-Thabit[2*], Onyinye J. Uwaezuoke[3], Joan O. Erebor[4], Margaret O. Ilomuanya[5], Riham R. Mohamed[6], Soliman M.A. Soliman[6], Mahmoud H. Abu Elella[6] and Noura A.A. Ebrahim[7]

1 Department of Pharmaceutics, Faculty of Pharmaceutical Sciences, University of Jos, Jos, Nigeria

2 Department of Chemical and Process Engineering Technology, Jubail Industrial College, Jubail Industrial City 31961, Saudi Arabia

3 Department of Pharmaceutics and Pharmaceutical Technology, Faculty of Pharmacy, Olabisi Onabanjo University, Ago-Iwoye, Ogun State, Nigeria

4 Department of Pharmacy Practice, College of Pharmacy and Pharmaceutical Sciences, University of Toledo, Toledo, Ohio, USA

5 Center for Biomedical Research, Population Council, New York, 10065, USA

6 Chemistry Department, Faculty of Science, Cairo University, Giza, Egypt

7 Pathology Department, National Cancer Institute, Cairo University, Giza, Egypt

*Address all correspondence to: ndidi.ngwuluka@biodrudel.com
and abuthabit_nidal@yahoo.com

IntechOpen

© 2021 The Author(s). Licensee IntechOpen. This chapter is distributed under the terms of the Creative Commons Attribution License (http://creativecommons.org/licenses/by/3.0), which permits unrestricted use, distribution, and reproduction in any medium, provided the original work is properly cited.

References

[1] Ngwuluka NC, Ochekpe NA, Aruoma OI. Naturapolyceutics: the science of utilizing natural polymers for drug delivery. polymers 2014;6(5):1312–1332.

[2] Vijeth S, Heggannavar GB, Kariduraganavar MY. Encapsulating wall materials for micro−/nanocapsules. In: Fabien Salaün (ed.). Microencapsulation-Processes, Technologies and Industrial Applications, IntechOpen 2019.

[3] Wandrey C, Bartkowiak A, Harding SE. Materials for encapsulation. In: Zuidam N., Nedovic V. (eds) Encapsulation Technologies for Active Food Ingredients and Food Processing. Springer, New York; 2010. p. 31–100.

[4] Aditya N, Macedo AS, Doktorovova S, Souto EB, Kim S, Chang P, et al. Development and evaluation of lipid nanocarriers for quercetin delivery: a comparative study of solid lipid nanoparticles (SLN), nanostructured lipid carriers (NLC), and lipid nanoemulsions (LNE). LWT-Food Science and Technology 2014;59 (1):115–121.

[5] Aguiar J, Estevinho BN, Santos L. Microencapsulation of natural antioxidants for food application–The specific case of coffee antioxidants–A review. Trends Food Sci Technol 2016; 58:21–39.

[6] Ahmad M, Qureshi S, Maqsood S, Gani A, Masoodi F. Micro-encapsulation of folic acid using horse chestnut starch and β-cyclodextrin: Microcapsule characterization, release behavior & antioxidant potential during GI tract conditions. Food Hydrocoll 2017;66: 154–160.

[7] Akolade JO, Oloyede HOB, Onyenekwe PC. Encapsulation in chitosan-based polyelectrolyte complexes enhances antidiabetic activity of curcumin. Journal of functional foods 2017;35:584–594.

[8] Augustin MA, Hemar Y. Nano-and micro-structured assemblies for encapsulation of food ingredients. Chem Soc Rev 2009;38(4):902–912.

[9] de Vos P, Faas MM, Spasojevic M, Sikkema J. Encapsulation for preservation of functionality and targeted delivery of bioactive food components. Int Dairy J 2010;20(4): 292–302.

[10] Belitz H, Grosch W, Schieberle P. Cabohydrates. In: Belitz H, Grosch W, Schieberle P, (eds). Food Chemistry. 4th Revised and Extended Edition ed.: Springer; 2009. p. 248–270.

[11] Nitta SK, Numata K. Biopolymer-based nanoparticles for drug/gene delivery and tissue engineering. International journal of molecular sciences 2013;14(1):1629–1654.

[12] Ngwuluka NC. Responsive polysaccharides and polysaccharides-based nanoparticles for drug delivery. In: Makhlouf ASH, Abu-Thabit N. (eds). Stimuli Responsive Polymeric Nanocarriers for Drug Delivery Applications: Volume 1: Types and triggers: Elsevier; 2018. p. 531–554.

[13] Wazarkar K, Patil D, Rane A, Balgude D, Kathalewar M, Sabnis A. Microencapsulation: an emerging technique in the modern coating industry. RSC advances 2016;6(108): 106964–106979.

[14] Abu-Thabit N, Judeh AA, Umar Y, Ahmad A, Hakeem AS, Ul-Hamid A. Isolation and characterization of microcrystalline cellulose from date seeds (*Phoenix dactylifera* L.). Int J Biol Macromol 2020;155:730–739.

[15] Abu-Thabit N, Makhlouf ASH. Historical development of drug delivery systems: From conventional macroscale to controlled, targeted, and responsive nanoscale systems. In: Makhlouf ASH, Abu-Thabit N. (eds). Stimuli Responsive Polymeric Nanocarriers for Drug Delivery Applications, Volume 1: Elsevier; 2018. p. 3–41.

[16] Efthimiadou EK, Theodosiou M, Toniolo G, Abu-Thabit N. Stimuli-responsive biopolymer nanocarriers for drug delivery applications. In: Makhlouf ASH, Abu-Thabit N. (eds). Stimuli Responsive Polymeric Nanocarriers for Drug Delivery Applications, Volume 1: Elsevier; 2018. p. 405–432.

[17] Emmanuel BD, Abu-Thabit N, Ngwuluka NC. Responsive polyelectrolyte complexes based on natural polysaccharides for drug delivery applications. In: Makhlouf ASH, Abu-Thabit N. (eds). Stimuli Responsive Polymeric Nanocarriers for Drug Delivery Applications, Volume 1: Elsevier; 2018. p. 267–287.

[18] Parmar V, Patel G, Abu-Thabit N. Responsive cyclodextrins as polymeric carriers for drug delivery applications. In: Makhlouf ASH, Abu-Thabit N. (eds). Stimuli Responsive Polymeric Nanocarriers for Drug Delivery Applications, Volume 1: Elsevier; 2018. p. 555–580.

[19] Mankala SK, Korla AC, Gade S. Development and evaluation of aceclofenac-loaded mucoadhesive microcapsules. J Adv Pharm Technol Res 2011;2(4):245–254.

[20] Dharmendra K, Manisha P, Kymonil KM, Awasthi SS. Aceclofenac delivery by microencapsulation using LBL self-assembly for delayed release. Pak.J.Pharm.Sci 2011;24(4):495–502.

[21] Kesharwani P, Gorain B, Low SY, Tan SA, Ling ECS, Lim YK, et al. Nanotechnology based approaches for anti-diabetic drugs delivery. Diabetes Res Clin Pract 2018;136:52–77.

[22] Cunha L, Rodrigues S, Rosa da Costa, Ana M, Faleiro L, Buttini F, Grenha A. Inhalable chitosan microparticles for simultaneous delivery of isoniazid and rifabutin in lung tuberculosis treatment. Drug Dev Ind Pharm 2019;45(8):1313–1320.

[23] Barbieri S, Buttini F, Rossi A, Bettini R, Colombo P, Ponchel G, et al. Ex vivo permeation of tamoxifen and its 4-OH metabolite through rat intestine from lecithin/chitosan nanoparticles. Int J Pharm 2015;491(1–2):99–104.

[24] Nagpal K, Singh S, Mishra D. Nanoparticle mediated brain targeted delivery of gallic acid: in vivo behavioral and biochemical studies for protection against scopolamine-induced amnesia. Drug Deliv 2013;20(3–4):112–119.

[25] Kahkeshani N, Farzaei F, Fotouhi M, Alavi SS, Bahramsoltani R, Naseri R, et al. Pharmacological effects of gallic acid in health and diseases: A mechanistic review. Iranian Journal of Basic Medical Sciences 2019; 22(3):225.

[26] Li J, Kim SY, Chen X, Park HJ. Calcium-alginate beads loaded with gallic acid: Preparation and characterization. LWT-Food Science and Technology 2016;68:667–673.

[27] Hajipour S, Sarkaki A, Farbood Y, Eidi A, Mortazavi P, Valizadeh Z. Effect of Gallic Acid on Dementia Type of Alzheimer Disease in Rats: Electrophysiological and Histological Studies. Basic Clin Neurosci 2016 Apr;7 (2):97–106.

[28] Bakhshi M, Ebrahimi F, Nazarian S, Zargan J, Behzadi F, Gariz DS. Nano-encapsulation of chicken immunoglobulin (IgY) in sodium alginate nanoparticles: In vitro

characterization. Biologicals 2017; 49:69–75.

[29] Alipour S, Montaseri H, Tafaghodi M. Preparation and characterization of biodegradable paclitaxel loaded alginate microparticles for pulmonary delivery. Colloids and Surfaces B: Biointerfaces 2010;81(2): 521–529.

[30] Blanco S, Peralta S, Morales ME, Martínez-Lara E, Pedrajas JR, Castán H, et al. Hyaluronate nanoparticles as a delivery system to carry neuroglobin to the brain after stroke. Pharmaceutics 2020;12(1):40.

[31] Martinelli F, Balducci AG, Kumar A, Sonvico F, Forbes B, Bettini R, et al. Engineered sodium hyaluronate respirable dry powders for pulmonary drug delivery. Int J Pharm 2017;517 (1–2):286–295.

[32] Park M, Lee D, Hyun J. Nanocellulose-alginate hydrogel for cell encapsulation. Carbohydr Polym 2015; 116:223–228.

[33] Morgen M, Bloom C, Beyerinck R, Bello A, Song W, Wilkinson K, et al. Polymeric nanoparticles for increased oral bioavailability and rapid absorption using celecoxib as a model of a low-solubility, high-permeability drug. Pharm Res 2012;29 (2):427–440.

[34] Singh P, Medronho B, Alves L, da Silva G, Miguel M, Lindman B. Development of carboxymethyl cellulose-chitosan hybrid micro-and macroparticles for encapsulation of probiotic bacteria. Carbohydr Polym 2017;175:87–95.

[35] Abdelbary A, El-Gendy NA, Hosny A. Microencapsulation Approach for Orally Extended Delivery of Glipizide: In vitro and in vivo Evaluation. Indian J Pharm Sci 2012 Jul; 74(4):319–330.

[36] Martoni C, Bhathena J, Urbanska AM, Prakash S. Microencapsulated bile salt hydrolase producing Lactobacillus reuteri for oral targeted delivery in the gastrointestinal tract. Appl Microbiol Biotechnol 2008; 81(2):225–233.

[37] Karan S, Choudhury H, Chakra BK, Chatterjee TK. Polymeric Microsphere Formulation for Colon Targeted Delivery of 5-Fluorouracil Using Biocompatible Natural Gum Katira. Asian Pac J Cancer Prev 2019 Jul 1;20 (7):2181–2194.

[38] Tekade BW, Jadhao UT, Mahajan YP, Patil VR. Formulation and Evaluation of Colon Specific Microsphere Containing Bicalutamide. International Journal of Pharmaceutical and Chemical Sciences 2017;6(4): 137–143.

[39] Li C, Li C, Le Y, Chen J. Formation of bicalutamide nanodispersion for dissolution rate enhancement. Int J Pharm 2011;404(1–2):257–263.

[40] Fisusi FA, Siew A, Chooi KW, Okubanjo O, Garrett N, Lalatsa K, et al. Lomustine nanoparticles enable both bone marrow sparing and high brain drug levels–a strategy for brain cancer treatments. Pharm Res 2016;33(5):1289–1303.

[41] Suganya V, Anuradha V. Microencapsulation and nanoencapsulation: A review. International Journal of Pharmaceutical and Clinical Research 2017;9(3):233–239.

[42] Lekshmi UD, Poovi G, Reddy PN. In-vitro observation of repaglinide engineered polymeric nanoparticle. Dig J Nanomater Bios 2012;7(1):1–18.

[43] Di Martino A, Pavelkova A, Maciulyte S, Budriene S, Sedlarik V. Polysaccharide-based nanocomplexes for co-encapsulation and controlled

release of 5-Fluorouracil and Temozolomide. European Journal of Pharmaceutical Sciences 2016;92:276–286.

[44] Derosa G, D'Angelo A, Romano D, Maffioli P. Effects of metformin extended release compared to immediate release formula on glycemic control and glycemic variability in patients with type 2 diabetes. Drug Des Devel Ther 2017;11:1481–1488.

[45] Bonnet F, Scheen A. Understanding and overcoming metformin gastrointestinal intolerance. Diabetes, Obesity and Metabolism 2017;19(4): 473–481.

[46] Nayak AK, Pal D, Santra K. Swelling and drug release behavior of metformin HCl-loaded tamarind seed polysaccharide-alginate beads. International Journal of Biological Macromolecules 2016 January 2016;82: 1023–1027.

[47] Sari RS, de Almeida AC, Cangussu AS, Jorge EV, Mozzer OD, Santos HO, et al. Anti-botulism single-shot vaccine using chitosan for protein encapsulation by simple coacervation. Anaerobe 2016;42:182–187.

[48] He P, Zou Y, Hu Z. Advances in aluminum hydroxide-based adjuvant research and its mechanism. Human vaccines & immunotherapeutics 2015;11 (2):477–488.

[49] Beck Z, Torres OB, Matyas GR, Lanar DE, Alving CR. Immune response to antigen adsorbed to aluminum hydroxide particles: Effects of co-adsorption of ALF or ALFQ adjuvant to the aluminum-antigen complex. Journal of Controlled Release 2018;275:12–19.

[50] Mandal S, Arfuso F, Sethi G, Dharmarajan A, Warrier S. Encapsulated human mesenchymal stem cells (eMSCs) as a novel anti-cancer agent targeting breast cancer stem cells: Development of 3D primed therapeutic MSCs. Int J Biochem Cell Biol 2019;110:59–69.

[51] Martínez-López AL, Carvajal-Millan E, Sotelo-Cruz N, Micard V, Rascón-Chu A, López-Franco YL, et al. Enzymatically cross-linked arabinoxylan microspheres as oral insulin delivery system. International Journal of Biological Macromolecules 2019;126:952–959.

[52] Cao J, Zhang N, Wang Z, Su J, Yang J, Han J, et al. Microneedle-Assisted Transdermal Delivery of Etanercept for Rheumatoid Arthritis Treatment. Pharmaceutics 2019;11(5): 235.

[53] Thomas LV, Rahul V, Nair PD. Effect of stiffness of chitosan-hyaluronic acid dialdehyde hydrogels on the viability and growth of encapsulated chondrocytes. Int J Biol Macromol 2017; 104:1925–1935.

[54] Ma F, Pang X, Tang B. Alginate/chondroitin sulfate based hybrid hydrogel with different molecular weight and its capacity to regulate chondrocytes activity. Carbohydr Polym 2019;206:229–237.

[55] Rapado-González Ó, Álvarez-Castro A, López-López R, Iglesias-Canle J, Suárez-Cunqueiro MM, Muinelo-Romay L. Circulating microRNAs as promising biomarkers in colorectal cancer. Cancers 2019;11(7):898.

[56] Chen B, Xia Z, Deng Y, Yang Y, Zhang P, Zhu H, et al. Emerging microRNA biomarkers for colorectal cancer diagnosis and prognosis. Royal Society Open Biology 2019;9(1):180212.

[57] Moraes FC, Antunes JC, Ramirez LMF, Aprile P, Franck G, Chauvierre C, et al. Synthesis of cationic quaternized pullulan derivatives for miRNA delivery. Int J Pharm 2020;577: 119041.

[58] Paulraj T, Wennmalm S, Riazanova AV, Wu Q, Crespo GA, Svagan AJ. Porous Cellulose Nanofiber-Based Microcapsules for Biomolecular Sensing. ACS applied materials & interfaces 2018;10(48):41146–41154.

[59] Qasemi S, Ghaemy M. Novel superabsorbent biosensor nanohydrogel based on gum tragacanth polysaccharide for optical detection of glucose. International Journal of Biological Macromolecules 2020;151:901–908.

[60] Chebl M, Moussa Z, Peurla M, Patra D. Polyelectrolyte mediated nano hybrid particle as a nano-sensor with outstandingly amplified specificity and sensitivity for enzyme free estimation of cholesterol. Talanta 2017; 169:104–114.

[61] Khattab TA, Fouda MM, Abdelrahman MS, Othman SI, Bin-Jumah M, Alqaraawi MA, et al. Co-encapsulation of enzyme and tricyanofuran hydrazone into alginate microcapsules incorporated onto cotton fabric as a biosensor for colorimetric recognition of urea. React Funct Polym 2019;142:199–206.

[62] Dalmoro A, Sitenkov AY, Lamberti G, Barba AA, Moustafine RI. Ultrasonic atomization and polyelectrolyte complexation to produce gastroresistant shell–core microparticles. J Appl Polym Sci 2016; 133(6):42976.

[63] Dhanka M, Shetty C, Srivastava R. Methotrexate loaded gellan gum microparticles for drug delivery. Int J Biol Macromol 2018 15 April 2018;110: 346–356.

[64] Miramontes-Corona C, Escalante A, Delgado E, Corona-González RI, Vázquez-Torres H, Toriz G. Hydrophobic agave fructans for sustained drug delivery to the human colon. React Funct Polym 2020 January 2020;146:104396.

[65] Wang S, Sun Y, Zhang J, Cui X, Xu Z, Ding D, et al. Astragalus Polysaccharides/Chitosan Microspheres for Nasal Delivery: Preparation, Optimization, Characterization, and Pharmacodynamics. Frontiers in pharmacology 2020;11:230.

[66] de Farias SS, Siqueira SMC, Cunha AP, de Souza CAG, dos Santos Fontenelle RO, de Araújo TG, et al. Microencapsulation of riboflavin with galactomannan biopolymer and F127: Physico-chemical characterization, antifungal activity and controlled release. Industrial Crops and Products 2018 August 2018;118:271–281.

[67] Ahmad M, Ashraf B, Gani A, Gani A. Microencapsulation of saffron anthocyanins using β glucan and β cyclodextrin: Microcapsule characterization, release behaviour & antioxidant potential during in-vitro digestion. Int J Biol Macromol 2018;109: 435–442.

[68] Monge Neto AÁ, Bergamasco RdC, de Moraes FF, Medina Neto A, Peralta RM. Development of a technique for psyllium husk mucilage purification with simultaneous microencapsulation of curcumin. PloS one 2017;12(8): e0182948.

[69] Estevinho BN, Mota R, Leite JP, Tamagnini P, Gales L, Rocha F. Application of a cyanobacterial extracellular polymeric substance in the microencapsulation of vitamin B12. Powder Technol 2019 1 February 2019; 343:644–651.

[70] Singh J, Kaur K, Kumar P. Optimizing microencapsulation of α-tocopherol with pectin and sodium alginate. Journal of food science and technology 2018;55(9): 3625–3631.

[71] Noor N, Shah A, Gani A, Gani A, Masoodi FA. Microencapsulation of caffeine loaded in polysaccharide based

delivery systems. Food Hydrocoll 2018; 82:312–321.

[72] Xiong W, Li L, Wang Y, Yu Y, Wang S, Gao Y, et al. Design and evaluation of a novel potential carrier for a hydrophilic antitumor drug: Auricularia auricular polysaccharide-chitosan nanoparticles as a delivery system for doxorubicin hydrochloride. Int J Pharm 2016;511(1):267–275.

[73] Wang H, Yang B, Sun H. Pectin-Chitosan polyelectrolyte complex nanoparticles for encapsulation and controlled release of nisin. American Journal of Polymer Science and Technology 2017;3(5):82–88.

[74] Mou J, Wu Y, Bi M, Qi X, Yang J. Polyanionic holothurian glycosaminoglycans-doxorubicin nanocomplex as a delivery system for anticancer drugs. Colloids and Surfaces B: Biointerfaces 2018;167:364–369.

[75] Jakki SL, Ramesh YV, Gowthamarajan K, Senthil V, Jain K, Sood S, et al. Novel anionic polymer as a carrier for CNS delivery of anti-Alzheimer drug. Drug Deliv 2016;23(9): 3471–3479.

[76] Hoseyni SZ, Jafari SM, Shahiri Tabarestani H, Ghorbani M, Assadpour E, Sabaghi M. Production and characterization of catechin-loaded electrospun nanofibers from Azivash gum- polyvinyl alcohol. Carbohydr Polym 2020;235:115979.

[77] Abreu CMWS, Paula HCB, Seabra V, Feitosa JPA, Sarmento B, de Paula RCM. Synthesis and characterization of non-toxic and thermo-sensitive poly(N-isopropylacrylamide)-grafted cashew gum nanoparticles as a potential epirubicin delivery matrix. Carbohydr Polym 2016;154:77–85.

[78] Kim ES, Lee J, Lee HG. Nanoencapsulation of red ginseng extracts using chitosan with polyglutamic acid or fucoidan for improving antithrombotic activities. J Agric Food Chem 2016;64(23):4765–4771.

[79] de Campo C, Dick M, Pereira dos Santos P, Haas Costa TM, Paese K, Stanisçuaski Guterres S, et al. Zeaxanthin nanoencapsulation with *Opuntia monacantha* mucilage as structuring material: Characterization and stability evaluation under different temperatures. Colloids Surf Physicochem Eng Aspects 2018;558: 410–421.

[80] Chan O, So K, Chan BP. Fabrication of nano-fibrous collagen microspheres for protein delivery and effects of photochemical crosslinking on release kinetics. J Controlled Release 2008;129 (2):135–143.

[81] Almine JF, Bax DV, Mithieux SM, Nivison-Smith L, Rnjak J, Waterhouse A, et al. Elastin-based materials. Chem Soc Rev 2010;39(9): 3371–3379.

[82] Matalanis A, Jones OG, McClements DJ. Structured biopolymer-based delivery systems for encapsulation, protection, and release of lipophilic compounds. Food Hydrocoll 2011;25(8):1865–1880.

[83] Fathi M, Donsi F, McClements DJ. Protein-based delivery systems for the nanoencapsulation of food ingredients. Comprehensive reviews in food science and food safety 2018;17(4):920–936.

[84] Ladjal-Ettoumi Y, Boudries H, Chibane M, Romero A. Pea, chickpea and lentil protein isolates: Physicochemical characterization and emulsifying properties. Food Biophysics 2016;11(1):43–51.

[85] Matejková M, Žídková J, Žídek L, Wimmerová M, Chmelík J, Sklenář V. Investigation of thermal denaturation of

barley nonspecific lipid transfer protein 1 (ns-LTP1b) by nuclear magnetic resonance and differential scanning calorimetry. J Agric Food Chem 2009;57 (18):8444–8452.

[86] Dhillon GS, Kaur S, Oberoi HS, Spier MR, Brar SK. Chapter 2 - Agricultural-Based Protein By-Products: Characterization and Applications. In: Dhillon GS (ed). Protein byproducts-transformation from environmental burden into value-added products: Academic Press 2016. P. 21–36.

[87] Sun C, Dai L, He X, Liu F, Yuan F, Gao Y. Effect of heat treatment on physical, structural, thermal and morphological characteristics of zein in ethanol-water solution. Food Hydrocoll 2016;58:11–19.

[88] Elmehdi HM, Scanlon MG, Page JH, Kovacs M. Probing thermal transitions and structural properties of gluten proteins using ultrasound. Journal of ultrasound 2013;16(3):101–110.

[89] Mession J, Roustel S, Saurel R. Interactions in casein micelle-pea protein system (part I): Heat-induced denaturation and aggregation. Food Hydrocoll 2017;67:229–242.

[90] Sadras V, Dreccer MF. Adaptation of wheat, barley, canola, field pea and chickpea to the thermal environments of Australia. Crop and Pasture Science 2015;66(11):1137–1150.

[91] El-Salam M, El-Shibiny S. Preparation and properties of milk proteins-based encapsulated probiotics: a review. Dairy science & technology 2015;95(4):393–412.

[92] Tarhini M, Greige-Gerges H, Elaissari A. Protein-based nanoparticles: From preparation to encapsulation of active molecules. Int J Pharm 2017;522 (1–2):172–197.

[93] Karaca AC, Low NH, Nickerson MT. Potential use of plant proteins in the microencapsulation of lipophilic materials in foods. Trends Food Sci Technol 2015;42(1):5–12.

[94] Tang C. Nanostructured soy proteins: Fabrication and applications as delivery systems for bioactives (a review). Food Hydrocoll 2019;91:92–116.

[95] Albano KM, Nicoletti V. Ultrasound impact on whey protein concentrate-pectin complexes and in the O/W emulsions with low oil soybean content stabilization. Ultrason Sonochem 2018; 41:562–571.

[96] Nishinari K, Fang Y, Guo S, Phillips GO. Soy proteins: A review on composition, aggregation and emulsification. Food Hydrocoll 2014;39: 301–318.

[97] Tang C. Emulsifying properties of soy proteins: A critical review with emphasis on the role of conformational flexibility. Crit Rev Food Sci Nutr 2017; 57(12):2636–2679.

[98] Nesterenko A, Alric I, Silvestre F, Durrieu V. Vegetable proteins in microencapsulation: A review of recent interventions and their effectiveness. Industrial crops and products 2013;42: 469–479.

[99] Delcour JA, Hoseney RC. Principles of cereal science and technology. 2010.

[100] Gil AM. Techniques for analysing wheat proteins. In: Cauvain SP (ed). Breadmaking: Elsevier; 2012. p. 77–99.

[101] Joye IJ. Cereal biopolymers for nano-and microtechnology: A myriad of opportunities for novel (functional) food applications. Trends Food Sci Technol 2019;83:1–11.

[102] Luo Y, Hu Q. Food-derived biopolymers for nutrient delivery. In: Grumezescu AM (ed). Nutrient Delivery: Elsevier; 2017. p. 251–291.

[103] Shafaei Z, Ghalandari B, Divsalar A, Saboury AA. Controlled release nutrition delivery based intelligent and targeted nanoparticle. In: Grumezescu AM (ed). Nutrient Delivery: Elsevier; 2017. p. 329–367.

[104] Lorenzo G, Sosa M, Califano A. Alternative Proteins and Pseudocereals in the Development of Gluten-Free Pasta. In: Holban AM, Grumezescu AM (eds). Alternative and Replacement Foods: Elsevier; 2018. p. 433–458.

[105] Elzoghby A, Freag M, Mamdouh H, Elkhodairy K. Zein-based nanocarriers as potential natural alternatives for drug and gene delivery: focus on cancer therapy. Curr Pharm Des 2017;23(35):5261–5271.

[106] Uthayakumaran S, Wrigley C. Wheat: grain-quality characteristics and management of quality requirements. In: Wrigley C (ed). Cereal grains: Elsevier; 2017. p. 91–134.

[107] Flambeau M, Redl A, Respondek F. Proteins From Wheat: Sustainable Production and New Developments in Nutrition-Based and Functional Applications. In: Nadathur SR, Wanasundara JPD, Scanlin L (eds). Sustainable Protein Sources: Elsevier; 2017. p. 67–78.

[108] Sun S, Song Y, Zheng Q. Rheological behavior of heat-induced wheat gliadin gel. Food Hydrocoll 2009; 23(3):1054–1056.

[109] Yalçın E, Çelik S, İbanoğlu E. Foaming properties of barley protein isolates and hydrolysates. European Food Research and Technology 2008; 226(5):967.

[110] Finnie C, Svensson B. Barley seed proteomics from spots to structures. Journal of proteomics 2009;72(3): 315–324.

[111] Wang C, Tian Z, Chen L, Temelli F, Liu H, Wang Y. Functionality of barley proteins extracted and fractionated by alkaline and alcohol methods. Cereal Chem 2010;87(6):597–606.

[112] Zhao J, Tian Z, Chen L. Effects of deamidation on structure and functional properties of barley hordein. J Agric Food Chem 2010;58(21):11448–11455.

[113] Roy F, Boye JI, Simpson BK. Bioactive proteins and peptides in pulse crops: Pea, chickpea and lentil. Food Res Int 2010;43(2):432–442.

[114] Ducel V, Richard J, Popineau Y, Boury F. Adsorption Kinetics and Rheological Interfacial Properties of Plant Proteins at the Oilâˆ' Water Interface. Biomacromolecules 2004;5 (6):2088–2093.

[115] Hall C, Hillen C, Garden Robinson J. Composition, nutritional value, and health benefits of pulses. Cereal Chem 2017;94(1):11–31.

[116] Liu S, Elmer C, Low NH, Nickerson MT. Effect of pH on the functional behaviour of pea protein isolate-gum Arabic complexes. Food Res Int 2010;43(2):489–495.

[117] Fan Y, Zeng X, Yi J, Zhang Y. Fabrication of pea protein nanoparticles with calcium-induced cross-linking for the stabilization and delivery of antioxidative resveratrol. Int J Biol Macromol 2020.

[118] Van der Spiegel M, Noordam MY, Van der Fels-Klerx H. Safety of novel protein sources (insects, microalgae, seaweed, duckweed, and rapeseed) and legislative aspects for their application in food and feed production. Comprehensive reviews in food science and food safety 2013;12(6):662–678.

[119] Ariyarathna IR, Karunaratne DN. Use of chickpea protein for encapsulation of folate to enhance nutritional potency and stability. Food Bioprod Process 2015;95:76–82.

[120] Puvvada N, Rajput S, Kumar BP, Sarkar S, Konar S, Brunt KR, et al. Novel ZnO hollow-nanocarriers containing paclitaxel targeting folate-receptors in a malignant pH-microenvironment for effective monitoring and promoting breast tumor regression. Scientific reports 2015;5:11760.

[121] Tomadoni B, Capello C, Valencia GA, Gutiérrez TJ. Self-assembled proteins for food applications: A review. Trends Food Sci Technol 2020.

[122] Rachwa-Rosiak D, Nebesny E, Budryn G. Chickpeas-composition, nutritional value, health benefits, application to bread and snacks: a review. Crit Rev Food Sci Nutr 2015;55 (8):1137–1145.

[123] Moser P, Ferreira S, Nicoletti V. Buriti oil microencapsulation in chickpea protein-pectin matrix as affected by spray drying parameters. Food Bioprod Process 2019;117:183–193.

[124] Ariyarathna IR, Karunaratne DN. Microencapsulation stabilizes curcumin for efficient delivery in food applications. Food Packaging and Shelf Life 2016;10:79–86.

[125] Brummer Y, Kaviani M, Tosh SM. Structural and functional characteristics of dietary fibre in beans, lentils, peas and chickpeas. Food Res Int 2015;67: 117–125.

[126] Jarpa-Parra M. Lentil protein: a review of functional properties and food application. An overview of lentil protein functionality. Int J Food Sci Tech 2018;53(4):892–903.

[127] Khazaei H, Subedi M, Nickerson M, MartÃ-nez-Villaluenga C, Frias J, Vandenberg A. Seed protein of lentils: Current status, progress, and food applications. Foods 2019;8(9):391.

[128] Chang C, Varankovich N, Nickerson MT. Microencapsulation of canola oil by lentil protein isolate-based wall materials. Food Chem 2016;212: 264–273.

[129] Dianawati D, Mishra V, Shah NP. Survival of Bifidobacterium longum 1941 microencapsulated with proteins and sugars after freezing and freeze drying. Food Res Int 2013;51(2):503–509.

[130] Livney YD. Milk proteins as vehicles for bioactives. Current opinion in colloid & interface science 2010;15(1–2):73–83.

[131] Tavares GM, Croguennec T, Carvalho AF, Bouhallab S. Milk proteins as encapsulation devices and delivery vehicles: Applications and trends. Trends Food Sci Technol 2014;37(1):5–20.

[132] Ghalandari B, Divsalar A, Eslami-Moghadam M, Saboury AA, Haertlé T, Amanlou M, et al. Probing of the interaction between Î²-lactoglobulin and the anticancer drug oxaliplatin. Appl Biochem Biotechnol 2015;175(2):974–987.

[133] Souza TSP, Luna AS, Barros DB, Pimentel TC, Pereira EPR, Guimarães JT, et al. Yogurt and whey beverages available in Brazilian market: Mineral and trace contents, daily intake and statistical differentiation. Food Res Int 2019;119:709–714.

[134] Botrel DA, de Barros Fernandes RV, Borges SV, Yoshida MI. Influence of wall matrix systems on the properties of spray-dried microparticles containing fish oil. Food Res Int 2014; 62:344–352.

[135] Bae EK, Lee SJ. Microencapsulation of avocado oil by spray drying using whey protein and maltodextrin. J Microencapsul 2008;25(8):549–560.

[136] Pérez-Masiá R, López-Nicolás R, Periago MJ, Ros G, Lagaron JM, López-Rubio A. Encapsulation of folic acid in food hydrocolloids through nanospray

drying and electrospraying for nutraceutical applications. Food Chem 2015;168:124–133.

[137] Katouzian I, Jafari SM. Nano-encapsulation as a promising approach for targeted delivery and controlled release of vitamins. Trends Food Sci Technol 2016;53:34–48.

[138] Oluk CA, Karaca OB. Functional Food Ingredients and Nutraceuticals, Milk Proteins as Nutraceuticals NanoScience and Food Industry. Nutraceuticals Nanoscience and Food Industry 2016:715–759.

[139] Boland M, Singh H. Milk proteins: from expression to food: Academic Press; 2019.

[140] Fox PF. Milk proteins: general and historical aspects. In: Fox PF, McSweeney PLH (eds). Advanced Dairy Chemistry-1 Proteins: Springer; 2003. p. 1–48.

[141] Yi J, Fan Y, Yokoyama W, Zhang Y, Zhao L. Characterization of milk proteins-lutein complexes and the impact on lutein chemical stability. Food Chem 2016;200:91–97.

[142] Elzoghby AO, El-Fotoh W, Elgindy NA. Casein-based formulations as promising controlled release drug delivery systems. J Controlled Release 2011;153(3):206–216.

[143] Penalva R, Esparza I, Agüeros M, Gonzalez-Navarro C, Gonzalez-Ferrero C, Irache JM. Casein nanoparticles as carriers for the oral delivery of folic acid. Food Hydrocoll 2015;44:399–406.

[144] Semo E, Kesselman E, Danino D, Livney YD. Casein micelle as a natural nano-capsular vehicle for nutraceuticals. Food Hydrocoll 2007;21(5–6):936–942.

[145] Sabaa MW, Hanna DH, Elella MHA, Mohamed RR. Encapsulation of bovine serum albumin within novel xanthan gum based hydrogel for protein delivery. Materials Science and Engineering: C 2019;94: 1044–1055.

[146] Li J, Yao P. Self-assembly of ibuprofen and bovine serum albumin-dextran conjugates leading to effective loading of the drug. Langmuir 2009;25 (11):6385–6391.

[147] Mainardes RM, Khalil NM. Nanoparticles of bovine serum albumin for encapsulation of food ingredients. In: Jafari SM (ed). Biopolymer Nanostructures for Food Encapsulation Purposes: Elsevier; 2019. p. 169–186.

[148] Raoufinia R, Mota A, Keyhanvar N, Safari F, Shamekhi S, Abdolalizadeh J. Overview of albumin and its purification methods. Advanced pharmaceutical bulletin 2016;6(4):495–507.

[149] Duconseille A, Astruc T, Quintana N, Meersman F, Sante-Lhoutellier V. Gelatin structure and composition linked to hard capsule dissolution: A review. Food Hydrocoll 2015;43:360–376.

[150] Albadran HA, Monteagudo-Mera A, Khutoryanskiy VV, Charalampopoulos D. Development of chitosan-coated agar-gelatin particles for probiotic delivery and targeted release in the gastrointestinal tract. Appl Microbiol Biotechnol 2020.

[151] Gullapalli RP, Mazzitelli CL. Gelatin and non-gelatin capsule dosage forms. J Pharm Sci 2017;106(6):1453–1465.

[152] Muhoza B, Xia S, Wang X, Zhang X. The protection effect of trehalose on the multinuclear microcapsules based on gelatin and high methyl pectin coacervate during freeze-drying. Food Hydrocoll 2020:105807.

[153] Vaziri AS, Alemzadeh I, Vossoughi M, Khorasani AC. Co-microencapsulation of Lactobacillus

plantarum and DHA fatty acid in alginate-pectin-gelatin biocomposites. Carbohydr Polym 2018;199:266–275.

[154] Yao M, Wu J, Li B, Xiao H, McClements DJ, Li L. Microencapsulation of Lactobacillus salivarious Li01 for enhanced storage viability and targeted delivery to gut microbiota. Food Hydrocoll 2017;72: 228–236.

[155] Weber C, Kreuter J, Langer K. Desolvation process and surface characteristics of HSA-nanoparticles. Int J Pharm 2000;196(2):197–200.

[156] Whitford D. Proteins: structure and function: John Wiley & Sons; 2013.

[157] Ezpeleta I, Irache JM, Stainmesse S, Chabenat C, Gueguen J, Popineau Y, et al. Gliadin nanoparticles for the controlled release of all-trans-retinoic acid. Int J Pharm 1996;131(2):191–200.

[158] Wen P, Zong M, Linhardt RJ, Feng K, Wu H. Electrospinning: A novel nano-encapsulation approach for bioactive ompounds. Trends Food Sci Technol 2017;70:56–66.

[159] Penalva R, González-Navarro CJ, Gamazo C, Esparza I, Irache JM. Zein nanoparticles for oral delivery of quercetin: Pharmacokinetic studies and preventive anti-inflammatory effects in a mouse model of endotoxemia. Nanomedicine: Nanotechnology, Biology and Medicine, 2017;13:103–110.

[160] Okagu OD, Verma O, McClements DJ, Udenigwe CC. Utilization of insect proteins to formulate nutraceutical delivery systems: Encapsulation and release of curcumin using mealworm protein-chitosan nano-complexes. Int J Biol Macromol 2020;151:333–343.

[161] Hu Q, Hu S, Fleming E, Lee J, Luo Y. Chitosan-caseinate-dextran ternary complex nanoparticles for potential oral delivery of astaxanthin with significantly improved bioactivity. Int J Biol Macromol 2020;151:747–757.

[162] Xiang C, Gao J, Ye H, Ren G, Ma X, Xie H, et al. Development of ovalbumin-pectin nanocomplexes for vitamin D3 encapsulation: Enhanced storage stability and sustained release in simulated gastrointestinal digestion. Food Hydrocoll 2020;106:105926.

[163] Ghasemi S, Jafari SM, Assadpour E, Khomeiri M. Nanoencapsulation of d-limonene within nanocarriers produced by pectin-whey protein complexes. Food Hydrocoll 2018;77:152–162.

[164] Assadpour E, Jafari S, Maghsoudlou Y. Evaluation of folic acid release from spray dried powder particles of pectin-whey protein nano-capsules. Int J Biol Macromol 2017;95: 238–247.

[165] Estrada LH, Chu S, Champion JA. Protein Nanoparticles for Intracellular Delivery of Therapeutic Enzymes, J Pharm Sci 2014;103(6):1863–1871.

[166] Noorani L, Stenzel M, Liang R, Pourgholami MH, Morris DL. Albumin nanoparticles increase the anticancer efficacy of albendazole in ovarian cancer xenograft model. Journal of Nanobiotechnology 2015;13(1):25.

[167] Verma D, Gulati N, Kaul S, Mukherjee S, Nagaich U. Protein Based Nanostructures for Drug Delivery. Journal of Pharmaceutics 2018;2018: 9285854.

[168] Melo MTd, Piva HL, Tedesco AC. Design of new protein drug delivery system (PDDS) with photoactive compounds as a potential application in the treatment of glioblastoma brain cancer. Materials Science and Engineering: C 2020;110:110638.

[169] Stein NC, Mulac D, Fabian J, Herrmann FC, Langer K. Nanoparticle

albumin-bound mTHPC for photodynamic therapy: Preparation and comprehensive characterization of a promising drug delivery system. Int J Pharm 2020;582:119347.

[170] Parveen S, Yadav N, Banerjee M. Nano-Based Drug Delivery Tools for Personalized Nanomedicine. In: Bhushan I, Singh VK, Tripathi DK (eds). Nanomaterials and Environmental Biotechnology: Springer; 2020. p. 189–199.

[171] Lee JH, Seo HS, Song JA, Koo KC, Lee EJ, Kim HJ, et al. Proteinticle engineering for accurate 3D diagnosis. ACS Nano. 2013;7(12):10879–10886.

[172] Ahmadian E, Dizaj SM, Sharifi S, Shahi S, Khalilov R, Eftekhari A, et al. The potential of nanomaterials in theranostics of oral squamous cell carcinoma: Recent progress. Trends in Analytical Chemistry 2019;116:167–176.

[173] Rohra N, Gore M, Dyawanapelly S, Tambe M, Gautam A, Suvarna M, et al. Emerging Trends in Nanotechnology for Diagnosis and Therapy of Lung Cancer. In: Dhawan A, Singh S, Kumar A, Shanker R (eds). Nanobiotechnology: Human health and environment. Taylor and Francis Group; 2018. p. 105–169.

[174] Wang R, Tian Z, Chen L. A novel process for microencapsulation of fish oil with barley protein. Food Res Int 2011;44(9):2735–2741.

[175] Can Karaca A, Low N, Nickerson M. Encapsulation of flaxseed oil using a benchtop spray dryer for legume protein–maltodextrin microcapsule preparation. J Agric Food Chem 2013;61(21):5148–5155.

[176] Wang Y, Liu W, Chen XD, Selomulya C. Micro-encapsulation and stabilization of DHA containing fish oil in protein-based emulsion through mono-disperse droplet spray dryer. J Food Eng 2016;175:74–84.

[177] Gómez-Mascaraque L,G., Perez-Masiá R, González-Barrio R, Periago MJ, López-Rubio A. Potential of microencapsulation through emulsion-electrospraying to improve the bioaccesibility of β-carotene. Food Hydrocoll 2017;73:1–12.

[178] Li K, Woo MW, Patel H, Selomulya C. Enhancing the stability of protein-polysaccharides emulsions via Maillard reaction for better oil encapsulation in spray-dried powders by pH adjustment. Food Hydrocoll 2017; 69:121–131.

[179] Silva DM, Vyas HKN, Sanderson-Smith M, Sencadas V. Development and optimization of ciprofloxacin-loaded gelatin microparticles by single-step spray-drying technique. Powder Technol 2018;330:201–209.

[180] Oliveira MB, da Silva JB, Montanha MC, Kimura E, Diniz A, Bruschi ML. Design and characterization of mucoadhesive Gelatin-Ethylcellulose microparticles for the delivery of curcumin to the bladder. Current drug delivery 2018;15 (8):1112–1122.

[181] Nouri-Felekori M, Khakbiz M, Nezafati N, Mohammadi J, Eslaminejad MB. Comparative analysis and properties evaluation of gelatin microspheres crosslinked with glutaraldehyde and 3-glycidoxypropyltrimethoxysilane as drug delivery systems for the antibiotic vancomycin. Int J Pharm 2019;557:208–220.

[182] Ye Q, Woo MW, Selomulya C. Modification of molecular conformation of spray-dried whey protein microparticles improving digestibility and release characteristics. Food Chem 2019;280:255–261.

[183] Paşcalău V, Tertis M, Pall E, Suciu M, Marinca T, Pustan M, et al. Bovine serum albumin gel/

polyelectrolyte complex of hyaluronic acid and chitosan based microcarriers for Sorafenib targeted delivery. J Appl Polym Sci 2020;137(34):49002.

[184] Schakowski KM, Linders J, Ferenz KB, Kirsch M. Synthesis and characterisation of aqueous haemoglobin-based microcapsules coated by genipin-cross-linked albumin. J Microencapsul 2020;37(3):193–204.

[185] Djoullah A, Saurel R. Controlled release of riboflavin encapsulated in pea protein microparticles prepared by emulsion-enzymatic gelation process. J Food Eng 2020;292:110276.

[186] Yang J, Zhou Y, Chen L. Elaboration and characterization of barley protein nanoparticles as an oral delivery system for lipophilic bioactive compounds. Food & function 2014;5(1): 92–101.

[187] Dong F, Dong X, Zhou L, Xiao H, Ho P, Wong M, et al. Doxorubicin-loaded biodegradable self-assembly zein nanoparticle and its anti-cancer effect: Preparation, in vitro evaluation, and cellular uptake. Colloids and Surfaces B: Biointerfaces 2016;140:324–331.

[188] Assadpour E, Maghsoudlou Y, Jafari S, Ghorbani M, Aalami M. Optimization of folic acid nano-emulsification and encapsulation by maltodextrin-whey protein double emulsions. Int J Biol Macromol 2016;86: 197–207.

[189] Cheng X, Wang X, Cao Z, Yao W, Wang J, Tang R. Folic acid-modified soy protein nanoparticles for enhanced targeting and inhibitory. Materials Science and Engineering: C 2017;71:298–307.

[190] De Queiroz J,Luana Carvalho, Costa RODA, Matias LLR, De Medeiros AF, Gomes AFT, Pais TDS, et al. Chitosan-whey protein nanoparticles improve encapsulation efficiency and stability of a trypsin inhibitor isolated from *Tamarindus indica* L. Food Hydrocoll 2018;84:247–256.

[191] Fonseca DP, Khalil NM, Mainardes RM. Bovine serum albumin-based nanoparticles containing resveratrol: Characterization and antioxidant activity. Journal of Drug Delivery Science and Technology 2017; 39:147–155.

[192] Gawde KA, Sau S, Tatiparti K, Kashaw SK, Mehrmohammadi M, Azmi AS, et al. Paclitaxel and di-fluorinated curcumin loaded in albumin nanoparticles for targeted synergistic combination therapy of ovarian and cervical cancers. Colloids and Surfaces B: Biointerfaces 2018;167:8–19.

[193] Shahgholian N, Rajabzadeh G. Preparation of BSA nanoparticles and its binary compounds via ultrasonic piezoelectric oscillator for curcumin encapsulation. Journal of Drug Delivery Science and Technology 2019;54:101323.

[194] Walia N. Pea Protein Based Nanoemulsions for Delivery of Vitamin D: Fabrication, Stability and In vitro Study using Caco-2 Cells (Master's thesis). University of Alberta, Alberta, Canada. 2019.

[195] Wei Y, Cai Z, Wu M, Guo Y, Wang P, Li R, et al. Core-shell pea protein-carboxymethylated corn fiber gum composite nanoparticles as delivery vehicles for curcumin. Carbohydr Polym 2020;240:116273.

[196] Madan JR, Ansari IN, Dua K, Awasthi R. Formulation and in Vitro Evaluation of Casein Nanoparticles as Carrier for Celecoxib. Advanced pharmaceutical bulletin 2020;10(3): 408–417.

[197] Chen L, Wei J, An M, Zhang L, Lin S, Shu G, et al. Casein nanoparticles as oral delivery carriers of mequindox

for the improved bioavailability. Colloids and Surfaces B: Biointerfaces 2020;195:111221.

[198] Das RP, Chakravarti S, Patel SS, Lakhamje P, Gurjar M, Gota V, et al. Tuning the pharmacokinetics and efficacy of irinotecan (IRI) loaded gelatin nanoparticles through folate conjugation. Int J Pharm 2020;586: 119522.

[199] Joachim E, Barakat R, Lew B, Kim KK, Ko C, Choi H. Single intranasal administration of 17β-estradiol loaded gelatin nanoparticles confers neuroprotection in the post-ischemic brain. Nanomedicine: Nanotechnology, Biology and Medicine 2020;29:102246.

Chapter 3

Nanoprecipitation: Applications for Entrapping Active Molecules of Interest in Pharmaceutics

Oscar Iván Martínez-Muñoz, Luis Fernando Ospina-Giraldo and Claudia Elizabeth Mora-Huertas

Abstract

Nanoprecipitation technique, also named solvent injection, spontaneous emulsification, solvent displacement, solvent diffusion, interfacial deposition, mixing-induced nanoprecipitation, or flash nanoprecipitation, is recognized as a useful and versatile strategy for trapping active molecules on the submicron and nanoscale levels. Thus, these particles could be intended among others, for developing innovative pharmaceutical products bearing advantages as controlled drug release, target therapeutic performance, or improved stability and organoleptic properties. On this basis, this chapter offers readers a comprehensive revision of the state of the art in research on carriers to be used for pharmaceutical applications and developed by the nanoprecipitation method. In this sense, the starting materials, the particle characteristics, and the *in vitro* and *in vivo* performances of the most representative of these carriers, i.e., polymer, lipid, and hybrid particles have been analyzed in a comparative way searching for a general view of the obtained behaviors.

Keywords: nanoprecipitation, nanoparticles, colloidal carriers, drug delivery systems, lipid carriers, hybrid nanoparticles

1. Introduction

Nanoprecipitation is a technique to incorporate active molecules into colloidal drug delivery systems, patented by Fessi et al. [1, 2], which attracts attention for developing pharmaceutical products mainly due to the simplicity of its procedure [3]. The obtained particles enable the optimization of the drug *in vivo* therapeutic performance exhibiting, for example, controlled release behaviors, target delivery, and better stability in biological fluids, which means major mean residence times, half-lives increased, and more efficient addressing of the actives toward the different body tissues. Consequently, less toxicity and minor secondary effects are expected.

Some of the research works undertaken during the last years have proposed the vectorization in nanoparticles, via nanoprecipitation, of hydrophobic active molecules, mainly exhibiting logP values higher than 3. They include antineoplastics (e.g., doxorubicin [4], paclitaxel [5, 6], docetaxel [7, 8], methotrexate [9], triptolide [6], cucurbitacin [10], and sorafenib [11]), antiretrovirals (e.g., efavirenz [12] and

IntechOpen

nevirapine [13]), immune suppressants (mycophenolate [14]), anti-inflammatories (clobetasol [15], fluticasone propionate [16], dexamethasone [17, 18], and diclofenac [19]), antimicrobial and antifungal agents (polymyxin B [20], amphotericin B [21], itraconazole [22], and linezolid [23]), antihyperlipidemics (fenofibrate [24, 25]), anesthetics (tetracaine [26] and ketamine [27]), antihypertensives (nimodipine [28] and atenolol [29]), vitamins or their precursors (β-carotene [30] and vitamin E [31]), and antioxidants (quercetin [14, 32]). Likewise, although in a much smaller number, hydrophilic active molecules such alendronate [33], N-acetylcysteine [34], and calcein [35], have been investigated. Moreover, natural extracts such as Brazilian red propolis extract [36] and essential oils [37] have also been incorporated into polymeric nanoparticles.

Practical matters as the possibility to use solvents of low toxic potential, the simple procedure, the low energy consumption required, and the feasibility to obtain particles from diverse compositions are also highlighted among the pros of the nanoprecipitation method when carriers at the submicron and nanometric scales are intended [3, 38]. Most of the nanoparticulated drug delivery systems reported as prepared by nanoprecipitation have been developed by using the physicochemical principles governing this technique, primarily those who underpin the precipitation of materials from the mixture of a solvent/non-solvent for the involved material. They include in their majority, polymer, lipid, and hybrid nanoparticles; therefore, this review will be fundamentally focused on them. Nevertheless, some interesting developments of nanoparticles prepared by nanoprecipitation have been reported as well. For example, Arizaga et al. [39] and Villela et al. [40] entrapped magnetic nanoparticles inside polymeric particles, Fan et al. [41] designed spatially controlled release multistage carriers via the complexation of dendrimers with gelatin, and Allen et al. [35] entrapped hydrophobic and hydrophilic active molecules into polymersomes. Likewise, modifications to facilitate the industrial scaling-up of the preparation process have been investigated by Charcosset et al. [42] and D'Oria et al. [43] who developed procedures based on the use of a membrane contactor. On its part, Valente et al. [44] and Tao et al. [45] propose controllable mixing devices such as microfluidic mixer systems that allow continuous and scalable processes for the synthesis of the particles.

Reviews published to date dealing with the nanoprecipitation technique provide valuable information from different standpoints. For example, regarding the role of the obtained particles as drug delivery systems and their applications in medicine, Martínez et al. [46] highlighted their ability for carrying either natural products or actives obtained via chemical synthesis. On the other hand, with respect to the study of nanoprecipitation as a physicochemical process, Mora-Huertas et al. [47] revised the influence of both the formulation and the work conditions used to prepare nanoparticles. In this case, data available in scientific reports supplemented with a systematic study of the nanoprecipitation method led to an approximation to the particle formation mechanisms and identify the factors influencing the particle properties. Recently, Saad and Prud'homme [48] deepened on the physicochemical principles of the nanoparticle formation when amphiphilic block copolymers are used as stabilizing agents (named flash nanoprecipitation). They focused on the key variables determining the nucleation and growth phenomena related to the particle formation, particularly the supersaturation condition, the mixing step, and the used solvents and stabilizing agents.

Based on the above, the present chapter revises the generalities of the nanoprecipitation technique such as the physicochemical aspects involved, some of the starting materials used to obtain polymer, lipid, and hybrid nanoparticles, and their characteristics. Then, the pharmacokinetic behaviors, safety evaluations, and efficacy tests are analyzed. It is our interest to provide readers with a comprehensive view about the nanoprecipitation as a technique to prepare nanocarriers and its potentialities for developing innovative pharmaceutical products.

2. Physicochemical fundamentals of the nanoprecipitation technique

To prepare nanoparticles via the nanoprecipitation technique, two miscible solvents are used, one of them being a good solvent (usually an organic solvent as ethanol, isopropanol, or acetone) and the other one acting as a non-solvent for the material that will form the particle (i.e., polymer, lipid, etc.), e.g., water. In general, as shown in **Figure 1**, the nanoprecipitation procedure requires the preparation of an organic phase and a non-solvent phase, frequently named aqueous phase, both guaranteeing the total solubility of all the starting materials. In this sense, the organic phase could contain polymers or solid and liquid lipids, surfactants of low HLB value, and active molecules dissolved in a solvent or mixture of organic solvents. The solubility in the solvent of the active molecule to be entrapped is one of the factors limiting the drug loading of the particles. On its part, the non-solvent phase mainly includes stabilizing agents solubilized in water, which allows the particle formation and the physical stability of the system [2]. Nonetheless, the preparation of particles without stabilizing agents has been reported. In these cases, for example, isoprenoid chains are linked to the active molecule making it easy to form the nanoparticle because of its amphiphilic nature [49].

Nanoparticles are spontaneously formed when the organic phase is dropped or added in a one-shot to the aqueous phase. Indeed, nanoprecipitation is a robust process and operational conditions used to prepare the particles do not seem to have a marked influence on the obtained particle size and polydispersity index. On the contrary, the variables linked to the used formulation appear as determinants of the characteristics of the nanosized system, mainly the nature and concentration of the starting materials [47]. This might be closely related to the proposed mechanisms to

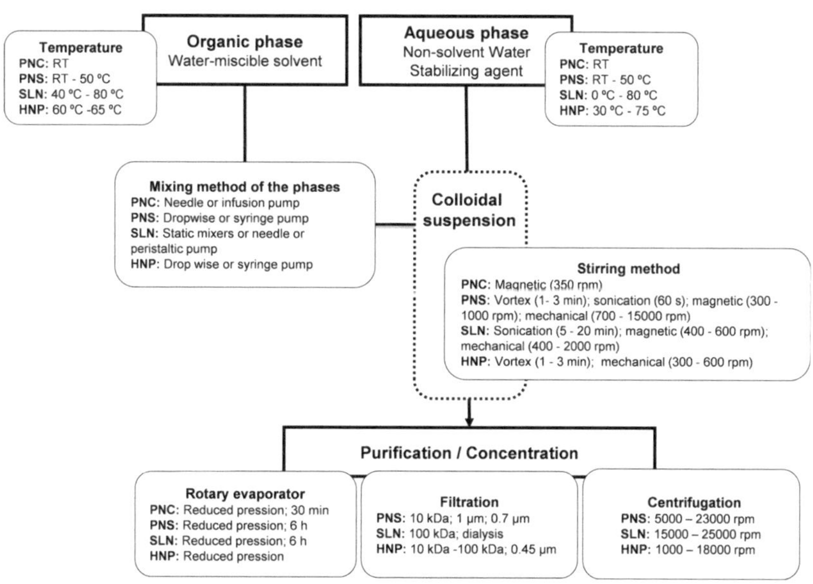

Figure 1.
General view of the preparation of polymer, lipid, and hybrid particles by nanoprecipitation summarizing the work conditions commonly reported (PNC: polymeric nanocapsules; PNS: polymeric nanospheres; SLN: solid lipid nanoparticles; HNP: hybrid nanoparticles; RT: room temperature).

form the particles by the nanoprecipitation technique. As a basic premise, only specific polymer/solvent/non-solvent ratios, where the polymer is in low concentrations and the solvent is in low proportion with respect to the nonsolvent, lead to particles at the nano- and submicron levels [50]. Thus, on the one hand, the mechanical approach states that when the phases are mixed, the organic phase is successively broken as drops within the aqueous phase due to the interfacial turbulence and thermal inequalities in the system because of the mutual miscibility between the solvent and the non-solvent and their different interfacial tensions (Gibbs-Marangoni effect) [51]. This fragmentation process will occur until the difference in interfacial tensions is minimized and the organic solvent migrates from the drops having a submicron size, which creates a non-solubility condition for the material causing the precipitation of the particles. On the other hand, a mechanism based on the chemical instability of the system has also been proposed ("ouzo effect"). In this case, when the phases are mixed, supersaturation of the molecules forming the particles is caused as the organic solvent migrates toward the aqueous phase, allowing the formation of "protoparticles" that grow following the classical nucleation-and-growth process [48, 52, 53]. It seems that depending on the formulation to prepare the nanoparticles, one of those mechanisms could predominate during the nanoprecipitation, and consequently, the adequate work conditions should be defined for allowing the spontaneous formation of submicron or nanoscale particle sizes exhibiting the smallest polydispersity indexes. Difficulties associated with the standardization of the procedure of nanoprecipitation result in the polymer aggregation yielding wide and asymmetric particle size distributions. For example, polymer aggregates are evidenced because of a concentrated organic phase, high organic phase ratio, low concentration of stabilizing agent, and poor mixing of the phases [47].

It is worth clarifying that in-depth studies on how particles are formed via the nanoprecipitation technique and the operating variables determining their characteristics have been carried out by using polymeric systems. Regarding lipid nanoparticles, only systematic studies have been reported to aid in understanding the variables that influence the preparation of the carriers; among them, the contributions of Martínez-Acevedo et al. [54] on the influence of the used recipe and Noriega-Pelaez [55] on the study of the particle preparation process are highlighted. Concerning the hybrid particles, research works to date have focused primarily on the impact of the starting materials on the particle characteristics [5, 9, 12, 23, 56].

Once the nanocarriers are formed, the particle dispersions are further processed to purified and concentrate them. To this end, rotary evaporation [14, 18, 22–24, 31, 55] and centrifugation [5, 6, 12, 13, 15, 16, 23, 25, 27–29, 36, 56, 57] are the most used methods; however, filtration [4, 6, 16, 18, 24] and dialysis [7–9, 21, 27, 34] have also been reported. Likewise, lyophilization is the preferred technique to stabilize the nanoparticles, although the storage to low temperatures has been used to preserve the aqueous dispersions [5, 8, 9, 13, 21, 29].

3. Starting materials and general characteristics of particles prepared by nanoprecipitation

As mentioned above, although different types of carriers intended for pharmaceutical applications can be prepared via nanoprecipitation, only polymer, lipid, and hybrid particles were chosen to be analyzed in detail because of the amount of reported research works to date. Polymeric nanoparticles are classified as polymeric nanospheres (PNS) and polymeric nanocapsules (PNC). The first ones correspond to a solid matrix conformed by the used polymers and other components, e.g., active molecules and lipophilic surfactants. On its part, the structure of the nanocapsules is proposed as an oil core surrounded by a polymeric shell. Approximately, 90% of the research works published on the preparation of polymeric nanoparticles via the nanoprecipitation technique are devoted to the obtention of nanospheres.

With respect to lipid nanoparticles, both solid lipid nanoparticles (SLN) and nanostructured lipid carriers (NLC) have been investigated, although almost 85% of the research works deal with SLN. Lipids nanoparticles are composed of a lipid matrix that is supposed to be surrounded by stabilizing agents. In the case of SLN, the lipid matrix is exclusively formed by solid lipids, while the lipid matrix of NLC is composed of solid and liquid lipids. It seems that the liquid lipid in NLC favors the entrapment efficiency of the active molecules [58].

Regarding hybrid nanoparticles, they are made from both polymers chemically modified with lipids (e.g., 1,2-distearoyl-sn-glycero-3-phosphoethanolamine-N-methoxy polyethylene glycol—DSPE-PEG) or the physical mixture between polymers and lipid components (e.g., PLGA and soy lecithin). Nevertheless, in the latter case, although the qualitative recipe is similar to that for polymeric particles, higher concentrations of solid lipids are used to prepare hybrid particles (i.e., lipid concentrations range between 20 and 50% for hybrid particles and between 1 and 5% for polymeric nanoparticles).

3.1 Starting materials

Figure 2 shows in a comparative way the reported starting materials used to prepare the different types of particles via nanoprecipitation. As can be seen, PLGA, PCL, and PLA are the most used polymers to prepare polymeric nanoparticles and when these polymers are chemically modified with, for example, PEG, stealth polymeric nanoparticles can be obtained [16, 17, 27]. Surfactants of low HLB value, e.g., soy phospholipids, could be added to the organic phase for facilitating the particle formation [19, 31] and, if nanocapsules are intended, castor oil, sesame oil, caprylic capric triglycerides, and caprylic capric triglyceride PEG-4 esters are part of the organic phase. Acetone appears as the preferred organic solvent of the organic phase and the non-solvent is water. Thus, the aqueous phases are solutions of stabilizing agents as poloxamer, polyvinyl alcohol, and polysorbate 80, which prevent the particle aggregation phenomena. Likewise, aqueous phases can only be water [16] or phosphate buffer [27, 59].

To prepare SLN, fatty acids and their glyceryl esters are frequently used as lipids (e.g., glyceryl monostearate, tristearate, behenate, and dilaurate); they are dispersed at a molecular level in organic solvents such as acetone and ethanol for obtaining the organic phase. As in the case of polymeric nanoparticles, phospholipids can be used to favor the particle formation and, to make NLC, liquid lipids as caprylic capric triglycerides are also dissolved in the organic phase. With respect to the non-solvent phase, aqueous solutions of stabilizing agents of varied nature are reported. Among them, surfactants as those mentioned for polymeric nanoparticles, proteins such as sodium caseinate and lactoferrin, and osmotic active compounds such as glucose and magnesium sulfate have been investigated.

Hybrid nanoparticles were designed to integrate the favorable characteristics of both polymeric and lipid systems and overcome their drawbacks [34]. These systems are proposed as an inner polymeric core surrounded by a lipid shell [60]. To obtain it, as is the rule in nanoprecipitation, organic and aqueous phases are designed so that solubility of the starting materials is guaranteed. As one of the strategies to prepare hybrid particles is employing polymers chemically modified with lipids (e.g., DSPE-PEG-NH2), they behave as amphiphilic compounds that

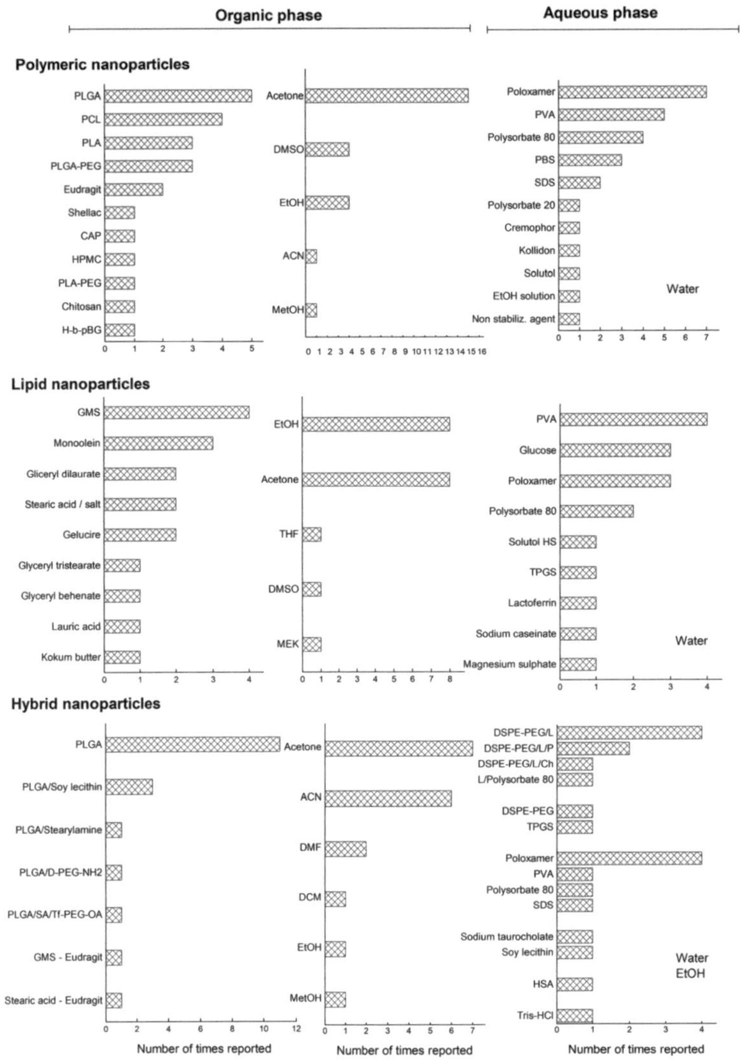

Figure 2.
Starting materials reported as used to prepare the organic and aqueous phases for obtaining polymer, lipid, and hybrid nanoparticles by the nanoprecipitation technique. Number of times reported for each starting material considering a total of 18, 11, and 13 research works for polymer, lipid, and hybrid particles, respectively [PLGA: poly(lactic-co-glycolic acid); PCL: polycaprolactone; PLA: poly(lactic acid); PEG: polyethylene glycol; HPMC: hydroxypropyl methylcellulose; DMSO: dimethyl sulfoxide; CAP: cellulose acetate phthalate; EtOH: ethanol; ACN: acetonitrile; MetOH: methanol; DMF: dimethylformamide; DCM: dichloromethane; THF: tetrahydrofuran; MEK: methyl ethyl ketone; H-b-pBG: hyaluronan poly(γ-benzyl-L-glutamate); PBS: phosphate-buffered saline; SDS: sodium dodecyl sulfate; GMS: glycerol monostearate; TPGS: tocopheryl polyethylene glycol succinate; PVA: polyvinyl alcohol; Tf-PEG-OA: transferrin-poly(ethylene glycol)-oleic acid; Tf: transferrin; HSA: human serum albumin; DSPE-PEG: 1,2-distearoyl-sn-glycero-3-phosphoethanolamine-N-[methoxy(polyethylene glycol)]].

could form part of any of the phases according to their solubility. On the contrary, if a physical mixture of polymer and lipid is used, they are dissolved in the organic phase. Unlike polymeric and lipid particles, acetonitrile is reported as the most used organic solvent for preparing hybrid nanoparticles. Another interesting matter of the recipe to prepare hybrid nanoparticles is the versatile composition of the aqueous phase. In this sense, for example, lecithin and cholesterol can be dissolved in ethanol and then incorporated in the aqueous phase that could contain surfactants such as polysorbate and poloxamer. Likewise, dispersions of surfactants, proteins, or buffers were tested as the aqueous phase.

3.2 General characteristics of the particles

Regardless of the type of particle, the shape, the particle size, the drug entrapment, and loading, and the zeta potential are among the crucial properties determining their pharmaceutical performance [61].

3.2.1 Shape

Polymeric and hybrid particles prepared by using the nanoprecipitation technique exhibit spherical shape as it is revealed by techniques of microscopy, mainly scanning electron (SEM), transmission electron (TEM), atomic force (AFM), and field emission scanning microscopies (FESEM). To investigate the shape of lipid nanoparticles in most cases, the same techniques were used, and spherical shapes were also reported. However, lipids might be melted during the sample examination destroying their native characteristics; consequently, controversial results could be obtained. For example, platelet shapes for SLN [62, 63] and structures with the liquid lipid located on the surface of the particles in the form of plates for NLC [64, 65] have been reported by using cryo-TEM and freeze-fracture TEM. Nevertheless, Dong et al. [24] report spherical shape from the analysis of SLN by using Cryo-FESEM.

3.2.2 Particle size

In general, the mean sizes, usually measured by dynamic light scattering, vary between less than 100 and 300 nm with PDI values below 0.4 (**Figure 3A** and **B**). It seems that polymeric nanocapsules and specially hybrid nanoparticles are the smallest; perhaps, any type of structural arrangement among the lipids and polymers could favor a better consolidation of the particle. With respect to lipid carriers, the platelet shapes as the lipids crystallize inside the particle could explain their high polydispersity [66].

3.2.3 Drug entrapment efficiency

Regarding the entrapment efficiency (**Figure 3C**), clear differences are identified among the carriers. Thus, polymeric nanocapsules entrap almost the totality of the active molecule in contrast with 40% attained by the SNL. As remarked by Westesen et al. [67], Pardeike et al. [68], and Weber et al. [69], when preparing SLN the solidification and the progressive crystallization of the lipid in more stable forms could lead the expulsion of the active substances whether during the particle formation or its consolidation. This results in eventual instabilities of the particle dispersions and, as evidenced in this case, low entrapment efficiency and loading of active molecules. On the other hand, as shown in **Figure 3D**, the best results of drug loading are reported for hybrid nanoparticles; active molecules could be located both in the polymeric core and the lipid layer of the particles maximizing their loading efficiency.

3.2.4 Physicochemical stability

Stability of the particle dispersions has been investigated by using refrigerated storage [6, 8, 13, 15, 21], room temperature at 25°C [8, 13, 14, 21, 57], and accelerated conditions varying between 35 and 40°C [8, 9, 11, 20, 27]. Particle size, PDI, and zeta potential are usually followed during the storage time, and the physical integrity of the dispersions is observed for up to 6 months. This good stability is expected for these nanosystems considering their colloidal nature and the absolute zeta potential values which are estimated varying between 15 and 40 mV.

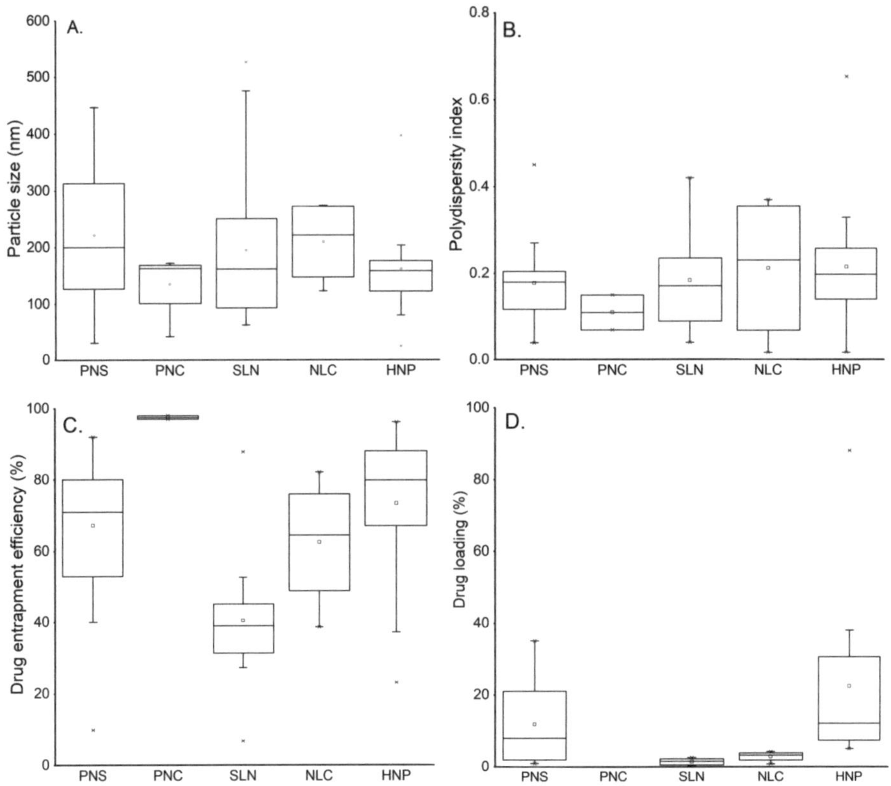

Figure 3.
General behaviors of particle size (A), polydispersity index (B), drug entrapment efficiency (C), and drug loading (D) for polymeric nanospheres (PNS), polymeric nanocapsules (PNC), solid lipid nanoparticles (SLN), nanostructured lipid carriers (NLC), and hybrid nanoparticles (HNP).

3.2.5 Release behavior

Table 1 summarizes the reported work conditions used to carry out the release tests. No matter what type of particles, dialysis is the most used technique to investigate their drug release behaviors, usually at 37°C in PBS media of pH 6.8 or 7.4. Comparisons of drug release data is risked because significant changes in the delivery behaviors are caused by the type of particle and its composition, the nature of the active molecule, and the work conditions associated with the release test, however, worth the risk for gaining a general view.

Thus, even though the mathematical modeling of the drug release data reported for the carriers of interest predicts Higuchi and Korsmeyer-Peppas kinetics, differences in the drug release patterns of polymeric, lipid, and hybrid particles are evidenced (**Figure 4**). In this way, biphasic release behaviors seem to be characteristic when nanoprecipitated polymeric particles, whether nanospheres or nanocapsules, are investigated. In these cases, the equilibrium is reached after 20 or 30 h of begun the study, and drug concentrations varying from 60 to 80% are released. Paclitaxel-loaded PLGA nanoparticles are the exception; in this case, a slow and constant drug release process occurs delivering hardly 40% of the active encapsulated after 60 h. Perhaps, the low entrapment efficiency of this molecule into the carriers makes the diffusion phenomena related to the active molecule delivery (37–70%) difficult.

On its part, the drug release patterns observed when lipid nanoparticles are tested seem to be those where the active molecule has faster delivery (before the

Nanoparticle	Drug release study				Reference
	Method	Medium	Stirring	Operating conditions	
Polymeric nanoparticles					
PNC	Directly added at the release medium	pH 6.8 PBS	Magnetic 25 rpm	37± 2°C	[19]
PNS	USP Apparatus I	pH 6.8 PBS	Mechanical 100 rpm	37± 2°C	[33]
PNS	Franz diffusion cells (sheep nasal mucosa)	pH 6.4 PBS	100 rpm	37± 0.5°C	[57]
PNS	Dialysis 12–14 kDa	pH 7.4 PBS	Mechanical 100 rpm	37± 1°C	[29]
PNS	Directly added at the release medium/ centrifugation	pH 7.4 PBS with 0.5% w/v polysorbate	Eppendorf thermomixer, gentle stirring	37°C	[16]
PNS	Dialysis	pH 7.4 PBS	Magnetic 100 rpm	37°C	[17]
PNS	Franz diffusion cells (dialysis 12–14 kDa)	pH 7.5 PBS	Magnetic 600 rpm	32°C	[18]
PNS	Dialysis 14 kDa	pH 7.4 PBS	Shaker 100 rpm	37± 2°C	[26]
PNS	Dialysis 10 kDa	pH 7.4 PBS	100 shakes/min	37°C	[27]
Lipid nanoparticles					
SLN/NLC	Directly added at the release medium	1% wt SDS solution	Shaker 60 strokes/min	37± 2°C	[15]
SLN/NLC	Directly added at the release medium/ centrifugation	0.2% wt SDS solution	Shaker 60 strokes/min	37± 2°C	[28]
SLN	Dialysis 50 kDa	pH 7.4 PBS	Shaker 50 rpm	37± 2°C	[24]
SLN	Dialysis 14 kDa	pH 7.4 PBS	Shaker 100 rpm	37± 2°C	[26]
SLN	Dialysis/USP Apparatus II	pH 7.4 PBS	Mechanical 100 rpm	37± 2°C	[13]
Hybrid nanoparticles					
HNP	Dialysis 3.5 kDa	pH 7.4 PBS	Gentle stirring	37 °C	[33]
HNP	Dialysis 12–14 kDa	pH 6.8 PBS (0.1 M)	Shaker 90 rpm	37 ± 2°C	[12]
HNP	Dialysis 10–12 kDa	pH 7.4. PBS with 0.1% (v/v) DMF	150 rpm	37 ± 0.5°C	[9]
HNP	Dialysis 12 kDa	pH 7.4 PBS	Shaker 100 rpm	37 ± 2°C	[4]
HNP	Dialysis 3.5 kDa	pH 7.4 PBS	100 rpm	37 °C	[6]
HNP	Dialysis 8–14 kDa	pH 7.4 PBS with 0.5% polysorbate 80	100 rpm	37°C	[56]
HNP	Dialysis 10 kDa	pH 7.4; 6.8 and 5.5 PBS	100 rpm	37 ± 1°C	[8]
HNP	Dialysis 12 kDa	pH 7.4 PBS	nr.	37 °C	[14]
HNP	Dialysis 100 kDa	pH 6.8 PBS, water, and HCl 0.1 M solution	nr.	nr.	[32]

Nanoparticle	Drug release study				Reference
	Method	Medium	Stirring	Operating conditions	
HNP	Dialysis 12 kDa	pH 7.4 PBS	Magnetic 200 rpm	37 ± 2°C	[5]
HNP	Dialysis 10 kDa	pH 7.4 PBS	nr.	37 °C	[23]
HNP	Dialysis 10–12 kDa	PBS with pH 7.4 FBS (10%)	100 rpm	37°C	[11]

PNS: polymeric nanospheres; PNC: polymeric nanocapsules; SLN: solid lipid nanoparticles; NLC: nanostructured lipid carriers; HNP: hybrid nanoparticles; SDS: sodium dodecyl sulfate; DMF: dimethylformamide; PBS: phosphate buffer solution; FBS: fetal bovine serum; nr.: non-reported data.

Table 1.
Summary of the work conditions used to investigate the drug release behavior of nanoparticles prepared by the nanoprecipitation technique.

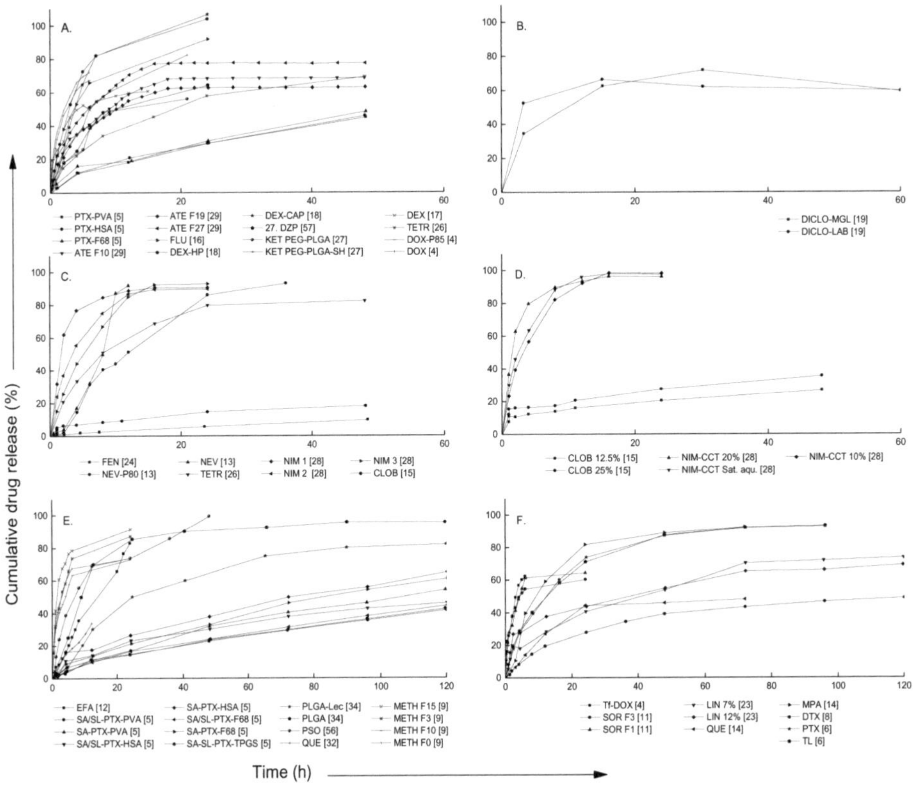

Figure 4.
Drug release behaviors for polymeric nanospheres (A), polymeric nanocapsules (B), solid lipid nanoparticles (C), nanostructured lipid carriers (D), hybrid nanoparticles obtained from the mixture of polymers and lipids (E), and hybrid nanoparticles obtained from chemically modified polymers with lipids (F) (PTX: paclitaxel; PVA: polyvinyl alcohol; ATE: atenolol; F: formulation; DEX: dexamethasone; CAP: cellulose acetate phthalate; HSA: human serum albumin; DZP: diazepam; TETR: tetracaine; F68: Pluronic 68; FLU: fluticasone propionate; KET: ketamine; SH: shellac; DOX: doxorubicin; P85: Pluronic 85; DICLO: diclofenac; MGL: Miglyol 810; LAB: labrafac; FEN: fenofibrate, NEV: nevirapine; NIM: nimodipine; P80: polysorbate 80; CLOB: clobetasol propionate; CCT: caprylic/capric triglycerides; EFA: efavirenz; SA: stearylamine, SL: soy lecithin; Lec: lecithin; METH: methotrexate; PSO: psoralen; TPGS: tocopheryl polyethylene glycol succinate; QUE: quercetin; Tf: transferrin; SOR: sorafenib; LIN: linezolid; DTX: docetaxel; MPA: mycophenolate; TL: triptolide).

first 20 h) and, at a rate, higher than 80%. Nimodipine reached delivered concentrations near 100% at 10 h, and other molecules such as tetracaine and nevirapine exhibit biphasic behaviors reaching drug deliveries higher than 80% at 25 h. NLC appear to be more efficient than SLN during the release process. The highest amounts of active molecule that could be encapsulated because of the oil component in the particle structure might have influence. Once again, there are exceptions to the general behavior. In this way, slow-release processes as in the case of clobetasol and fenofibrate, lead to less than 40% of active molecule released even at 100 h. It is important to keep in mind that fenofibrate has a high logP value (~5.2) and that clobetasol propionate was the starting material to prepare the nanoparticles. Thus, a high affinity of the active molecules for the lipid matrix of the particle would difficult its delivery process.

Hybrid nanoparticles, irrespective of whether the particles are obtained from the mixture of polymers and lipids (**Figure 4E**) or by using chemically modified polymers with lipids (**Figure 4F**), characterize by a very slow release of the active molecule where, for example, some carriers deliver above 90% of the drug after 50 h of started the test. It should be noted that in this case, the data are reported twice the set time for the other carriers. For some active molecules such as methotrexate, N-acetylcysteine, psoralen, quercetin, and paclitaxel, the prolonged drug release could be related to the uniform distribution presumed for the drug into the matrix and the core-shell structure of the particle, which difficult the diffusion of the drug toward the release medium [9]. Likewise, the hydrolysis and erosion processes of the polymeric core could be hindered by the lipid layer surrounding the polymeric core [34] or, perhaps, the hydrophobic interactions of the active molecule with the polymer might result of relevance for the drug release [5]. These effects offset, for example, the favorable solubility gained because of the precipitation of amorphous active during the preparation of the particles, which is expected to facilitate the drug delivery [9].

4. *In vivo* performance of carriers prepared by nanoprecipitation

Drug delivery systems such as the polymeric, lipid, and hybrid nanoparticles have been promoted for use in therapeutics as an interesting approach to facilitate uptake of drugs at the desired site of action, particularly when free drugs might give rise to significant off-site toxicities or characterize by poor bioavailability because of their molecular and physicochemical properties. Accordingly, knowing the bioavailability behaviors, including the pharmacokinetic parameters and the biodistribution of the carriers obtained via the nanoprecipitation technique, as well as the stability of the carriers in biological fluids and their cellular uptake, result of paramount importance to investigate their applicability in pharmaceutics.

Considering that submicron sizes for most particles prepared by nanoprecipitation range between 200 and 300 nm, which are larger than pores between endothelial cells, it is expected that, in the absence of specific affinity for receptors, their distribution is limited to the vascular space. Nevertheless, for example, larger endothelial pores such as the fenestrations in the liver and the spleen might lead to the uptake of the particles by these tissues via bulk fluid flow. Once in the bloodstream, particles are coated with a layer of plasma proteins (opsonization or protein corona formation) facilitating their elimination by immune cells. Besides, dynamic interactions between nanoparticles and blood cells, e.g., erythrocytes, platelets, and leukocytes, could occur. Then, the carriers are entrapped in the microvasculature and clearing compartments of the reticuloendothelial system like the liver, the spleen, the bone marrow, and the lung, via phagocytic uptake by cells accessible from the vascular space such us the hepatic Kupffer cells. This allows the elimination of the particles from the organism via the bile ducts into the feces or in the urine [70].

To provide a therapeutic response, nanoparticles must overcome these physiological clearance mechanisms and distributional barriers. The objective is to guarantee a high mean residence time for the carriers in the systemic circulation while their drug release delivery is modulated. Some alternatives in this way include the development of particles exhibiting sizes less than 100 nm or a positive surface charge. Stealth particles by using nonionic polymers or mimic the outer surface of blood cells by locating mixtures of phospholipids, cholesterol, sphingomyelin, and ganglioside molecules on the particle surface have also been proposed, and the modification of the particle surface with specific ligands appears as the best strategy for the target delivery of active substances up to now [61, 70].

Regarding the carriers prepared by nanoprecipitation, among the reported developments of particles that could theoretically allow them a better *in vivo* performance are: (i) particle sizes lesser than 100 nm for polymeric nanospheres [25, 26, 34], solid lipid nanoparticles [71], and hybrid nanoparticles [7, 34, 56], (ii) positively charged polymeric nanospheres by using chitosan [72] and Eudragit® RL 100 [18] as polymers or positively charged hybrid nanoparticles prepared from lipids as the stearylamine [5], (iii) stealth polymeric nanospheres [17, 27] and stealth hybrid particles [4–8], and (iv) targeted cancer hybrid particles [7, 59].

4.1 Pharmacokinetic parameters

An approach to the pharmacokinetic aspects of the particles prepared via nanoprecipitation is made from the reported studies where carrier dispersions were administered by the intravenous, oral, and intranasal routes to animal models as Sprague-Dawley rats, Wistar rats, and BALB/c mice (**Table 2**). First, the slow-release patterns previously discussed appear to be maintained in the *in vivo* behavior, i.e., nanoparticles extend in some way the drug delivery regardless of the administration route and the carrier properties. Thus, mean residence times (MRT) in the systemic circulation between 1.2 and 20 folds higher than that for the free drug and elimination half-lives between 5 and 10 folds higher than free drug are achieved. Likewise, larger values of area under curve (AUC) are reported which, provided that the amount of drug that is released allows the therapeutic dose required, are attractive for treating chronic diseases where less frequent dosing regimens are convenient.

A general view depending on the administration route (**Figure 5**, where solid and dashed lines correspond to carriers and free-drug plasma profiles, respectively) shows that polymeric particles orally administered increase the T_{max}, C_{max}, and $AUC_{0\text{-}t}$ values compared with free drugs administered in suspension or, as in the case of lipid nanoparticles, with an intravenously administered solution of the drug. The slow drug release behavior characteristic of lipid particles, where T_{max} is abruptly reached after 20 h of administration is interesting. On the other hand, although T_{max}, C_{max} and, AUC are increased when using hybrid particles, it must be noted that drug could be rapidly or slowly delivered to the serum which might be related to the location of the active molecule into the particle. For example, if the active molecule is located at the lipid shell surrounding the polymeric core, the drug might be easily released; on the contrary, if the active molecule locates at the polymeric core, more extended drug release behaviors could be obtained. Zhu et al. [4] and Godara et al. [5] demonstrate the usefulness of the lipid layer covering the polymeric core in the hybrid particles to prolong the circulation time of the particles. Probably, the lipid shell restricts the plasma protein adsorption reducing the opsonization phenomena. Moreover, the modifications of the particle with cholate enhance the drug absorption by the oral route. Likewise, developments as that of mycophenolate particles containing quercetin, where the antioxidant activity of

Active molecule—carrier	Active ingredient	Route of administration	Animal model	Equivalent dose of active molecule	T_{max} (h)	C_{max}	AUC_{0-t}	MRT (h)	$t_{1/2}$ (h)	Reference
Polymeric nanoparticles										
PNS	Itraconazole	Parenteral	Sprague-Dawley rats	5 mg/kg	7.7	nr.	1.2 µg h/mL	12.4	nr.	[22]
PNS (PEG-PLGA)	Ketamine	Parenteral	Male C57BL/6 J mice	1 mg/kg	nr.	20.1 µg/mL	88.6 µg h/mL	nr.	103.1	[27]
PNS (PEG-PLGA:SH)					nr.	19.6 µg/mL	86.8 µg h/mL	nr.	79.7	
PNS	Paclitaxel	Oral	Wistar rats	10 mg/kg	6.0	3.6–4.2 µg/mL	nr.	nr.	nr.	[5]
PNS	Diazepam	Intranasal	Sprague-Dawley rats	0.2–0.25 mg/kg	2.0	2.4%/g	13.9% h/g	nr.	nr.	[57]
Lipid nanoparticles										
SLN (P80)	Nevirapine	Parenteral	Wistar rats	20 mg/kg	4.0	9.3 µg/g	2.9 µg h/g	17.4	27.6	[13]
SLN					4.0	5.8 µg/g	1.1 µg h/g	8.6	7.2	
SLN	Amphotericin B	Oral	Sprague-Dawley rats	3.6 mg/kg	24.0	1.1 µg/mL	27.9 µg h/mL	nr.	15.9	[21]
Hybrid nanoparticles										
HNP	Doxorubicin	Parenteral	Male Sprague-Dawley rats	20 mg/kg	nr.	17.5 µg/mL	62.9 µg h/mL	9.5	6.4	[4]
HNP (P85)					nr.	17.8 µg/mL	75.4 µg h/mL	10.82	7.1	
HNP (Tf-P85)					nr.	19.9 µg/mL	107.1 µg h/mL	11.43	8.0	
HNP	Docetaxel	Parenteral	BALB/c female mice	10 mg/kg	nr.	8.0 µg/mL	198.5 µg h/mL	34.9	25.7	[8]
HNP	Mycophenolate	Oral	Sprague-Dawley rats	25 mg/kg equivalent to MPA and QC	nr.	1.2 µg/mL	27.4 µg h/mL	34.0	24.1	[14]
HNP	Mycophenolate + quercetin				nr.	1.2 µg/mL	35.9 µg h/mL	46.0	28.4	
HNP	Quercetin	Oral	Sprague-Dawley rats	25 mg/kg	1.0	8.8 µg/mL	33.3 µg h/mL	nr.	3.4	[32]
HNP	Paclitaxel	Oral	Wistar rats	10 mg/kg	6.0	6.8–7.6 µg/mL	nr.	nr.	nr.	[5]

PNS: polymeric nanospheres; SLN: solid lipid nanoparticles; NLC: nanostructured lipid carriers; HNP: hybrid nanoparticles; Tf: transferrin; P85: Pluronic 85; T_{max}: time taken to reach peak plasma concentration; $t_{1/2}$: half-life; C_{max}: maximum concentration; AUC_{0-t}: area under the curve of a plasma concentration versus time profile; MRT: mean residence time; P80: polysorbate 80; PEG: poly(ethylene glycol), PLGA: poly (D,L-lactic-coglycolic acid), SH: shellac, nr.: non-reported data.

Table 2.
Summary of the pharmacokinetic parameters reported in research works on nanoparticles prepared by the nanoprecipitation technique.

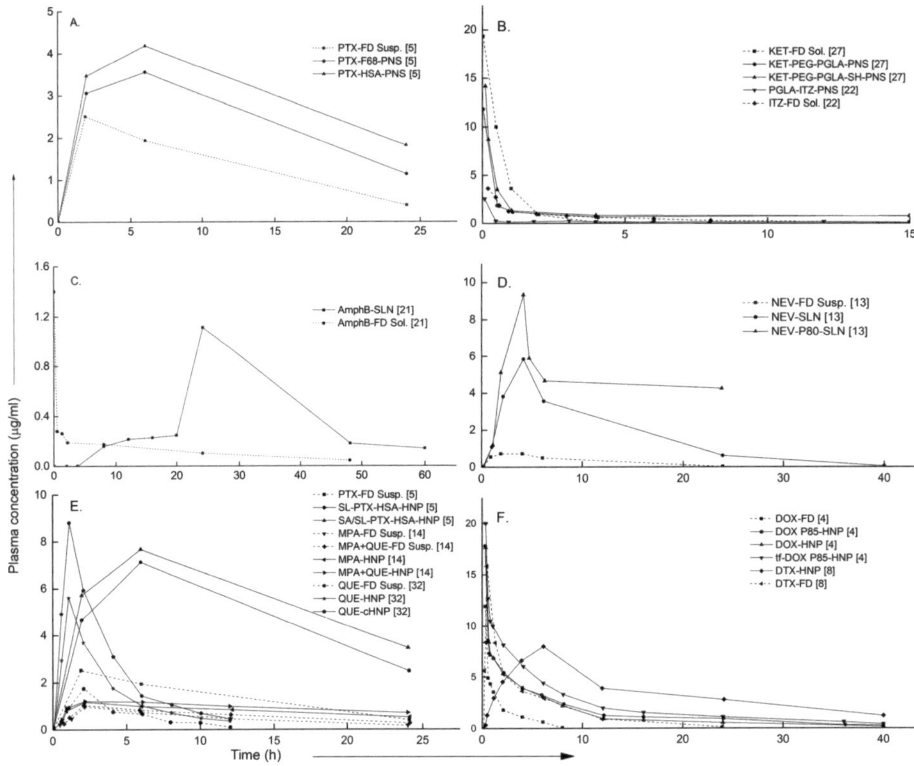

Figure 5.
General behaviors of plasma concentration reported for polymeric nanoparticles (A and B), lipid nanoparticles (C and D), and hybrid nanoparticles (E and F). Oral administration (A, C, and E); intravenous administration (B, D, and F) (PTX: paclitaxel; FD: free drug; F68: Pluronic 68; HSA: human serum albumin; KET: ketamine; SH: shellac; ITZ: itraconazole; NEV: nevirapine; AmphB: amphotericin B; P80: polysorbate 80; SA: stearylamine; SL: soy lecithin; P: PLGA; MPA: mycophenolate; PVA: polyvinyl alcohol; QUE: quercetin; cHNP: cholate-modified hybrid nanoparticle; DOX: doxorubicin; DTX: docetaxel; P85: Pluronic 85; tf: transferrin).

quercetin inhibits the mycophenolate metabolism through cytochrome P450, are highlighted. This, together with the slow-release pattern of the particles, improves in a significant way the *in vivo* performance of the hybrid nanoparticles [14].

Concerning the administration of carriers by the intravenous route, pharmacokinetic advantages were also evidenced compared to the free drug administration. As reported by Bian et al. [22] and Han et al. [27], even if a fraction of the polymeric nanoparticles are quickly removed by the reticuloendothelial system during the first 4 h after the administration, the remaining particles into the systemic circulation allow a sustained drug delivery for more than 20 h achieving $AUC_{0\text{-}t}$ values from 2 to 10 times higher than free drug. As intended, pegylation of polymeric nanoparticles extends the elimination half-life by ~100 h and increases in 84% the AUC regarding the free drug [27]. With respect to lipid carriers, Lahkar et al. [13] evidence a significant increase of their $AUC_{0\text{-}t}$ which could remain in the blood circulation four times more than the free drug. Moreover, modifications to the particle surface providing some hydrophilicity with polysorbate 80 result in an MRT eight times higher than that of the free drug. Regarding the hybrid nanoparticles, Zhu et al. [4] provide evidence on their extended drug delivery pattern that is improved as modifications on the particle surface are introduced. Thus, plasma circulation of the particles and their corresponding $AUC_{0\text{-}t}$ could be prolonged up to six and seven times, respectively, compared with that for the free drug. Jadon and Sharma [8] illustrate results in the same direction where drug delivery from the hybrid particles continues to be detected 72 h after the administration with AUC_{0-t} values around 3.6 times higher than free drug.

4.2 Biodistribution

Figure 6 shows an overview of the organ distribution patterns of the carriers under study as an approximation of their *in vivo* transport and metabolism processes depending on the route of administration. Perhaps, these behaviors would better correspond to the carried drug since the concentration of the active molecule in the tissues of interest is the measure commonly used to follow the particles in this kind of experiments. Once again, it is the intention to illustrate general behaviors; therefore, the punctual analyses on the particular work conditions used by each research team such as the animal models, the sampling times, and the way as the samples were analyzed are not considered. Thus, caution must be taken to do statements that lead to misinterpretations.

As can be seen in **Figure 6**, after 8 h of oral administration of both lipid and hybrid carriers, the liver, the spleen, and the kidney appear as the organs where lipid and hybrid particles are located. This could be attributed to the important role of the liver in the clearance of the particles and the blood filtration function of spleen within the immune system which might also remove the particles of the bloodstream. On its part, drug concentration in the kidney could mean the normal transit of the carrier because of the systemic circulation and the high irrigation of this organ. Nonetheless, the elimination process of intact carriers would also be happening.

On the other hand, as expected, the brain accumulates substantial amounts of lipid nanoparticles administered via intranasal because of the closeness of this organ to the nasal mucosa and its high blood perfusion. This behavior should be harnessed to improve therapies targeted to the brain as those for the treatment of diseases of the central nervous system. Likewise, particles intended for lung cancer therapies, prepared from a hyaluronan-modified polymer, and administered via

Intravenous

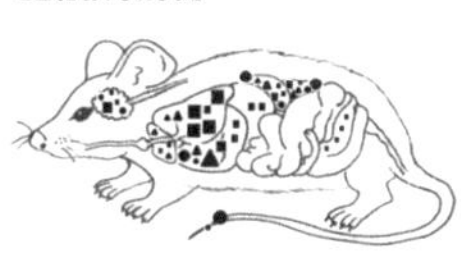

Nanoparticle /Active ingredient	Animal model	Sampling period (h)	Organ concentration (%)									Reference
			Liver	Kidney	Lung	Heart	Brain	Spleen	Blood	Gut	Stomach	
PNS (KET)	C57BL/6J mice	120	25	20	15	nr.	25	15	nr.	nr.	nr.	[27]
PNS 30 nm	NMRI mice	24	5	5	58	5	5	5	nr.	5	12	[59]
PNS 300 nm		24	5	5	53	5	5	5	nr.	5	15	[59]
PNS 30 nm	Balb/c mice	24	10	5	55	5	5	5	nr.	5	10	[59]
PNS 300 nm		24	10	10	50	5	5	5	nr.	5	10	[59]
SLN (NEV)	Wistar rat	24	27	32	nr.	nr.	4.5	32	4.5	nr.	nr.	[13]
SLN P80 (NEV)			9	14	nr.	nr.	23	14	40	nr.	nr.	[13]
HNP (DTX)	CD1 mice	24	73	9	4.5	4.5	nr.	9	nr.	nr.	nr.	[7]
HNP (DTX)	Balb/c mice	24	19	25	19	12	nr.	25	nr.	nr.	nr.	[8]

Intranasal - Intrapulmonar

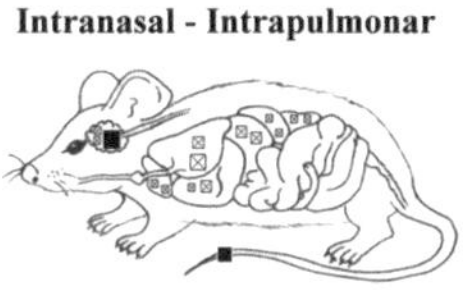

Nanoparticle - Active ingredient	Animal model	Sampling period (h)	Organ concentration (%)								Reference
			Liver	Kidney	Lung	Heart	Brain	Spleen	Blood	Stomach	
PNS (DZP)	Sprague-Dawley rats	24	nr.	nr.	nr.	nr.	60	nr.	40	nr.	[57]
PNS 30 nm	NMRI mice	24	10	5	44	5	5	5	nr.	26	[59]
PNS 300 nm		24	5	5	69	nr.	5	nr.	nr.	16	[59]
PNS 30 nm	Balb/c mice	24	20	4	52	4	4	8	nr.	8	[59]
PNS 300 nm		24	12	12	50	4	4	9	nr.	9	[59]

Oral

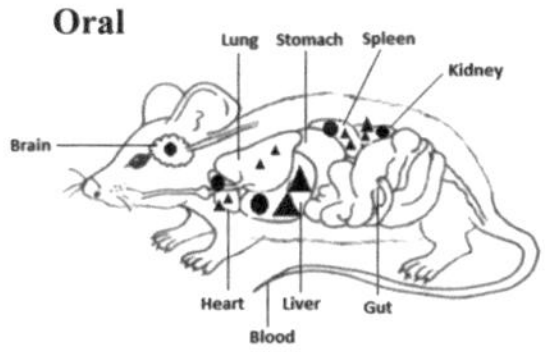

Nanoparticle - Active ingredient	Animal model	Sampling period (h)	Organ concentration (%)						Reference
			Liver	Kidney	Lung	Heart	Brain	Spleen	
SLN (AmphB)	Sprague-Dawley rats	8	24	19	nr.	19	19	19	[21]
HNP (MPA)	Sprague-Dawley rats	720	64	7	7	7	nr.	15	[14]
HNP (QUE)			73	12	5	3	nr.	7	[14]

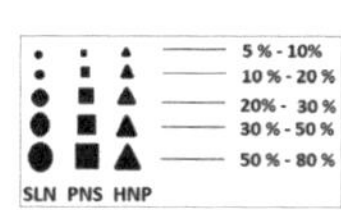

Figure 6.
General behavior of biodistribution for polymer, lipid, and hybrid nanoparticles after administration by oral, intranasal, intrapulmonary, and intravenous routes. Administration by intravenous, intranasal and oral routes (black-filled symbols) and by intrapulmonary route (crossed symbols) (KET: ketamine; NEV: nevirapine; DTX: docetaxel; DZP: diazepam; AmphB: amphotericin B; MPA: mycophenolate; QUE: quercetin).

intrapulmonary route, directly locate on lung up to 24 h [59]. This finding confirms the ability of hyaluronan to be recognized by cancer lung receptors allowing the particle concentration in this tissue and consequently, avoiding the waste of active substance in other organs.

Regarding the intravenous administration, it seems that after 24 h, polymeric nanoparticles mainly locate at the lung, liver, and brain; lipid particles are distributed in blood, liver, kidney, and spleen; and hybrid particles accumulate in the liver. However, it should be noted that regardless of the kind of particle and compared with the oral and intranasal administration, when carriers are administered by intravenous route, drug is found in low levels in all the investigated organs. In addition, after extended periods (e.g., 120 h), particles are more homogeneously distributed among the investigated tissues [27]. This is a natural consequence of the systemic circulation and the irrigation of the different organs. Besides, as previously mentioned, there is a high probability that the concentration of carriers on the liver occurs due to the ability of the hepatic Kupffer cells to phagocyte them. Likewise, the phagocytic activity of the alveolar macrophages could explain why high concentrations of the drug are found in the lung. In addition, to find carriers or active molecules in the stomach might also be possible considering that the pH of this tissue could favor the retention of active molecules exhibiting a basic nature.

It is important to highlight the efficacy of targeted carriers to reach the intended tissues. As it has been evidenced by Jeannot et al. [59], working with polymeric nanoparticles, the functionalization of the polymer with polysaccharide hyaluronan, known for its affinity toward certain cancer cells receptors, allows high concentrations of particles on the lung offering an interesting alternative for the lung cancer treatment. In the same direction, Dehaini et al. [7] demonstrate the ability of docetaxel-loaded hybrid nanoparticles functionalized with folate to reach cancerous tumors.

4.3 Stability in biological fluids

Knowing if nanoparticles aggregate after their *in vivo* administration is of crucial importance for their application as drug delivery systems. To this end, the colloidal stability of the particulate systems dispersed in biological fluids has been investigated by monitoring variables such as the particle size and the drug encapsulation. Thus, Lazzari et al. [73] demonstrated that polymeric nanospheres prepared by flash nanoprecipitation from PMMA were stable up to 60 h in synthetic saliva, gastric juice, intestinal fluid, and lysosomal fluid while PLA nanoparticles aggregate in gastric juice. Likewise, Dehaini et al. [7] report the aggregation of PLGA nanoparticles in fetal bovine serum (FBS). On the other hand, polymeric nanocapsules coated with brush layers of an oligo ethylene glycol derived methacrylate polymer exhibit major stability in human serum albumin solution, FBS, and human blood plasma, that those non-coated [74]. This evidences the usefulness of designing stealth nanoparticles as a strategy to prevent the particle aggregate formation in blood avoiding their rapid removal from the systemic circulation by the immune system. Regarding SLN, Liu et al. [26] verified their colloidal stability in FBS reporting increases in particle size of approximately 50%, although encapsulation efficiency does not vary. Chaudhari et al. [21] delved into the stability of SLN in simulated gastric fluid confirming that after 2 h, amphotericin B remains encapsulated favoring its stability. With respect to hybrid nanoparticles, contradictory results of aggregation [23] and non-aggregation [7] have been reported when the particle dispersions are mixed with FBS. This can be attributed to the experimental conditions used. In the first case, aggregation is reported after 2 days of storage of the samples at 37°C; in the second one, aggregation was investigated immediately

Nanoparticle	Assay	Experimental conditions				General results	Reference
		Cellular model	Tracer molecule concentration	Interaction—cellular model (some work conditions)	Technique of analysis		
PNS	CD44 expression levels	Human H322, H358, and A549 NSCLC cell lines	8 μg/mL	30 min at 37 C	Flow cytometry FITC	Dose-dependent binding of NP 30 nm and NP 300 nm, was observed in the three cell lines, with a higher intensity for A549 cells compared with H322 and H358 cells.	[59]
HNP	Cellular uptake	The MDA-MB-231 breast cancer cells; human prostate cancer PC3 cells	10, 300, and 500 μg/mL	24 h	CLSM	High internalization of the HNP in the cells at the highest concentrations.	[9]
HNP	Cellular uptake	A549 human lung adenocarcinoma cells	20 μg/mL	24 h	Flow cytometry	Functionalization of HNP plays a key role in the uptake of drugs in *in vitro* lung cancer cells.	[6]
HNP	Cellular uptake Qualitative study	Human breast adenocarcinoma MDA-MB-231 cells	1 μg/mL	12 h	CLSM	The improved cell uptake efficiency of HNP is attributed by cytosolic delivery of the drug.	[8]
HNP	Cellular uptake Quantitative study	Human breast adenocarcinoma MDA-MB-231 cells	Equivalent to 10, 20, 30, and 40 μg/mL	24 h	CLSM	HNP exhibit improved cellular uptake efficiency (45–48%) compared with free drug (37–39%).	[8]
HNP	Cellular uptake analysis	MCF-7 human breast cancer cell	1 μg/mL	2 h	Differential interference contrast microscopy	High internalization of HNP inside the cells after 2 h of incubation with respect to reference nanoparticles.	[14]
HNP	Cellular uptake	Caco-2 cells	25 μg/mL	0.5–2 h	Protein quantification: BCA protein assay kit Drug quantification: HPLC	HNP exhibited improved cellular uptake of quercetin relative to its free form, showing a time-dependent uptake accumulation.	[32]

Nanoparticle	Assay	Experimental conditions				General results	Reference
		Cellular model	Tracer molecule concentration	Interaction—cellular model (some work conditions)	Technique of analysis		
HNP	Internalization into osteoblasts	MC3T3-E1 osteoblasts	2, 4, and 8 μg/mL	6 h at 37°C	CLSM	HNP were more effective in reducing the intracellular MRSA counts than the free linezolid.	[23]
HNP	Cellular internalization	Prostate cancer cells (PC3-MM2) and human breast cancer cells (MDA-MB-231)	100–300 μg/mL	3 min at 37°C	CLSM FITC	Cellular uptake ability depends on particle concentration.	[11]

PNS: polymeric nanospheres; HNP: hybrid nanoparticles; NP: nanoparticle; MTX: methotrexate; FITC: fluorescein isothiocyanate; HPLC: high-performance liquid chromatography; CLSM: confocal laser scanning microscope; MRSA: methicillin-resistant Staphylococcus aureus*; nr.: non-reported data.*

Table 3.
Summary of experimental conditions and general results reported in research works on cellular uptake of nanoparticles prepared by the nanoprecipitation technique.

the particle dispersions were diluted. On the other hand, when the stability of hybrid particles was tested in human plasma, interactions of particle and serum proteins were evidenced which increased the carrier size. But what is more interesting is that those interactions seem to be related to the type of stabilizing agent used. As reported by Godara et al. [5], by using PVA or stearylamine as stabilizing agents, particle sizes increased ~15% that contrast with an increase of ~50% when particles were stabilized with human serum albumin. Maybe, the protein layer covering the particle surfaces promote their interaction with the serum proteins.

4.4 Cellular uptake

Regarding cellular uptake, **Table 3** reports the experimental conditions and general results. Indeed, researches on this regard have been mostly carried out for the hybrid nanoparticles by using human cancer cells taken in their majority from the breast. Nevertheless, some research works have also investigated on prostate and lung cancer cells. Other used cell lines include Caco-2 and MC3T3-E1 osteoblasts. In general terms, the analyses by flow cytometry and confocal laser scanning microscopy reveal that the functionalization of the hybrid particles favors the *in vitro* cellular uptake when compared to the free drugs and the pattern of cellular uptake correlates with the carrier drug loading.

On the other hand, the ability of nanoparticles to penetrate the different physiological barriers and reside in the target tissues has also been demonstrated. For example, SLN could provide efficient *in vivo* skin permeation [26], polymeric nanoparticles might penetrate mucus also exhibiting mucoadhesive behavior [16], and hybrid nanoparticles would cross the enterocyte walls [32] or reach bone tissue [23].

5. Safety and efficacy of carriers prepared by nanoprecipitation

5.1 Safety

A revision of the starting materials used to prepare particles via nanoprecipitation shows that the polymers and lipids present in the different recipes are recognized as safe considering their biocompatibility. Likewise, most organic solvents are classified as with low toxic potential according to ICH [75]. In the cases where acetonitrile, dichloromethane, tetrahydrofuran, dimethylformamide, and even methanol are used as solvents, the obtained particles should meet the specific requirements of limited concentrations of residual solvent because of their inherent toxicity. Traces of organic solvents would remain in the nanoparticle dispersions after the stage of solvent removal during their preparation. For example, up to 2300 ppm of tetrahydrofuran can be detected in lipid nanoparticles, which exceed the limit of 720 ppm established by the ICH [75]. However, as shown in **Table 4**, the safety tests including hematological studies on mice [27], hemolysis assays on human blood [8] or with erythrocytes [5], MTT assay on alveolar epithelial cells [34] or osteoblasts [23], cell viability on cancer cells [9, 11], and histological examination of mice [56], evidence concerns on the safety of that particles, and in general, neither of the particles were prepared via nanoprecipitation. Moreover, nanoparticles reduce the toxicity of the active molecules [8, 57].

5.2 Efficacy

One of the promising applications of nanoparticles, including those obtained by nanoprecipitation, is the therapy against cancer. As shown in **Table 5**, hybrid

Nanoparticle	Experimental conditions for toxicity testing					General results	Reference
	Cellular/animal model	Assay	Drug concentration or dosage used	Time of interaction—cellular model (h)	Technique of analysis		
Polymeric nanoparticles							
PNS	Vero cell line (green monkey kidney epithelial cells)	MTT assay	3.12–100 μg/mL	24 h	ELISA microplate reader	Nanoparticles reduce cytotoxicity of the active molecule.	[57]
PNS	Normal human keratinocytes	MTT assay	0.05 and 0.5 mg/mL	48 h	Microplate reader	No cytotoxic effect was detected after exposure of the NHK for 24 and 48 h to the nanoparticles.	[18]
PNS	Normal human keratinocytes	(H2DCFDA) assay	0.5 mg/mL	1 h	FITC fluorescence	The nanoparticles have no oxidative stress induction potential.	[18]
PNS	Male C57BL/6 J mice	Hematological studies	1 mg/kg	5 days	Hematology analyzer	All hematological parameters assessed at study remained in the normal range for mice.	[27]
Lipid nanoparticles							
SLN	Sprague-Dawley rats	Renal toxicity assessment	3.6 mg/kg	72 h	UV-visible	Freeze-dried nanoparticles are considered as a safe oral alternative.	[21]
SLN	Wistar rats	(OECD) guidelines, 423	5–2000 mg/kg	14 days	LD_{50} by Karber method	None of the animals showed any sign of toxicity. The lethal dose (LD_{50}) of KB is higher than 2000 mg/kg.	[13]
SLN/PNS	BALB/c 3T3	MTT assay	50–200 μM	24 h	Microplate reader	A moderate effect on cell viability, no obvious changes were found.	[26]
Hybrid nanoparticles							
HNP	Normal L929 alveolar epithelial cells	MTT assay	0.1–30 mg/mL	48 h	Spectrophotometric	No significant cytotoxicity against normal alveolar cells.	[34]

Nanoparticle	Experimental conditions for toxicity testing					General results	Reference
	Cellular/animal model	Assay	Drug concentration or dosage used	Time of interaction—cellular model (h)	Technique of analysis		
HNP	MDA-MB-231 breast cancer cells; human prostate cancer PC3 cells; colon cancer HT29 cells	Cell viability	50 to 300 μg/mL	Over night	Fluorescence intensity	No cytotoxic effects were observed for the particles tested.	[9]
HNP	BALB/c female mice	Side effects on vital organs	3 mg/kg	21 days	Histological examination	No significant toxicity to the heart, liver, spleen, lung, or kidney.	[56]
HNP	Whole human blood (from a healthy person)	Hemolysis assay	1 μL of suitably diluted free DTX and HNP	0.5 h	Spectrophotometric	The hemolysis of nanoparticle formulation was lesser than free drug.	[8]
HNP	Sprague-Dawley rats	In vivo toxicity	25 mg/kg	30 days	Spectrophotometric	Concentration of hepatotoxicity biomarkers (ALT and AST) was insignificant as compared to control.	[14]
HNP	MC3T3-E1 osteoblasts	MTT assay	0.5–40 μg/mL	16 h	Microplate reader	All groups showed minimum cytotoxicity against osteoblasts.	[23]
HNP	Erythrocytes	Hemolysis assay	0.7 mg/mL	1 h	Spectrophotometric	The average percentage hemolysis rate of nanoparticles was found between 7 and 16%.	[5]
HNP	Prostate cancer cells (PC3-MM2) and human breast cancer cells (MDA-MB-231)	In vitro cytotoxicity studies	25, 50, 100, 150, 200, and 300 μg/mL	48 h	Measure the luminescence	No cytotoxic effects were observed.	[11]

PNS: polymeric nanospheres; SLN: solid lipid nanoparticles; HNP: hybrid nanoparticles; MTT: 3-(4,5-dimethylthiazol-2-yl)-2,5-diphenyltetrazolium bromide; OECD: Organisation for Economic Co-operation and Development; KB: kokum butter; H2DCFDA: 6-carboxy-2′,7′-dichlorodihydrofluorescein diacetate; NHK: normal human keratinocytes; FITC: fluorescein isothiocyanate; PLGA: poly(D,L-lactide-co-glycolide); ALT: alanine transaminase; AST: aspartate transaminase; DTX: docetaxel; nr.: non-reported data.

Table 4.
Summary of experimental conditions and general results reported in research works on safety testing of nanoparticles prepared by the nanoprecipitation technique.

Nanoparticle	Experimental conditions for efficacy testing					General results	Reference
	Assay	Cellular/animal model	Drug concentration	Time of interaction—cellular model	Technique of analysis		
Polymeric nanoparticles							
PNS (Brazilian red propolis extract)	Antioxidant activity by using DPPH method	—	80 μg/mL	30 min	Spectrophotometry UV	The PNS displayed good antioxidant activity with inhibition values higher than 75%.	[36]
	Antileishmanial *in vitro* assay	L. (V.) braziliensis culture	5–100 μg/mL	24 h	Inverted microscopy	Nanoparticles containing between 30 and 40% of EEP maintained antileishmanial activity like the EEP in its original form.	
PNS (fluticasone propionate)	Mucus mobility by multiple particle tracking	Human cervicovaginal mucus	0.2–0.5 μL (nanosuspension)	30 min	Fluorescent microscopy	Particles exhibit rapid mucus penetration and mucoadhesive behavior.	[16]
	Anti-inflammatory action	Lewi rats	~0.1 mg of FP/kg	24 h	Total and differential cell counts on an automated cell counter.	Inhibition of bronchoalveolar lavage fluid (BAL) lavage neutrophils between 50 and 70% in 24 h.	
	Duration of residence in mouse lung	CF-1 mouse	10 μg of FP per animal	24 h	HPLC/MS	Upon deposition onto respiratory tissue, solution formulations or non-encapsulated drugs are rapidly removed through absorption into systemic circulation compared with nanoparticles.	
Lipid nanoparticles							
L-βCD-C10 L-βCD-C10/DOPE-PEG L-βCD-C10/stabilizer (nr.)	Complement protein C3 activation	Polyclonal anti C3 antibody	Topical	75 min	Immuno-electrophoretic	L-βCD-C10/DOPE-PEG shows a low level of complement C3 activation.	[71]

Nanoparticle	Experimental conditions for efficacy testing					General results	Reference
	Assay	Cellular/animal model	Drug concentration	Time of interaction—cellular model	Technique of analysis		
SLN/PNS (tetracaine)	Franz diffusion cell	Hairless abdominal full-thickness skins of Sprague-Dawley rats	Corresponding to 5 mg of tetracaine	72 h	Spectrophotometry UV	SLN provides an efficient *in vitro* permeation and sustained performance up to 72 h.	[26]
	Tail-flick test	Sprague-Dawley rats	0.25 mg/mL	4 h	Response threshold (seconds to withdraw the tail before the thermal stimulus).	PNS exhibited prolonged antinociceptive effect showing efficiency until 3.5 h of study.	
	Paw pressure test	Sprague-Dawley rats	0.25 mg/mL	8 h	Response threshold (amount of pressure supported by the animal before removing the paw).	The analgesic effects are maintained for a longer period. Greater than 50% pain control was still found at 6 and 4 h for PNS and SLN, respectively.	
SLN (polymyxin B)	Antimicrobial evaluation	Strain of *E. coli*	6.6 μg/mL	2–18 h	Turbidimetry	Activity (% inhibition of growth) by the plain drug and SLN were 52.7 and 56.7%, respectively.	[20]
SLN (amphotericin B)	*In vitro* antifungal efficacy	*C. albicans*	0.5–250 μg/mL	48 h	Change in original blue color of resazurin to pink.	Minimum inhibitory concentration value of 7.812 μg/mL attributed to controlled release of drug from the nanoparticulate matrix.	[21]
Hybrid nanoparticles							
HNP (docetaxel)	Targeting studies	KB cells	0.25 mg/mL	30 min	Flow cytometry	The targeted hybrid nanoparticles were found much deeper within the tumor and further away from the vasculature.	[7]
	In vivo tumor treatment efficacy	Female nude mice	4 mg/kg	35 days	Tumor width, length, and size	Half of the mice were still alive at 64 days after tumor challenge. As an indicator of global health, body weights were monitored over the course of the study.	

Nanoparticle	Experimental conditions for efficacy testing					General results	Reference
	Assay	Cellular/animal model	Drug concentration	Time of interaction—cellular model	Technique of analysis		
HNP (methotrexate)	Antiproliferation assay	MDB-MB-231 breast cancer and PC3 prostate cancer cells	5, 10, 20, 50, 100, 150, and 200 μg/mL	72 h	ATP-based cell viability kit	MTX encapsulated in the HNP preserve its anticancer activity.	[9]
HNP (doxorubicin)	Cytotoxicity evaluation	HL-60 cells and HL-60/DOX. MTT assay	0.25, 0.5, 1, 2, 5, 10, and 20 μg/mL	70 h	Microplate reader	The cytotoxicity activity of HNP was superior to DOX solution. The IC_{50} of HNP was lower than DOX solution.	[4]
	Tumor growth inhibition	Male BALB/c mice	20 mg/kg	18 days	Xenograft model	The tumor growth inhibition was (68.9–89.6%). The body weight of the mice in any of HNP treatments groups showed no obvious decrease in comparison with untreated groups.	
HNP (paclitaxel)	Cytotoxicity (MTT assay)	A549 human lung adenocarcinoma cells	0.5–10 mg/mL	48 h	Microplate reader	Drugs loaded HNP exhibited marked cytotoxicity on cells in a dose-dependent way and showed higher cytotoxicity compared with their free drug counterparts.	[6]
	Synergistic effects	A549 human lung adenocarcinoma cells	0.5–10 mg/mL	48 h	The results of cytotoxicity were evaluated via the Combination Index	The *in vivo* and *in vitro* results show synergetic effect of the two drugs incorporated in HNP against the lung cancer.	
	In vivo antitumor efficacy	BALB/c-nude mice	5 mg/kg of paclitaxel and 3 mg/kg of triptolide	18 days	Tumor width, length, and size	The inhibition of the *in vivo* tumor growth was lesser than that of the control group.	

Nanoparticle	Experimental conditions for efficacy testing					General results	Reference
	Assay	Cellular/animal model	Drug concentration	Time of interaction—cellular model	Technique of analysis		
HNP (psoralen)	Antitumor efficacy	MCF-7 cells	3 mg/kg	21 days	Changes in the tumor volume and final tumor weight	HNP show more efficient antitumor effects respect to other formulations.	[56]
HNP (docetaxel)	Cytotoxicity (MTT assay)	Human breast adenocarcinoma MDA-MB-231 cells	0.05, 0.1, 1, 10, and 20 μg/mL	24, 48, and 72 h	ELISA plate reader	Cytotoxicity activity of HNP could be attributed to lipid-mediated cytosolic delivery of the drug which is dose dependent.	[8]
	Annexin V-FITC/ propidium iodide apoptosis assay	MDA-MB-231 cells	10 μg/mL	24 h	Flow cytometry	Injured cells (including early apoptosis, late apoptosis, and necrotic cells) with HNP are greater (87%) as compared with free drug (51%).	
	Antitumor efficiency	BALB/c female mice	10 mg/kg	3 weeks	Tumor width, length and size	The repeated dosing of HNP exhibit less mortality (33%) than with free drug.	
HNP (mycophenolate; quercetin)	Annexin V apoptosis assay	MCF-7	10, 20, 40, and 60 μg/mL	6 h	CLSM	Apoptosis indices of MPA-NP and QC-NP are higher compared to respective free drugs. Moreover, the apoptosis index is significantly higher when combination MPA-NP + QC-NP is used.	[14]
	Inosine-5′-monophosphate dehydrogenase (IMPDH) assay	MCF-7	1 μM MPA NP	24 h	IMPDH assay kit	Significantly higher enzyme inhibition was observed in MPA-NP than free MPA.	

Nanoparticle	Experimental conditions for efficacy testing					General results	Reference
	Assay	Cellular/animal model	Drug concentration	Time of interaction —cellular model	Technique of analysis		
	In vivo antitumor efficacy	Sprague-Dawley rats	25 mg/kg	30 days	Tumor width, length, and size	Combination therapy of MPA and QC loaded LPN demonstrates significant suppression of tumor growth as compared to other groups.	
	Cytotoxicity (MTT assay)	MCF-7 human breast cancer cell	10, 20, 40, and 60 μg/mL	nr.	Optical density	Combination treatment of nanoparticles (MPA-NP + QC-NP) shows significantly higher cytotoxic effect compared with individual nanopreparation (MPA-NP and QC-NP).	
HNP (quercetin)	Cellular internalization	Caco-2 cells	25 mg/kg	0.5 h	CLSM	Excellent affinity and permeability to enterocytes allows HNP to be efficiently transported.	[32]
	Cytotoxic evaluation on P388 cells (MTT assay)	Lymphoblastic leukemia P388 cells	5, 10, and 20 μM	24 h	Spectrophotometry UV	HNP have higher cellular approachability that accords well with the cellular uptake by Caco-2 cells.	
	In vivo antileukemic effect	DBA/2 mice	25 mg/kg	21 days	Automatic blood counter	HNP can enhance the oral bioavailability of QC.	
HNP (paclitaxel)	Plasma protein binding study	Blood sample from a healthy volunteer	0.7 mg/mL	2 h	Bradford assay	The protein binding of HNP was found between 15.1 and 33.7%. The interaction between the biological environment and HNP can be controlled by surfactant.	[5]

DOI: http://dx.doi.org/10.5772/intechopen.93338

Nanoparticle	Experimental conditions for efficacy testing					General results	Reference
	Assay	Cellular/animal model	Drug concentration	Time of interaction—cellular model	Technique of analysis		
HNP (linezolid)	Minimum inhibitory concentration (MIC)	Strains of USA300-0114, CDC-587, and RP-62A	500 μg/mL stock solution in TSB, and serially diluted for the assay	24 h	Broth dilution method Microplate reader	The MIC50 and MIC90 values of free linezolid were approximately 40–50% of the values of HNP.	[23]
	Biofilm microplate assay	*S. aureus*	32, 64, 128, 164, and 256 μg/mL	12 h	Microplate reader	HNP were more effective than free linezolid for eradicating the MRSA biofilm.	
	Biofilm microplate assay	*S. aureus*	32, 64, 128, 164, and 256 μg/mL	12 h	CLSM	Extensive retention of the nanoparticles in the biofilms even after multiple buffer washing.	
	Drug's levels in animals' bones	Sprague-Dawley rats	32, 64, 128, 164, and 256 μg/mL	24 h	HPLC	Bone linezolid levels from HNP increase to over four-folds those of the free drug.	
HNP (sorafenib)	Cell growth inhibition assay	Prostate cancer cells (PC3-MM2) and human breast cancer cells (MDA-MB-231)	5, 10, 20, 50, 100, 150, and 200 μg/mL	72 h	Cell viability kit	The inhibition of the tumor cell growth was found to be time- and dose dependent for drug solution as well as HNP.	[11]

PNS: polymeric nanospheres; SLN: solid lipid nanoparticles; NLC: nanostructured lipid carriers; HNP: hybrid nanoparticles; CD: cyclodextrin; IC50: half-maximal inhibitory concentration; MPA: mycophenolate; Nv: nevirapine; QC: quercetin; MIC: minimum inhibitory concentration; MTS: 3-(4,5-dimethylthiazol-2-yl)-5-(3-carboxymethoxyphenyl)-2-(4-sulfophenyl)-2H-tetrazolium; LRP: luciferase reporter phage; CFU: colony-forming units; MTT: 3-(4,5-dimethylthiazol-2-yl)-2,5-diphenyltetrazolium bromide; DOX: doxorubicin; MTX: methotrexate; HL-60: human leukemia cell line; DPPH: 2,2-diphenyl-1-picryhydrazyl; EEP: ethanolic extract of propolis; NSCLCs: non-small cell lung cancers; NMRI: Naval Medical Research Institute; MS: mass spectrometer; HPLC: high-performance liquid chromatography; CLSM: confocal laser scanning microscopy, nr.: non-reported data.

Table 5.
Summary of experimental conditions and general results reported in research works on efficacy testing of nanoparticles prepared by the nanoprecipitation technique.

nanoparticles give good results in this sense. First, the incorporation of the active molecules into the carriers preserve the anticancer activity [9] and nanoparticles offer better performance compared with the free drug [4, 14, 56], in some cases being dose dependent [6, 8, 11]. Besides, significant improvements in the *in vivo* anticancer performance were achieved by the encapsulation of both an anticancer molecule (mycophenolate) and an antioxidant agent (quercetin) into the same hybrid nanoparticle, as quercetin prevents mycophenolate of its hepatic metabolism via the oxygenase enzymes [14]. Moreover, it was demonstrated that the *in vivo* tumor treatment in mice prolongs the life of the animals [7].

Taken advantage of the slow-release patterns that could be obtained with nanoparticulated systems, the development of carriers exhibiting antimicrobial and anesthetic activities are also of interest in research. Thus, the lowest values of minimum inhibitory concentrations of SLN containing polymyxin B or amphotericin B [20, 21] with respect to the free drugs contribute to support the applicability of nanoparticles prepared by nanoprecipitation in this area. In line with this, polymeric nanoparticles containing Brazilian red propolis extract have also shown antileishmanial activity [36], and linezolid-loaded hybrid nanoparticles demonstrated their ability to be retained in biofilms optimizing their antibacterial performance [23]. Regarding the behavior of nanoparticles in anesthetic and anti-inflammatory tests, tetracaine-loaded SLN exhibited prolonged antinociceptive effect leading to better control of pain [26].

Finally, the possibilities to get target particles prepared by the nanoprecipitation technique have been opened from the research works of Jeannot et al. [59] and Dehaini et al. [7] who investigate hyaluronan and folate as receptors chemically bonded to the polymer obtaining promising results for cancer therapies.

6. Conclusions

Nanoprecipitation is a simple, energy-efficient, and versatile method to entrap active molecules into carriers at the submicron and nanometric levels being the most common developments those oriented to obtain polymer, lipid, and hybrid particles. As the knowledge on the *in vivo* behavior of nanocarriers progresses and the need to produce them at the industrial scale demands for greater efficiency, the technique and the used starting materials have been optimized to improve the characteristics of the carriers and the control and standardization of continuous processes. In this way, sophisticated devices have been proposed to get sizes lower than 100 nm and the procedure has been refined, either through the chemical modification of polymers or through the careful definition of the work conditions, leading to particles entrapping hydrophobic and hydrophilic molecules, or exhibiting a targeted performance, a positive charge on their surface, or behaviors as stealth carriers. Moreover, the hybrid nanoparticles are promising drug delivery systems where the advantages of both polymeric and lipid particles are harnessed in their design to offer major drug loadings, slow drug-release patterns, and better pharmacokinetic properties. Regardless of the type of carrier, nanoprecipitation seems to be appropriate to obtain safe particles. Even using solvents characterized by inherent toxicity, the satisfactory results achieved by safety tests support their applicability in pharmaceutics. On this basis, it is expected that research on nanoprecipitation will continue looking for innovative solutions to the challenges facing current and future medicine. Some of the findings reported by different research teams and summarized in this chapter provide valuable insights regarding the potentialities of this technique in this respect.

Author details

Oscar Iván Martínez-Muñoz, Luis Fernando Ospina-Giraldo
and Claudia Elizabeth Mora-Huertas*
Departamento de Farmacia, Facultad de Ciencias, Universidad Nacional de
Colombia Sede Bogotá, Bogotá, Colombia

*Address all correspondence to: cemorah@unal.edu.co

IntechOpen

© 2020 The Author(s). Licensee IntechOpen. This chapter is distributed under the terms of the Creative Commons Attribution License (http://creativecommons.org/licenses/by/3.0), which permits unrestricted use, distribution, and reproduction in any medium, provided the original work is properly cited. (cc) BY

References

[1] Fessi H, Puisieux F, Devissaguet JP. Procédé de préparation de systèmes colloïdaux dispersibles d'une substance sous forme de nanocapsules. European Patent 1988;274961 A1, 20 July

[2] Fessi H, Puisieux F, Devissaguet JP, Ammoury N, Benita S. Nanocapsule formation by interfacial polymer deposition following solvent displacement. International Journal of Pharmaceutics. 1989;**55**:R1-R4. DOI: 10.1016/0378-5173(89)90281-0

[3] Schubert S, Delaney JT, Schubert US. Nanoprecipitation and nanoformulation of polymers: From history to powerful possibilities beyond poly (lactic acid). Soft Matter. 2011;**7**:1581-1588. DOI: 10.1039/c0sm00862a

[4] Zhu B, Zhang H, Yu L. Novel transferrin modified and doxorubicin loaded Pluronic 85/lipid-polymeric nanoparticles for the treatment of leukemia: In vitro and in vivo therapeutic effect evaluation. Biomedicine & Pharmacotherapy. 2017; **86**:547-554. DOI: 10.1016/j. biopha.2016.11.121

[5] Godara S, Lather V, Kirthanashri VS, Awasthi R, Pandita D. Lipid-PLGA hybrid nanoparticles of paclitaxel: Preparation, characterization, in vitro and in vivo evaluation. Materials Science and Engineering C. 2020;**109**: 110576. DOI: 10.1016/j. msec.2019.110576

[6] Liu J, Cheng H, Han L, Qiang Z, Zhang X, Gao W, et al. Synergistic combination therapy of lung cancer using paclitaxel- and triptolide-coloaded lipid–polymer hybrid nanoparticles. Drug Design, Development and Therapy. 2018;**12**:3199-3209. DOI: 10.2147/dddt.s172199

[7] Dehaini D, Fang RH, Luk BT, Pang Z, Hu CMJ, Kroll AV, et al. Ultra-small lipid–polymer hybrid nanoparticles for tumor-penetrating drug delivery. Nanoscale. 2016;**8**:14411-14419. DOI: 10.1039/c6nr04091h

[8] Jadon RS, Sharma M. Docetaxel-loaded lipid-polymer hybrid nanoparticles for breast cancer therapeutics. Journal of Drug Delivery Science and Technology. 2019;**51**: 475-484. DOI: 10.1016/j. jddst.2019.03.039

[9] Tahir N, Madni A, Balasubramanian V, Rehman M, Correia A, Kashif PM, et al. Development and optimization of methotrexate-loaded lipid-polymer hybrid nanoparticles for controlled drug delivery applications. International Journal of Pharmaceutics. 2017;**533**:156-168. DOI: 10.1016/j. ijpharm.2017.09.061

[10] Alshamsan A. Nanoprecipitation is more efficient than emulsion solvent evaporation method to encapsulate cucurbitacin I in PLGA nanoparticles. Saudi Pharmaceutical Journal. 2014;**22**: 219-222. DOI: 10.1016/j.jsps.2013.12.002

[11] Tahir N, Madni A, Li W, Correia A, Khan MM, Rahim MA, et al. Microfluidic fabrication and characterization of sorafenib-loaded lipid-polymer hybrid nanoparticles for controlled drug delivery. International Journal of Pharmaceutics. 2020;**581**:119275. DOI: 10.1016/j.ijpharm.2020.119275

[12] Raina H, Kaur S, Jindal AB. Development of efavirenz loaded solid lipid nanoparticles: Risk assessment, quality-by-design (QbD) based optimisation and physicochemical characterisation. Journal of Drug Delivery Science and Technology. 2017;**39**:180-191. DOI: 10.1016/j.jddst.2017.02.013

[13] Lahkar S, Das MK. Surface modified kokum butter lipid nanoparticles for the brain targeted delivery of nevirapine.

Journal of Microencapsulation. 2018;**35**: 680-694. DOI: 10.1080/02652048.2019.1573857

[14] Patel G, Thakur NS, Kushwah V, Patil MD, Nile SH, Jain S, et al. Mycophenolate co-administration with quercetin via lipid-polymer hybrid nanoparticles for enhanced breast cancer management. Nanomedicine: Nanotechnology, Biology and Medicine. 2020;**24**:102147. DOI: 10.1016/j.nano.2019.102147

[15] Hu FQ, Jiang SP, Du YZ, Yuan H, Ye YQ, Zeng S. Preparation and characteristics of monostearin nanostructured lipid carriers. International Journal of Pharmaceutics. 2006;**314**:83-89. DOI: 10.1016/j.ijpharma.2006.01.040

[16] Popov A, Schopf L, Bourassa J, Chen HB. Enhanced pulmonary delivery of fluticasone propionate in rodents by mucus-penetrating nanoparticles. International Journal of Pharmaceutics. 2016;**502**:188-197. DOI: 10.1016/j.ijpharm.2016.02.031

[17] Albisa A, Piacentini E, Sebastian V, Arruebo M, Santamaria J, Giorno L. Preparation of drug-loaded PLGA-PEG nanoparticles by membrane-assisted nanoprecipitation. Pharmaceutical Research. 2017;**34**:1296-1308. DOI: 10.1007/s11095-017-2146-y

[18] Sahle FF, Gerecke C, Kleuser B, Bodmeier R. Formulation and comparative in vitro evaluation of various dexamethasone-loaded pH-sensitive polymeric nanoparticles intended for dermal applications. International Journal of Pharmaceutics. 2017;**516**:21-31. DOI: 10.1016/j.ijpharm.2016.11.029

[19] Mora-Huertas CE, Garrigues O, Fessi H, Elaissari A. Nanocapsules prepared via nanoprecipitation and emulsification-diffusion methods: Comparative study. European Journal of Pharmaceutics and Biopharmaceutics. 2012;**80**:235-239. DOI: 10.1016/j.ejpb.2011.09.013

[20] Pattani AS, Mandawgade SD, Patravale VB. Development and comparative anti-microbial evaluation of lipid nanoparticles and nanoemulsion of polymyxin B. Journal of Nanoscience and Nanotechnology. 2006;**6**: 2986-2990. DOI: 10.1166/jnn.2006.459

[21] Chaudhari MB, Desai PP, Patel PA, Patravale VB. Solid lipid nanoparticles of amphotericin B (AmbiOnp): In vitro and in vivo assessment towards safe and effective oral treatment module. Drug Delivery and Translational Research. 2016;**6**:354-364. DOI: 10.1007/s13346-015-0267-6

[22] Bian X, Liang S, John J, Hsiao CH, Wei X, Liang D, et al. Development of PLGA-based itraconazole injectable nanospheres for sustained release. International Journal of Nanomedicine. 2013;**8**:4521-4531. DOI: 10.2147/IJN.S54040

[23] Guo P, Buttaro BA, Xue HY, Tran NT, Wong HL. Lipid-polymer hybrid nanoparticles carrying linezolid improve treatment of methicillin-resistant *Staphylococcus aureus* (MRSA) harbored inside bone cells and biofilms. European Journal of Pharmaceutics and Biopharmaceutics. 2020;**151**:189-198. DOI: 10.1016/j.ejpb.2020.04.010

[24] Dong Y, Ng WK, Shen S, Kim S, Tan RBH. Solid lipid nanoparticles: Continuous and potential large-scale nanoprecipitation production in static mixers. Colloids and Surfaces B: Biointerfaces. 2012;**94**:68-72. DOI: 10.1016/j.colsurfb.2012.01.018

[25] Torres-Flores G, Nazende GT, Emre TA. Preparation of fenofibrate loaded Eudragit L100 nanoparticles by nanoprecipitation method. Materials Today: Proceedings. 2019;**13**:428-435. DOI: 10.1016/j.matpr.2019.03.176

[26] Liu X, Zhao Q. Long-term anesthetic analgesic effects: Comparison of tetracaine loaded polymeric nanoparticles, solid lipid nanoparticles, and nanostructured lipid carriers in vitro and in vivo. Biomedicine & Pharmacotherapy. 2019;**117**:109057. DOI: 10.1016/j.biopha.2019.109057

[27] Han FY, Liu Y, Kumar V, Xu W, Yang G, Zhao CX, et al. Sustained-release ketamine-loaded nanoparticles fabricated by sequential nanoprecipitation. International Journal of Pharmaceutics. 2020;**581**:119291. DOI: 10.1016/j.ijpharm.2020.119291

[28] Hu FQ, Zhang Y, Du YZ, Yuan H. Nimodipine loaded lipid nanospheres prepared by solvent diffusion method in a drug saturated aqueous system. International Journal of Pharmaceutics. 2008;**348**:146-152. DOI: 10.1016/j.ijpharma.2007.07.025

[29] Chourasiya V, Bohrey S, Pandey A. Formulation, optimization, characterization and in-vitro drug release kinetics of atenolol loaded PLGA nanoparticles using 33 factorial design for oral delivery. Materials Discovery. 2016;**5**:1-13. DOI: 10.1016/j.md.2016.12.002

[30] Oliveira DRB, Furtado GF, Cunha RL. Solid lipid nanoparticles stabilized by sodium caseinate and lactoferrin. Food Hydrocolloids. 2019;**90**:321-329. DOI: 10.1016/j.foodhyd.2018.12.025

[31] Khayata N, Abdelwahed W, Chehnaa MF, Charcosset C, Fessi H. Preparation of vitamin E loaded nanocapsules by the nanoprecipitation method: From laboratory scale to large scale using a membrane contactor. International Journal of Pharmaceutics. 2012;**423**:419-427. DOI: 10.1016/j.ijpharma.2011.12.016

[32] Lee MK, Lim SJ, Kim CK. Preparation, characterization and in vitro cytotoxicity of paclitaxel-loaded sterically stabilized solid lipid nanoparticles. Biomaterials. 2007;**28**:2137-2146. DOI: 10.1016/j.biomaterials.2007.01.014

[33] Miladi K, Sfar S, Fessi H, Elaissari A. Encapsulation of alendronate sodium by nanoprecipitation and double emulsion: From preparation to in vitro studies. Industrial Crops and Products. 2015;**72**:24-33. DOI: 10.1016/j.indcrop.2015.01.079

[34] Ahmaditabar P, Momtazi-Borojeni AA, Rezayan AH, Mahmoodi M, Sahebkar A, Mellat M. Enhanced entrapment and improved in vitro controlled release of N-acetyl cysteine in hybrid PLGA/lecithin nanoparticles prepared using a nanoprecipitation/self-assembly method. Journal of Cellular Biochemistry. 2017;**118**:4203-4209. DOI: 10.1002/jcb.26070

[35] Allen S, Osorio O, Liu YG, Scott E. Facile assembly and loading of theranostic polymersomes via multi-impingement flash nanoprecipitation. Journal of Controlled Release. 2017;**262**:91-103. DOI: 10.1016/j.jconrel.2017.07.026

[36] Do Nascimento TG, Da Silva PF, Azevedo LF, Da Rocha LG, Porto ICCM, Moura TFAL, et al. Polymeric nanoparticles of Brazilian red propolis extract: Preparation, characterization, antioxidant and leishmanicidal activity. Nanoscale Research Letters. 2016;**11**:301. DOI: 10.1186/s11671-016-1517-3

[37] Lammari N, Louaer O, Meniai AH, Elaissari A. Encapsulation of essential oils via nanoprecipitation process: Overview, progress, challenges and prospects. Pharmaceutics. 2020;**12**:431. DOI: 10.3390/pharmaceutics12050431

[38] Mora-Huertas CE, Fessi H, Elaissari A. Polymer-based nanocapsules for drug delivery. International Journal of Pharmaceutics. 2010;**385**:113-142. DOI: 10.1016/j.ijpharm.2009.10.018

[39] Arizaga A, Ibarz G, Piñol R, Urtizberea A. Encapsulation of magnetic nanoparticles in a pH-sensitive poly (4-vinyl pyridine) polymer: A step forward to a multi-responsive system. Journal of Experimental Nanoscience. 2014;**9**: 561-569. DOI: 10.1080/ 17458080.2012.678393

[40] Villela AL, Martynek D, Bautkinová T, Šoó M, Ulbrich P, Raquez J-M, et al. Self-assembly of poly(L-lactide-co-glycolide) and magnetic nanoparticles into nanoclusters for controlled drug delivery. European Polymer Journal. 2020;**133**:109795. DOI: 10.1016/j.eurpolymj.2020.109795

[41] Fan Y, Yuan S, Huo MM, Chaudhuri AS, Zhao M, Wu Z, et al. Spatial controlled multistage nanocarriers through hybridization of dendrimers and gelatin nanoparticles for deep penetration and therapy into tumor tissue. Nanomedicine: Nanotechnology, Biology and Medicine. 2017;**13**:1399-1410. DOI: 10.1016/j. nano.2017.01.008

[42] Charcosset C, El-Harati A, Fessi H. Preparation of solid lipid nanoparticles using a membrane contactor. Journal of Controlled Release. 2005;**108**:112-120. DOI: 10.1016/j.jconrel.2005.07.023

[43] D'oria C, Charcosset C, Barresi AA, Fessi H. Preparation of solid lipid particles by membrane emulsification-influence of process parameters. Colloids and Surfaces A: Physicochemical and Engineering Aspects. 2009;**338**:114-118. DOI: 10.1016/j.colsurfa.2009.01.003

[44] Valente I, Celasco E, Marchisio DL, Barresi AA. Nanoprecipitation in confined impinging jets mixers: Production, characterization and scale-up of pegylated nanospheres and nanocapsules for pharmaceutical use. Chemical Engineering Science. 2012;**77**:217-227. DOI: 10.1016/j. ces.2012.02.050

[45] Tao J, Chow SF, Zheng Y. Application of flash nanoprecipitation to fabricate poorly water-soluble drug nanoparticles. Acta Pharmaceutica Sinica B. 2019;**9**:4-18. DOI: 10.1016/j. apsb.2018.11.001

[46] Martínez Rivas CJ, Tarhini M, Badri W, Miladi K, Greige-Gerges H, Nazari QA, et al. Nanoprecipitation process: From encapsulation to drug delivery. International Journal of Pharmaceutics. 2017;**532**:66-81. DOI: 10.1016/j.ijpharm.2017.08.064

[47] Mora-Huertas CE, Fessi H, Elaissari A. Influence of process and formulation parameters on the formation of submicron particles by solvent displacement and emulsification-diffusion methods. Advances in Colloid and Interface Science. 2011;**163**:90-122. DOI: 10.1016/ j.cis.2011.02.005

[48] Saad WS, Prud'homme RK. Principles of nanoparticle formation by flash nanoprecipitation. Nano Today. 2016;**11**:212-227. DOI: 10.1016/j. nantod.2016.04.006

[49] Couvreur P, Stella B, Reddy LH, Hillaireau H, Dubernet C, Desmaële D, et al. Squalenoyl nanomedicines as potential therapeutics. Nano Letters. 2006;**6**:2544-2548. DOI: 10.1021/ nl061942q

[50] Stainmesse S, Orecchioni AM, Nakache E, Puisieux F, Fessi H. Formation and stabilization of a biodegradable polymeric colloidal suspension of nanoparticles. Colloid & Polymer Science. 1995;**273**:505-511. DOI: 10.1007/BF00656896

[51] Quintanar-Guerrero D, Allémann E, Fessi H, Doelker E. Preparation techniques and mechanisms of formation of biodegradable nanoparticles from preformed polymers. Drug Development and Industrial Pharmacy. 1998;**24**(12):

1113-1128. DOI: 10.3109/03639049809108571

[52] François G, Katz JL. Nanoparticles and nanocapsules created using the ouzo effect: Spontaneous emulsification as an alternative to ultrasonic and high-shear devices. ChemPhysChem. 2005;**6**:209-216. DOI: 10.1002/cphc.200400527

[53] Lepeltier E, Bourgaux C, Couvreur P. Nanoprecipitation and the "ouzo effect": Application to drug delivery devices. Advanced Drug Delivery Reviews. 2014;**71**:86-97. DOI: 10.1016/j.addr.2013.12.009

[54] Martínez-Acevedo L, Zambrano-Zaragoza M, Vidal-Romero G, Mendoza-Elvira S, Quintanar-Guerrrero D. Evaluation of the lubricating effect of magnesium stearate and glyceryl behenate solid lipid nanoparticles in a direct compression process. International Journal of Pharmaceutics. 2018;**545**:170-175. DOI: 10.1016/j.ijpharm.2018.05.002

[55] Noriega-Pelaez EK, Mendoza-Muñoz N, Ganem-Quintanar A, Quintanar-Guerrero D. Optimization of the emulsification and solvent displacement method for the preparation of solid lipid nanoparticles. Drug Development and Industrial Pharmacy. 2011;**37**:160-166. DOI: 10.3109/03639045.2010.50180

[56] Du M, Ouyang Y, Meng F, Zhang X, Ma Q, Zhuang Y, et al. Polymer-lipid hybrid nanoparticles: A novel drug delivery system for enhancing the activity of Psoralen against breast cancer. International Journal of Pharmaceutics. 2019;**561**:274-282. DOI: 10.1016/j.ijpharm.2019.03.006

[57] Sharma D, Sharma RK, Sharma N, Gabrani R, Sharma SK, Ali J, et al. Nose-to-brain delivery of PLGA-diazepam nanoparticles. American Association of Pharmaceutical Scientists. 2015;**16**: 1108-1121. DOI: 10.1208/s12249-015-0294-0

[58] Jenning V, Thünemann AF, Gohla SH. Characterisation of a novel solid lipid nanoparticle carrier system based on binary mixtures of liquid and solid lipids. International Journal of Pharmaceutics. 2000;**199**:167-177. DOI: 10.1016/S0378-5173(00)00378-1

[59] Jeannot V, Mazzaferro S, Lavaud J, Laetitia V, Henry M, Arboléas M, et al. Targeting CD44 receptor-positive lung tumors using polysaccharide-based nanocarriers: Influence of nanoparticle size and administration rout. Nanomedicine: Nanotechnology, Biology and Medicine. 2015;**12**:921-932. DOI: 10.1016/j.nano.2015.11.018

[60] Tahara K, Karasawa K, Onodera R, Takeuchi H. Feasibility of drug delivery to the eye's posterior segment by topical instillation of PLGA nanoparticles. Asian Journal of Pharmaceutical Sciences. 2017;**12**:394-399. DOI: 10.1016/j.ajps.2017.03.002

[61] Zhao J, Stenzel MH. Entry of nanoparticles into cells: The importance of nanoparticle properties. Polymer Chemistry. 2018;**9**:259-273. DOI: 10.1039/C7PY01603D

[62] Yin J, Hou Y, Song X, Wang P, Li Y. Cholate-modified polymer-lipid hybrid nanoparticles for oral delivery of quercetin to potentiate the antileukemic effect. International Journal of Nanomedicine. 2019;**14**:4045-4057. DOI: 10.2147/ijn.s210057

[63] Helgason T, Awad TS, Kristbergsson K, McClements DJ, Weiss J. Effect of surfactant surface coverage on formation of solid lipid nanoparticles (SLN). Journal of Colloid and Interface Science. 2009;**334**:75-81. DOI: 10.1016/j.jcis.2009.03.012

[64] Bunjes H, Drechsler M, Koch MHJ, Westesen K. Incorporation of the model

drug ubidecarenone into solid lipid nanoparticles. Pharmaceutical Research. 2001;**18**:287-293. DOI: 10.1023/A:1011042627714

[65] Jores K, Mehnert W, Drechsler M, Bunjes H, Johann C, Mäder K. Investigations on the structure of solid lipid nanoparticles (SLN) and oil-loaded solid lipid nanoparticles by photon correlation spectroscopy, field-flow fractionation and transmission electron microscopy. Journal of Controlled Release. 2004;**95**:217-227. DOI: 10.1016/j.jconrel.2003.11.012

[66] Gordillo-Galeano A, Mora-Huertas CE. Solid lipid nanoparticles and nanostructured lipid carriers: A review emphasizing on particle structure and drug release. European Journal of Pharmaceutics and Biopharmaceutics. 2018;**133**:285-308. DOI: 10.1016/j.ejpb.2018.10.017

[67] Westesen K, Bunjes H, Koch MHJ. Physicochemical characterization of lipid nanoparticles and evaluation of their drug loading capacity and sustained release potential. Journal of Controlled Release. 1997;**48**:223-236. DOI: 10.1016/S0168-3659(97)00046-1

[68] Pardeike J, Hommoss A, Müller RH. Lipid nanoparticles (SLN, NLC) in cosmetic and pharmaceutical dermal products. International Journal of Pharmaceutics. 2009;**366**:170-184. DOI: 10.1016/j.ijpharm.2008.10.003

[69] Weber S, Zimmer A, Pardeike J. Solid lipid nanoparticles (SLN) and nanostructured lipid carriers (NLC) for pulmonary application: A review of the state of the art. European Journal of Pharmaceutics and Biopharmaceutics. 2014;**86**:7-22. DOI: 10.1016/j.ejpb.2013.08.013

[70] Glassman PM, Muzykantov VR. Pharmacokinetic and pharmacodynamic properties of drug delivery systems. The Journal of Pharmacology and Experimental Therapeutics. 2019;**370**:570-580. DOI: 10.1124/jpet.119.257113

[71] Nguyễn CH, Putaux JL, Santoni G, Tfaili S, Fourmentin S, Coty JB, et al. New nanoparticles obtained by co-assembly of amphiphilic cyclodextrins and nonlamellar single-chain lipids: Preparation and characterization. International Journal of Pharmaceutics. 2017;**531**:444-456. DOI: 10.1016/j.ijpharm.2017.07.007

[72] Luque-Alcaraz A, Lizardi-Mendoza J, Goycoolea FM, Higuera-Ciapara I, Argüelles-Monal W. Preparation of chitosan nanoparticles by nanoprecipitation and their ability as a drug nanocarrier. RSC Advances. 2016;**6**:59250-59256. DOI: 10.1039/c6ra06563e

[73] Lazzari S, Moscatelli D, Codari F, Salmona M, Morbidelli M, Diomede L. Colloidal stability of polymeric nanoparticles in biological fluids. Journal of Nanoparticle Research. 2012;**14**:920-930. DOI: 10.1007/s11051-012-0920-7

[74] Rodriguez-Emmenegger C, Jäger A, Jäger E, Stepanek P, Alles AB, Guterres SS, et al. Polymeric nanocapsules ultra stable in complex biological media. Colloids and Surfaces B: Biointerfaces. 2011;**83**:376-381. DOI: 10.1016/j.colsurfb.2010.12.013

[75] International Council for Harmonisation of Technical Requirements for Pharmaceuticals for Human Use. Impurities: Guideline for residual solvents Q3C (R6). 2016

Chapter 4

Nano/Microparticles Encapsulation Via Covalent Drug Conjugation

Victoria Fasiku, Edith K. Amuhaya, Kingo M. Rajab and Calvin A. Omolo

Abstract

Advancement in chemistry holds a great promise in improving drug encapsulation that leads to superior drug delivery efficiency and the therapeutic efficacy of nano/micro-delivery systems. Drugs are being designed to specifically access the infection sites via covalent conjugation to nano/micro-delivery systems. This chapter focuses on techniques for achieving covalent encapsulation of drugs in nano/micro-delivery systems, how conjugation is applied to selectively influence pharmacokinetic profile, intracellular, and extracellular uptake, specific targeting to disease sites, binding to specific receptors, and controlled/sustained release. In addition, the effect of conjugation on drug efficacy and biosafety of the micro/nanoparticulate drug delivery systems are discussed.

Keywords: covalent conjugation, sustained release, smart responsive, targeted delivery

1. Introduction

For drugs to execute their effective mechanism of action, they require to reach its targeted site of action so that they can exert their intended action [1]. While conventional dosage formulations of drugs can achieve desired therapeutic concentrations, they are unable to effectively maintain the desired therapeutic concentrations, conferring a limited half-life thereby leading to ineffective treatment by the drugs [2]. Therefore, the development of novel drug delivery systems with the ability to improve on this limitation of the conventional drug delivery systems is needed.

Micro- and nano-carrier systems are among the approaches that have been successfully utilized for encapsulation of various types of drugs such as peptides, proteins, and low-molecular weight drugs [3–5]. These systems have been found to overcome limitations of conventional dosages forms such as improving solubility [6], bioavailability, and biodistribution of drugs [7], and targeting disease sites [8], hence contributing to a high proportion of the active drug reaching the targeted site. In addition, drug carrier systems protect the loaded drugs from premature degradation in the biological environment, thus enhancing bioavailability and cellular uptake. For effective delivery of drugs to occur, they have to be successfully loaded onto drug delivery systems as payloads. Two techniques are employed in encapsulating drugs onto drug delivery systems. They include noncovalent physical encapsulation and covalent linking of the drugs to drug delivery systems.

Physical encapsulation of drugs into a carrier system involves hydrophobic interactions, electrostatic ionic interactions, and physical entrapping of drugs in the carrier matrix [9]. While the physical encapsulation of drugs into a carrier system is a popular technique, certain disadvantages are associated with it. For example, ionic complexation precipitation and dose dumping may take place if the effective attractions between the drug and the delivery system are reduced due to charge fluctuations and short-range attractions between monomers [10]. For hydrophobic drugs entrapped in the core of micelles, dose dumping may occur if micelles undergo hemodilution below the critical micelle concentration [11]. Moreover, challenges have been encountered in entrapping hydrophilic drugs in carrier systems using physical encapsulation [12]. These challenges have resulted in physical encapsulation with low loading efficiencies. Due to this, drug delivery scientists are resorting to covalently linking drugs to nano/micro-drug delivery system as an alternative method to physical encapsulation. This chapter discusses the techniques of covalent drug encapsulation, the mechanism of drug release from the covalent linkages, efficacy, and biosafety of drugs due to covalent conjugation and how disease site targeting via covalent conjugation is achieved.

2. Techniques of covalent drug encapsulation

Covalent drug conjugation involves attaching the drug into drug delivery systems via a physiologically labile bond [13]. A greater control over drug release is achieved by the covalent attachment of drugs to the drug delivery systems. Targeting and release of the drug from such systems is achieved through hydrolysable or biodegradable linkages between the payload and the micro/nanosystems [14]. Most commonly employed bio-hydrolysable bonds include amide, disulfide, ester, thiol, and carbamate bonds [15]. Conjugation of the drug to a delivery system may also include covalent linkers. The choice of a covalent linkers used is determined by its selectivity for drug release and the environment in which the drug should be released. Covalently conjugated drugs have exhibited the ability to release drugs by cleaving conjugated bonds under internal or external stimuli such as pH, redox potential, enzyme, light, and thermal energy [16].

The main advantages of covalent linking over physical encapsulation include the enhanced residence time of the drug in the body, slow release, improved biodistribution, and therapeutic efficacy, as well as reduced systemic toxicity [16, 17]. Covalent drug conjugation to micro and nanosystems is achieved via special bonds that are biodegradable or cleaved inside the body or a special environment at disease sites. Special linker moieties and functional groups of the drug dictate the success of conjugation on a nano/microsystem [18]. Based on the functional groups available on the delivery system and the drug being conjugated, several conjugation methods have been devised (**Figure 1**). The section below discusses the techniques of drug conjugations and their application in drug delivery.

2.1 Ester-linked drug conjugates

Ester bonds are widely used in conjugating drugs to drug delivery systems [19]. The ester bond is formed when a hydroxyl group and a carboxylic acid group react. Drugs with carboxylic groups can therefore be conjugated to hydroxyl groups of the drug delivery system and vice versa (**Figure 2**). Linkers or spacers such as a succinic anhydride may be employed to facilitate the conjugation [20]. Esterification of

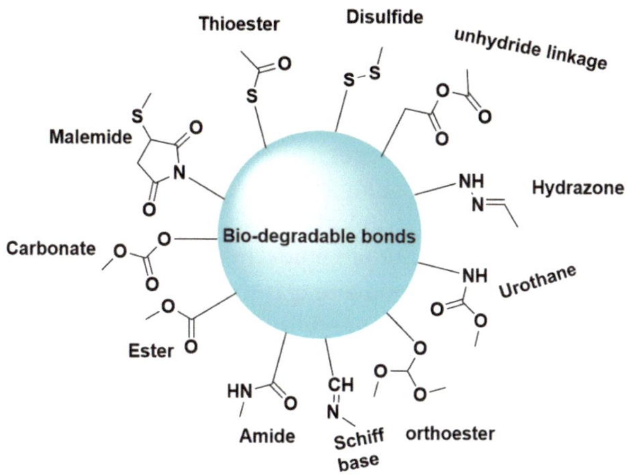

Figure 1.
Biodegradable bonds employed in covalent drug conjugation.

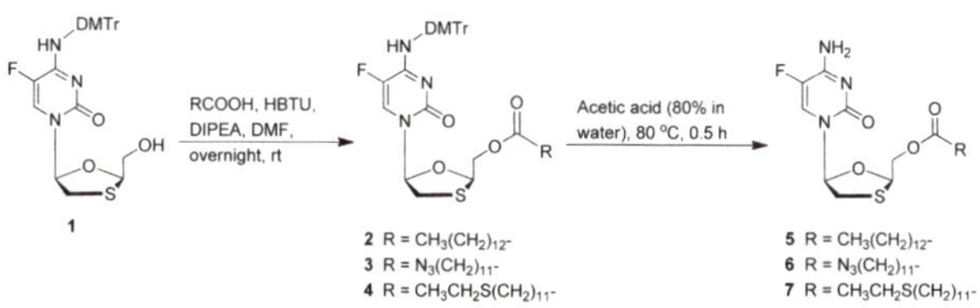

Figure 2.
Synthesis of the fatty acid ester-linked Emtricitabine. Adapted from [21]. DTMTr, 4,4′-dimethoxytrityl chloride; HBTU, hexafluorophosphate benzotriazole tetramethyl uronium; DPEA, N,N-diisopropylethylamine; DMF, dimethylformamide.

hydrophilic drugs with fatty acid is a popular technique to formulate self-assembling particulate prodrugs. This conjugation has shown to improve cellular uptake of hydrophilic drugs [22]. While viruses are intracellular obligate microorganisms, most of the drugs employed for their treatment are DNA nucleosides analogs which are highly hydrophilic with poor cellular uptake. Improving cellular uptake of these drugs usually improves their activity [23]. Agarwal et al. reported that conjugation of Emtricitabine (FTC) with myristic acid resulted to an analog that had 35.2 times higher activity than the nonconjugated drug against multidrug-resistant HIV viruses strain B-NNRTI and B-K65R [21]. These results indicated that antiretroviral ester conjugation with fatty acids could generate more potent analogs with a better resistance profile than its parent compound [24]. Similar results have been reported via esterification of fatty acids with lamivudine (3TC) [21] and acyclovir [25].

2.2 Amide and linked drug conjugates

Amide linkages can be used to covalently attach drugs to Nano/microcarriers using an anchor functionalized with carboxylic acid end groups [26]. Among the covalent linkages, amide bonds are the most widely used linkages to conjugate drugs to drug delivery systems. The conjugation is usually catalyzed by 1-ethyl-3-(3-(dimethylamino)propyl)carbodiimide hydrochloride (EDC) or N, N′-dicyclohexylcarbodiimide (DCC) chemistry [27, 28]. The process involves reacting a carboxylic group with EDC and N-hydroxysuccinimidyl (NHS) to form an acyl amino ester that is subsequently reacted with an amine to create the amide bond.

EDC has good water solubility enabling its direct application in aqueous solutions without the addition of any organic compounds, thus making it suitable for the attachment of bioactive molecules to the carrier surface [29].

Several nano/micro-delivery systems with amide-linked drug conjugates have been widely reported with a great success. Such a system was reported by Yousefpour et al. (**Figure 3**) who conjugated doxorubicin and monoclonal antibody, trastuzumab to chitosan to form nanoparticles with high conjugation capacity, enhanced and selective uptake by human epidermal growth factor receptor 2 (Her2+) on cancer cells compared with the nonconjugated drug. Similar conjugation was reported by Kurtoglu et al. who conjugated Ibuprofen to PAMAM dendrimer and mPEG via amide linkages [30]. The drug conjugates showed better results when compared to bare drugs.

Monoclonal antibodies and derived therapeutics have also been linked with adverse effects and toxicity. The associated toxic effects of monoclonal antibodies

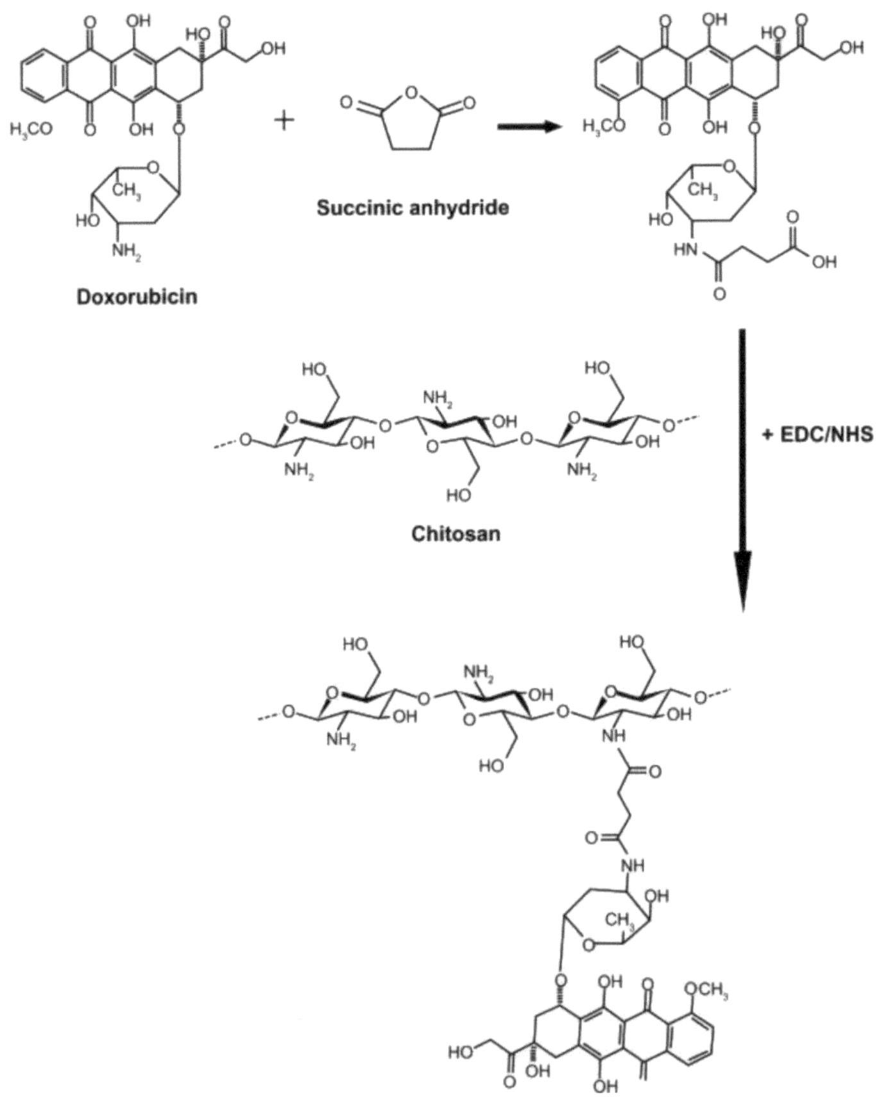

Figure 3.
Schematic description of the procedures for the amide conjugation between chitosan and doxorubicin to form a self-assembling nano-drug delivery system [29].

Drug	Drug delivery system	Main findings	Reference
Doxorubicin (DOX)	Self-assembled prodrugs	• Greater antitumor efficacy than free DOX. • High drug loading • Sustained drug release	[31]
Adriamycin	Micelles	• *In vivo* high anticancer activity • Low side effects	[32]
Camptothecin and Capecitabine	Nanofibers and spherical nanoaggregates	• Synergism of the co-conjugated drugs	
Penicillin V and Cephradine	Aggregates	• Similar activity to bare drugs • Low on side effects • Sustained release of the drug	[33]
DOX and trastuzumab	Nanoparticles	• Enhanced and selective uptake • High loading capacity • Reduction of drug side effects in Her2+ breast and ovarian cancers.	[29]
Gemcitabine	Self-assembled prodrug	• High loading capacity • Increased biological half-life of the loaded drug • Better activity than the bare drug	[34]

Table 1.
Drug loading via amide conjugation functionalized for varied clinical and research applications.

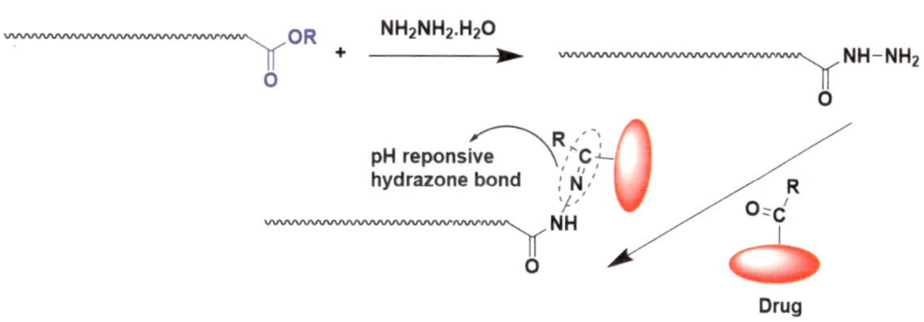

Figure 4.
Illustration of linking drugs to the delivery system via hydrazine bond.

(mAb) have limited their therapeutic application. However, antibody/drug covalent (ADC) conjugation-based platform has enabled selective delivery of a potent cytotoxic payload to target diseased cells, resulting in improved efficacy, reduced systemic toxicity, and preferable pharmacokinetics (PK), pharmacodynamics (PD), and biodistribution compared to traditional chemotherapy [35]. The success of such conjugations includes FDA approved Adcetris® which is a drug conjugate of Dolastatin 10 and monomethyl auristatin E (MMAE). The link between Dolastatin 10 and MMAE is N-terminal amine via the amide bond linked to a self-immolating spacer, p-aminobenzyloxycarbonyl (PABC).

Apart from ADCs, amide bonds have been employed to link mAb to other drug delivery surfaces such as liposomes. Liposomes with 1,2-distearoyl-sn-glycero-3-phosphoethanolamine-N-[carboxy(polyethylene glycol) (DSPE-PEG-COOH) linked with mAb have been reported to prepare immunoliposomes. The attachment of mAb to the liposomes was achieved via surface —COOH on the surface of liposomes and $—NH_2$ of the mAB. This conjugation enhanced significantly the blood residence time of the mAb [36]. Another amide conjugation between targeted ligand and liposome was reported where the peptide was covalently attached to the carboxylic groups on the PEGylated liposomes to form a nanoparticulate system able to target the infarcted heart. The system was effective in *in vitro* testing against cardiac cells [37]. Due to their stability, the rate of hydrolysis of amide bonds is lower when compared to ester bonds. This slower rate of hydrolysis affects the release of drugs, thus affecting the activity of the conjugated drugs [31]. The amide conjugation of drugs to drug delivery systems is summarized in **Table 1**.

2.3 Hydrazones conjugates

Hydrazones are formed by the action of hydrazine on ketones or aldehydes functional groups [38]. Their basic structure is $R_1R_2C{=}NNH_2$ which is formed when oxygen in ketones and aldehydes is replaced with the $-NNH_2$ functional group. pH-sensitivity attributes of hydrazones bond have been used in the formation of stimuli responsive nano/micro-drug delivery system. At a lower pH, the bond decomposes efficiently while at basic pH, hydrazones are usually stable [39]. The instability of hydrazone bonds in acidic mean molecules can be cleaved in acidic intracellular environment of endosomes or lysosomes, tumor tissues, and bacterial infection sites. Hydrazone bonds have been successfully used to covalently load drugs into delivery systems resulting to pH-responsive nano/micro-dosage forms that can effectively target a disease that alters physiological pH to acidic (**Figure 4**) [38, 40, 41].

2.4 Thioether linkage

Thioether bond is formed from the reaction between the thiol group containing SH group and first carbon of maleimide that is attached to the drug carrier [42]. Conjugation via thioether bonds is favored technique as the bond is formed under mild conditions, at room temperature, and in aqueous solution [26]. Thioether linkage makes it possible to link peptides to a delivery system or drugs to peptide (**Figure 5**). Several drug delivery systems have been reported to employ thioether linkage as a means of covalently loading drug on to them. mAb trastuzumab and nanoparticle doped with doxorubicin were successfully loaded in a drug delivery system via thioether linkage [43]. DOX was conjugated to a drug delivery system via thioether bond through poly(ethylene glycol) polymer having two linkers of maleimide and n-hydroxysuccinimide (nhs). The conjugates showed better cancer uptake when compared to free DOX. The better uptake was attributed to better affinity of the system to the HER2 receptor of breast cancer cells. When compared to the free drug, the conjugated delivery system had a longer blood circulation with less toxic effects when compared to the free drug [28]. Similar results were reported by Park et al. who formulated immunoliposomes conjugated with monoclonal antibodies (mAB) [44]. Additionally, another liposomal covalent system has also been reported by Kirpotin et al.; in the system, a free thiol group was used to conjugate antibodies to the nanocarriers. The carrier showed increased cellular uptake resulting in better tumor reduction [45]. Thioether linkage has also been applied successfully on carbon nanotubes functionalized by folic acid. The system employed in targeted delivery of DOX against cancer [46]. From literature reports, thioether-

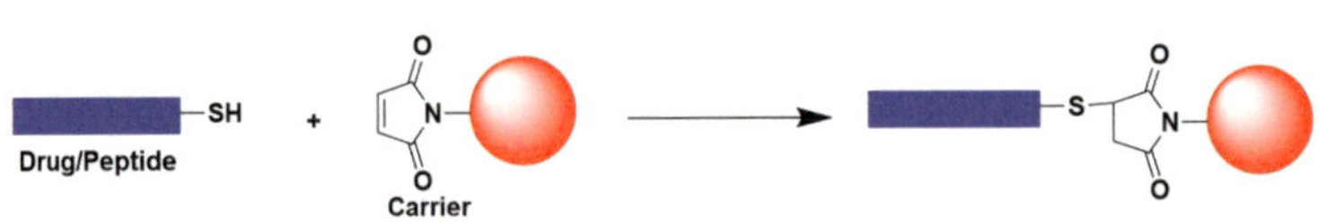

Figure 5.
Illustration showing maleimide thiol covalent linkage to drug delivery systems.

linked drug delivery systems can be effectively employed in targeted delivery of the conjugated drugs.

2.5 Disulfide linkage

Two thiol groups' conjugation results in the formation of a disulfide bond. One group originates from a nanocarrier and the other from a ligand [47]. Disulfide drug conjugates have shown to be stable in the extracellular environments but easily broken down in intracellular reductive intracellular environment. There is an increasing number of drug formulations that incorporate disulfide bonds being reported, for nano/micro-drug delivery system. Disulfide bonds are being designed to exploit differences in the reduction potential at disease location and the whole body at large [18]. Formulating environmentally responsive drug delivery systems has been made possible due to the desirable attribute of disulfide bonds. Lu et al. using a disulfide-bridged created mesoporous silica nanoparticle covalently loaded with folic acid (FA) and decorated bull serum albumin (BSA) for improved tissue biocompatibility and effective dual pH/glutathione (GSH) response drug releasing drug delivery system. Disulfides have also been employed as cleavable linkers in drug conjugates or to formulate stimuli-responsive carriers, and this has resulted in disulfides linker-based mAb drug covalent linkages (ADCs) in clinical trials [48].

2.6 Other covalent linkages

Other covalent linkages that include carbamate linkage, Schiff bases, and polycyclic linkages have also been employed to form covalent linkages between the drug and delivery systems. Reaction between a diene and dienophile results to cycloaddition via the Diels-Alder chemistry which forms bicyclic compounds. This chemistry can be utilized to form polycyclic linkages between the drug and the delivery system [49]. Whereas other hydrolyzable linkages include carbamate [50, 51], oximes [52], and Schiff bases [53, 54]. These types of linkages are specifically designed to make drug delivery systems have targeting ability due to the physiological changes brought about by the diseases.

3. Self-assembly of covalent conjugated drugs

Roughly 70% of new drug discoveries have shown poor aqueous solubility, while approximately 40% of the marketed immediate-release drugs are practically insoluble [55]. Additionally, the drugs that are highly soluble have been found to have membrane penetration difficulties [56]. Covalent modification of therapeutic compounds is therefore a strategy that enhances efficacies of the conjugated drugs by solving physicochemical problems associated with the drugs [57]. When hydrophobic drug molecules are attached to hydrophilic material or when hydrophilic drugs are attached to hydrophobic biomaterial or delivery systems, an amphiphilic system is formed. The resulting amphiphilic system can self-assemble into stable core-shell aggregates such as vesicles, classical micelles, unimolecular micelles, and nanorods [2, 58].

When amphiphiles are dispersed in water, the hydrophilic component of the amphiphile preferentially interacts with the aqueous phase (shell) while the hydrophobic portion tends to reside in the air or in the nonpolar solvent (core) in order to form stable assemblies [59]. Self-assemblies of drug conjugates are usually governed by forces such as hydrogen bonds, Van der Waals interactions, hydrophobic interactions, and electrostatic interactions [2]. Self-assembled drug conjugates often

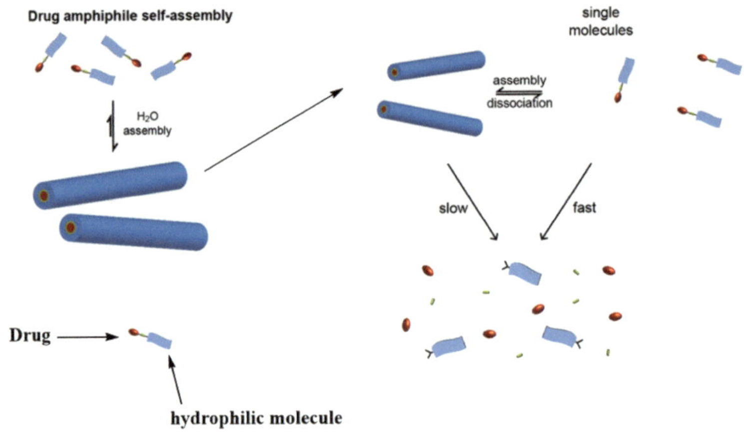

Figure 6.
Schematic representation of self-assembly of drug conjugates and subsequent release mechanism of the drug from the self-assembly. Adapted with permission from [60].

result to effective therapies as they possess better physicochemical properties that lead to enhanced drug penetration for highly hydrophilic and charged drug molecules [61], enhanced solubility for highly insoluble drugs, and increased residence time for drugs that are easily eliminated via the kidney [62]. For instance, most of anticancer drugs are hydrophobic in nature, and therefore, to produce self-assembled nanostructures with better therapeutic and formulation aspects, hydrophilic molecules or polymers are usually attached to them via a degradable linker to induce amphiphilicity and self-assembly (**Figure 6**) [61]. Self-assembly widely occurs in nature and has been borrowed by science to formulate self-assembled nano/micro-drug delivery systems with better therapeutic outcomes than original drug molecules [63].

4. Mechanism of drug release from drug conjugates

Covalent linkages alter the absorption, distribution, metabolism, and elimination (ADME) properties of an active drug [64]. Before conjugation, it is paramount to have a complete understanding of the physicochemical, structural relationship activity of the drug candidates. It is also important to understand the ability of the attached groups to cleave, leaving and exposing the functional groups responsible for the activity of the drug [65]. Moreover, once the drug is cleaved from the delivery system, the delivery system should be inactive and nontoxic [66]. Most of the drawbacks from covalent linkages of drugs to the delivery systems are the inability of the drug to cleave from the delivery system. The inability of the drug to detach from the drug delivery system may lower the activity of the drug due to poor bioavailability [67]. Therefore, the chosen covalent linking technique should have the ability to easily cleave to enable the release of the drug.

Esterification is a common technique for conjugation because esterases are widely distributed in body tissues that easily cleave the ester bonds leaving the free drug to act. Esterase is a hydrolase enzyme that splits esters into an acid and alcohol in a chemical reaction with water called hydrolysis [68]. The easy cleaving of esters makes the use of ester linkages as an attractive technique. Breakage of amide bonds is via hydrolysis of the carbon-nitrogen bond, and this results in a carboxylic acid and either ammonia or an amine [69]. This cleavage of amides is responsible for the drug release from the drug delivery systems. It is important to note that amides are stable bonds, which do not hydrolyze at physiological pH and body temperature.

Disulfide bonds usually exploit differences in the reduction potential at different locations within and upon cells to release the conjugated drugs. Due to this, different delivery platforms have been designed to achieve different targeted delivery strategies. Redox enzymes reduce disulfide bonds on and inside the cells resulting in drug release [18]. Other bonds like hydrazones, Schiff bases hydrolysis is catalyzed by acid environment. In an acid environment, the bond between the drug delivery system and the drug is broken to release the drug. Apart from direct drug linkage to the delivery systems [70], suitable linkers that are self-immolating such as p-aminobenzyloxycarbonyl (PABC) can also be involved in the reaction. The purpose of the linkers is to situate the cleavable delivery system away from the drug to allow facile release. Upon cleavage, the linkers rapidly fragment, leading to the release of the drug in a chemically unmodified form [71, 72] (**Table 2**).

5. Efficacy and biosafety of drugs due to covalent conjugation

Particulate drug delivery systems have recorded significant progress in the delivery of small molecular drugs; however, some challenges such as poor drug loading, formulation instability, premature drug leakage, and poor blood circulation are still encountered. This has led to the discovery of newer strategies that can be used to overcome these challenges. Over the years, various research groups have explored the efficacy and biosafety of drugs that were covalently conjugated to nano/micro-delivery systems [73]. These include systems developed from polymers, dendrimers, and peptides among others; usually, the drug is bond to the biomaterial via a linker. The efficacy of drugs covalently conjugated has been significantly improved in terms of drug loading capacity and stability amongst other benefits. Biomaterials such as polymers that are covalently bonded to drugs have shown to be useful drug carriers which help to hold drugs and are tunable to increase the efficacy of the drug [74, 75].

The other advantages drug conjugation provides include increased solubility of the drugs that are insoluble in water, thus enhancing a controlled release of the drug as there will be increased permeability through lipophilic tissues. This will, in turn, lead to an increased effective concentration of the drug at the targeted site [75]. Additionally, drug conjugated covalently to biomaterials are shielded from degradation or deactivation as well as increases the circulation time of the drug [76]. One or more of these advantages offered by drug conjugation has been reported by various groups of researchers. For instance, the efficacy of different poly(ethylene glycol) (PEG)-based anticancer drug conjugates has been extensively explored [73, 77, 78]. The details of the importance of nano/micro-delivery systems such as lysosomes, polymeric micelles, and polymeric nanoparticles in drug delivery applications have also been discussed [79].

In a study [80], hydrazine-based doxorubicin-polymer conjugates were synthesized into doxorubicin-loaded nanoparticles. It was reported that the bioactivity of the drug was largely retained *in vitro*, and there was a tremendous reduction in systemic toxicity of doxorubicin upon nanoparticle conjugation *in vivo* when compared to the physical formulation of the drug. In addition, the nanoparticles prevented the drug from disassembling upon interaction with serum proteins in the blood [81, 82]. The *in vitro* study showed that the doxorubicin-nanoparticle conjugate accelerated the release of the drug in acidic conditions and killed the cancer cell. In the same vein, Modarassi and colleagues investigated the drug release

Bond	Mechanism of cleavage	Method of hydrolysis	References
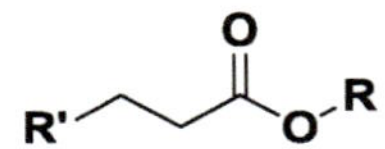 Esters	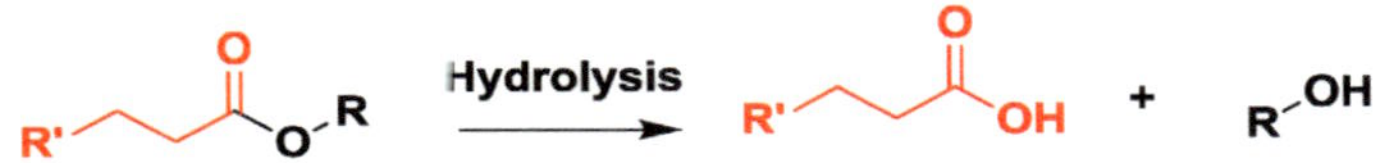	Cleavage in the body is catalyzed by esterases	[83]
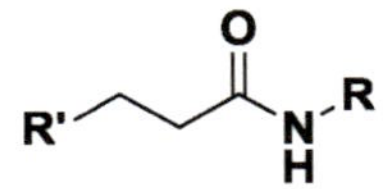 Amides	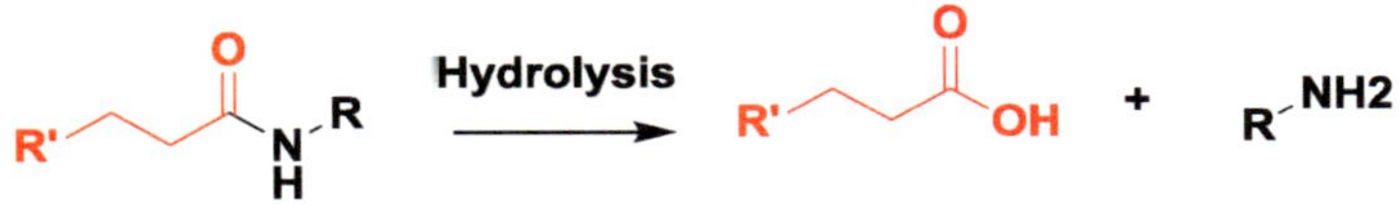	The bond is cleaved via hydrolysis. Sometimes catalyzed by enzymes like esterase, hydrolase, serine and cysteine proteases, peptidases, antibody Fab-BL 125 and RNA	[84–90]
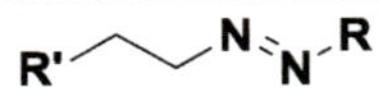 Hydrazones	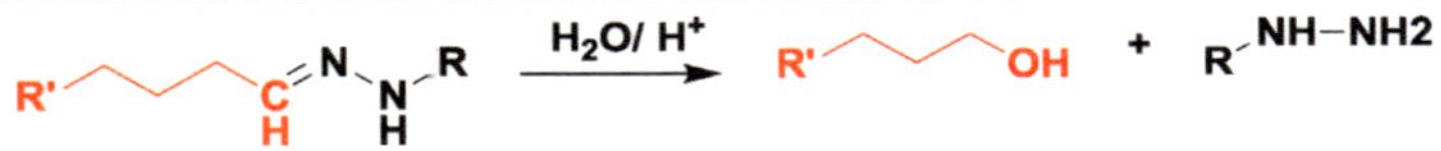	Cleavage is via acid-catalyzed hydrolysis	[91]
Disulfide 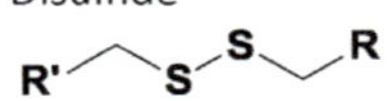	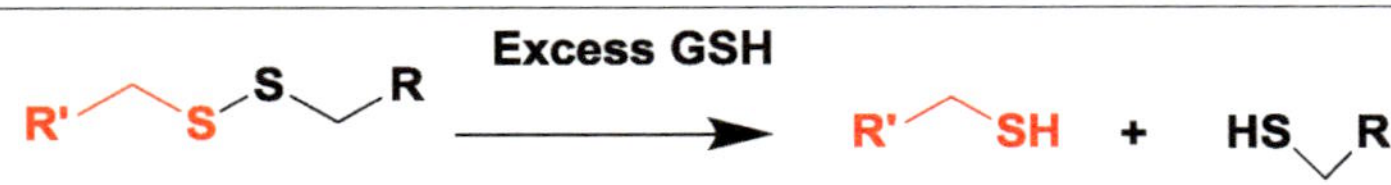	Bond cleavage is achieved via acid and base catalysis and redox potential hydrolysis catalyzed by various classes of reductases enzyme in the presence of excess reduced glutathione (GSH) and thioredoxin Reductase	[18]
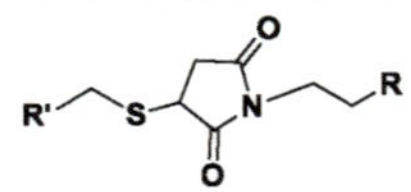 Thiol-maleimide	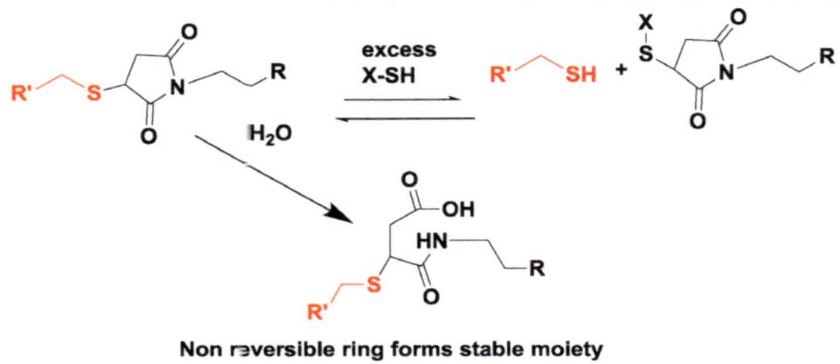	Drug release is via ring-opening hydrolysis and thiol exchange	[92, 93]

Table 2.
Cleavage mechanism resulting in drug release of common bonds employed in covalent conjugation.

behavior of doxorubicin that was conjugated onto the structure of nanoparticles. The conjugation was achieved via an acid-labile hydrazone linkage, and the effect of conjugation was compared with the nonconjugated drug [94] (**Figure 7**). The results of the *in vitro* investigation revealed that the release of doxorubicin was dependent on the amount of crosslinker. The higher the amount of crosslinkers, the lower the cumulative drug release in the physically loaded drug. On the other hand, drug conjugation showed that an increase in the amount crosslinker within the structure led to an increased rate and amount of drug released. This implies that the efficacy of drug conjugation with respect to drug release is superior to nonconjugated drugs.

Another drug PEG conjugate that has shown enhanced drug efficacy is the paclitaxel (PTX) conjugated with polyethylene glycol (PEG-B-PTX), synthesized by Dong et al. [95]. The antitumor efficacy of the stable micelle of about 50 nm, and 13.3 wt% drug load content was investigated against human glioma and breast cancer cells *in vitro*. The conjugate micelle exhibited improved antitumor effects when compared to the clinically used taxol. This result suggests that the drug conjugate can be a superior alternative for current clinically used PTX nanoformulations which has limitations such as poor *in vivo* stability, premature release, and little improvements in its antitumor efficacy [96, 97]. A detailed *in vivo*

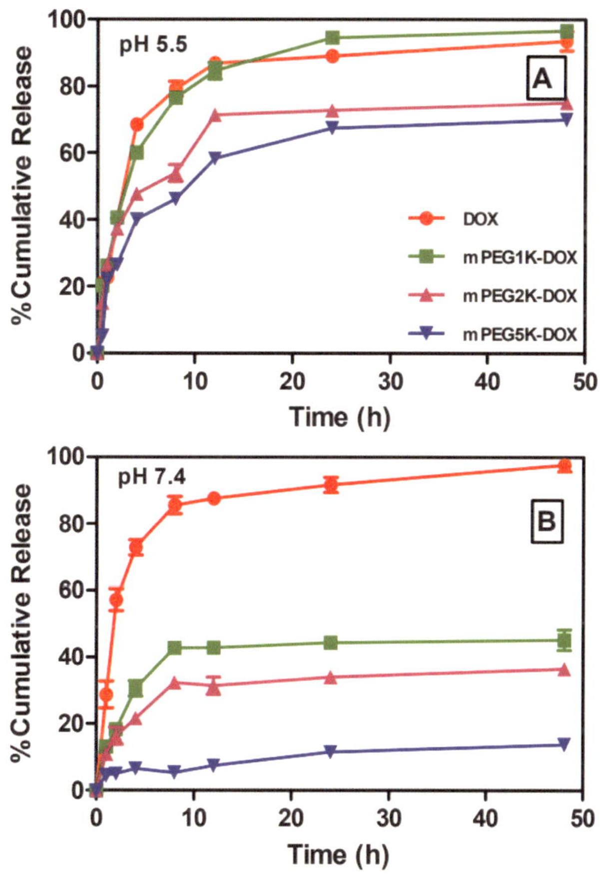

Figure 7.
A) The hydrazone acid-labile DOX release behavior from nano/microparticles at pH 7.4. (B) The hydrazone acid-labile DOX release behavior from nano/microparticles at pH 5.5. Sustained release slow drug release at pH 7.4 when compared to acidic pH. Overall slower release when compared to nonconjugated DOX. Adapted with permission from [98].

experiment by the same research group further revealed that PEG-B-PTX showed prolonged circulation time as well as enhanced *in vivo* antitumor efficacy (tumor inhibition rate of 89.4%) with low side effects. This observation can be attributed to the favorable pharmacokinetic profile and tumor-specific release of the drug from the drug conjugate. This promising study has prompted other groups of researchers to investigate the efficacy of other stimuli responsive PTX conjugates [99–103]. This same set of researchers [95] went further to demonstrate that hydrophobic drugs can be conjugated with a short water-soluble polymer or peptide chain to make the drug amphiphilic. It was proven that the self-assembled nanovehicles are suitable for the delivery of the drug and even co-delivery of other drugs as reported by other research groups [104, 105]. The effects of this approach are well-characterized chemical structures, accurate and reproducible drug loading efficiency (i.e., 100%), fixed, and high drug loading contents. Also, burst release of drugs associated with physically drug-loaded micelles can be prevented [106]. These attributes are very important and favorable for clinical translation; therefore, these conjugates have great potential for clinical application.

Furthermore, other studies have buttressed the potential excellent effect of drug conjugates in combating diseases as seen in the experiment done by Li et al. [107]. Camptothecin and doxorubicin were loaded onto a polymer, and the efficiency of the drug conjugate was explored. A synergistic drug delivery which improved the anti-cancer efficiency of the drugs was reported. The *in vitro* stability study showed that the drugs were stable with 80% drug loading after 4 weeks at a storage temperature of 4°C. In addition, the *in vitro* studies showed an approximately 30% increase in the cellular uptake of the conjugated drugs into the cancer cells when compared to the free drugs. It is noteworthy that a superior anticancer efficacy was observed in the combined drug conjugate, and the enhanced synergistic effects of about 23.9% was attributed to the good better stability profile, internalization by cells and pH response. Other benefits of the drug conjugate observed from this study include suitable sizes and good water solubility. This led to the greater penetration of the drugs into the solid tumors, thus improving the overall efficacy of the drug conjugate when compared to the free drugs. From these results, it is suggested that DOX-CPT conjugated to nano-delivery systems has the potential to provide synergistic anticancer treatment.

The superior efficacy of drug-conjugated covalently compared to nonconjugated drugs has also been proven by Tang and coworkers via conjugating sorafenib with polyethylene glycol (PEG) nanoparticles. The efficacy of the drug conjugate (SFP) was evaluated on cancer cells in an *in vitro* antitumor experiment [108]. The result showed that SFP had an excellent antitumor activity due to the self-immolative release of the intact drug inside tumor cells caused by the GSH-responsive disulfide linker thus suggests that SFP may be a potential candidate for cancer treatment. Additionally, it was reported that the covalent drug conjugation prevented drug leakage and improved drug stability. SFP is therefore a promising nano/micro-carrier for safe drug delivery which may pave room for new opportunities to explore other drug conjugates. Among other studies, Daniel et al. have reported that drug conjugates especially polymer conjugates are potentially suitable for the delivery of antiviral drugs [109, 110]. A typical example is the synthesis of poly(lactide-co-glycolide) nanoparticles loaded with a combination of reverse transcriptase and protease inhibitors. Such drug conjugates have been reported to be effective in preventing the replication process of HIV replication [111, 112]. This implies that drug conjugates are a promising approach in improving the therapeutic efficacy of therapeutic agents, and this may encourage their clinical translation.

Irrespective of the excellent efficacy of any drug conjugates, before their application, it is very important that the biosafety is proven and confirmed to be harmless to the human system. Hence, it has become necessary that developed drug conjugates are evaluated for its biosafety. This has led to the investigation of the toxicity of different drug conjugates by various researchers. For instance, an *in vitro* cytotoxicity study was carried out by Tang and fellow workers, and the cytotoxicity of the drug-conjugate was assessed using the MTT assay method [108]. The study investigated the cytotoxicity effect of sorafenib-polyethylene glycol (PEG) nanoparticles conjugate (SFP) on Hela and HepG2, respectively, after incubation for 48 h at 37°C. The result showed a dose-dependent cytotoxic effect of free sorafenib (SF) and SFP on both cell lines, and no significant difference in cytotoxicity was observed for SF and SFP on both cell lines. Nonetheless, a higher cytotoxicity of SFP was displayed between the concentration ranges of 5–15 μM when compared to free SF. The higher *in vitro* cytotoxicity of SFP observed at those concentrations may be due to the increased intracellular localization of SFP nanoparticles. This suggests that the conjugation of sorafenib with a polyethylene glycol (PEG) nanoparticle does not have a negative influence on the toxicity as seen in the favorably cytotoxic effect on both cell lines. Also, the ability of SFP to serve as a biosafe anticancer therapeutic agent was further confirmed in the hemocompatibility and histological safety results. These nontoxic properties of the drug conjugate can be attributed to the outer PEG shell of SFP.

Furthermore, drawbacks such as dose-dependent toxicity have been reported with drug conjugates; therefore, in an attempt to minimize toxicity, Li et al. have evaluated the effect of combining drugs onto a nano-drug delivery system on toxicity [107]. The cell cytotoxicity of the DOX and CPT conjugate versus the free drugs showed enhanced uptake in the cancer cells but reduced in the normal cells exposed to the drug-conjugate. Additionally, it was reported that the side effects of the drugs (doxorubicin and camptothecin) employed in the study decreased by reducing the dosage of the drugs. The toxic side effects of the drugs were alleviated, and it was also observed that the multidrug resistance (MDR) was reversed. This may be attributed to the synergistic effects of multiple therapeutic agents [113, 114]. Remarkably, to assess the general biosafety of drug conjugates, Ibrahim et al. have gone further into *in vivo* investigation of the drug conjugates developed by their group [115]. The organs of mice exposed to these drug conjugates for 21 days were sliced and analyzed histologically. It was noted that exposure to the tissues (heart, liver, spleen, lung, and kidney) did not result in any tissue damage; hence, the biocompatibility of the formulations was confirmed. Other studies that reported little or no toxic side effects of drug conjugates are Dong and Lu with their co-workers, respectively [96, 116].

In the cytotoxicity study carried by Lu et al., pullulan which is a natural biocompatible polysaccharide was used to synthesize a novel pH-sensitive nanoparticle drug delivery system for the delivery of doxorubicin (DOX) [116]. The chemical structure of the pullulan/DOX conjugate nanoparticles was assessed using FTIR and 1H NMR and further investigated for *in vitro* drug release and cytotoxicity activities, respectively. The result of the release behavior *in vitro* showed that a faster release of DOX was released from the drug delivery at pH 5.0 than at pH 7.4. It was observed that lower concentrations of the drug (DOX) were more cytotoxic to 4 T1 cells than pullulan/DOX conjugate nanoparticles at a concentration range of 0.01–5 mg/l. This may be due to the ability of free DOX to readily transport into the cells via passive diffusion [117]. On the other hand, low cytotoxicity was reported for DOX released from the nanoparticle. This may be due to a time-consuming DOX release from nanoparticles and delayed nuclear uptake in 4 T1 cells [118]. Lin et al.

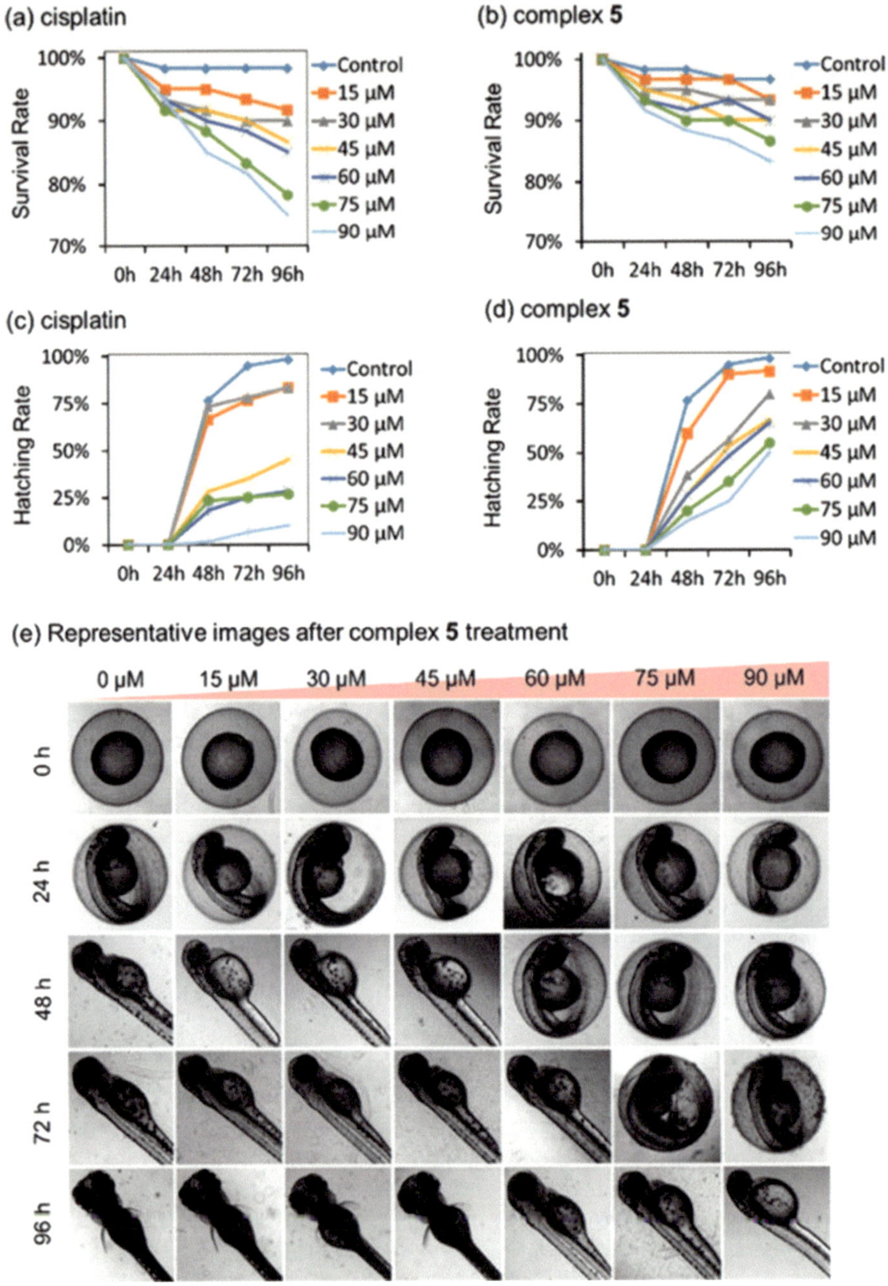

Figure 8.
Biosafety evaluation of free cisplatin and prodrug cisplatin using zebrafish embryos. Survival rates of embryos in the presence of (a) the bare drug and (b) prodrug. Hatching rates of zebrafish embryos after the exposure to (c) the bare drug (d) prodrug. (e) Pictogram representation the embryos with treatment of prodrug at different concentrations over a period of 96 hours.

improved biosafety of profile of cisplatin by converting it a prodrug. The prodrug has higher survival rate of the zebrafish embryos [119] (**Figure 8**).

From the observations made in these studies, it is clear that drug conjugation impacts positively on the efficacy of the drug as well as its biosafety/toxicity. The biosafety concerns are greatly eliminated or minimized by conjugating drugs to biomaterials. Some unwanted side effects, toxicity, and organ damage associated with the fluctuations that arise from periodic drug administration can be avoided by drug conjugation [120]. Surprisingly, it appears that a substantial number of anti-cancer drugs and polymers are the most explored in covalent drug conjugation compared to other therapeutic drugs and biomaterials. This may be because polymer-drug conjugates provide more advantages in enhancing stability, increasing water solubility, and prolonging blood circulation [121–123]. Despite these advantages, certain drawbacks such as difficulty to accurately control the reaction site and the degree of conjugation have been associated with polymer-drug conjugates. Thus, the ability to reduce the heterogeneity and batch-to-batch difference of the product remains a challenge [75, 124]. It is therefore suggested that more studies to be done to overcome these challenges; this will provide more information on the efficacy and biosafety of drug conjugates (**Figure 9**). Furthermore, reports from these studies revealed that the efficacy and biosafety of the drugs conjugated onto various nano/micro-delivery systems were significantly enhanced when compared to the free drugs. Other nano/micro-delivery systems and drugs that have been explored are summarized in **Table 3**. The table highlights the key findings of various nano/micro-delivery systems that have been reported by different groups of scientists.

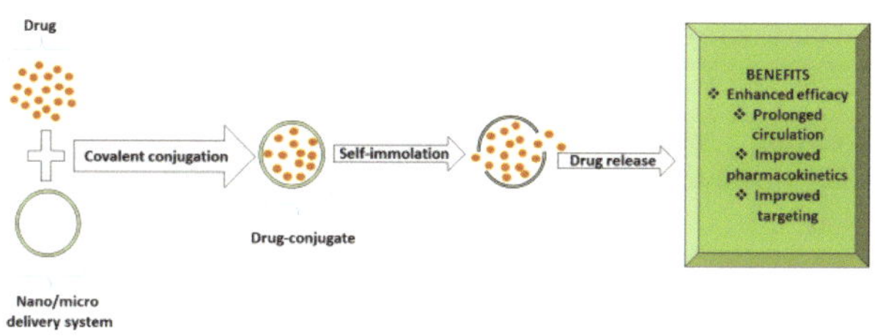

Figure 9.
Key benefits derived from drug conjugation.

Nano/micro-delivery system	Drug	Target	Outcome	References
Polyglutamic acid	Paclitaxel	Nonsmall-cell lung cancer (NSCLC)	Paclitaxel poliglumex reduced the systemic exposure to peak concentrations of free paclitaxel. In addition, the drug-conjugate produced similar survival to docetaxel as second-line treatment in NSCLC with less febrile neutropenia and alopecia and greater ease of administration.	[125]
PEG-b-PCC poly(2-methyl-2-carboxyl-propylene carbonate) polymer	Gemcitabine and dodecanol	Pancreatic cancer	*In vivo* studies showed a significant increase in the effectiveness of drug-conjugate when compared to the free drug.	[126]
Hyaluronic acid (HA)	Cisplatin	H1299, H358 cell lines and mice	HA-cisplatin conjugate bounded to CD44 expressing cancer cell lines (H1299 and H358). The drug-conjugate was more effective in killing lung tumors in mice when compared to the free drug	[127]

Nano/micro-delivery system	Drug	Target	Outcome	References
Poly(styrene-comaleic acid	Neocarzinostatin	Liver and renal cancer	Arterial infusion therapy with poly(styrene-co-maleic acid)-conjugated neocarzinostatin SMANCS/ Lpd showed to be effective for large renal cell carcinoma	[128]
Poly(methyl methacrylate) (PMMA) polymer	Gemcitabine	A549 cell-derived xenograft murine model	*In vivo* experiment showed that the Gem-conjugates reduced tumor growth by 68% with little toxicity while free Gem had no effect but significant toxicity.	[129]
PEG	Interferon α2a/b	Hepatitis B	The HBsAg clearance rate was significantly greater in the group treated with drug-conjugate compared to the standard therapy group at 24 and 48 weeks post-treatment (33.3% vs. 10.5% and 35.7% vs. 10.5%, respectively; $P < 0.05$ for both).	[130]
Glycol chitosan (GC)	Heparin	Lungs, mice	GC-heparin conjugates were safe in the lungs and revealed comparable blood coagulation times compared to free heparin	[131]
Chimeric peptides (CPs)	Doxorubicin	4 T1 and Lewis lung cancers	Increased intratumoral accumulation of the conjugate with a curative effect in 60% of the treated mice was observed	[132]
Poly(amidoamine) (PAMAM)	Doxorubicin	Mice bearing melanoma (B16-F10) lung metastases	Prolonged lung retention of drug-dendrimer conjugate compared to free drug. Improved chemotherapeutic activity on the lung of mice compared to the free drug	[133]
Poly(2-ethyl-2-oxazoline)	Rotigotine	Parkinson disease	POZ-conjugated rotigotine showed the potential to be viable for subcutaneous treatment for PD patients.	[134]
Glycol chitosan	Doxorubicin		Drug-conjugate accumulated within tumors via the EPR effect, and a significant antitumor activity was observed compared to free doxorubicin	[135]
Carbopol®(CP)	Calcitonin	A549 cells; rats	Drug-conjugate showed no signs of toxicity and maximally lowered blood calcium levels when compared to calcitonin alone	[136]
Carboxymethylcellulose	Docetaxel	EMT-6 breast cancer	Biodistribution studies showed a 5.5-fold greater tumor accumulation of drug-	[137]

Nano/micro-delivery system	Drug	Target	Outcome	References
			conjugate compared to the clinically administered DTX formulation (Taxotere). Drug-conjugate also showed a two-fold improvement in anticancer activity in a murine EMT-6 breast cancer model compared to Taxotere.	
Hyaluronic acid,	Paclitaxel (PTX)	Breast cancer	PTX conjugate showed more enhanced *in vivo* tumor inhibition effects compared to free PTX.	[138, 139]
PEG-b-poly(glutamic acid) micelle	Oxaliplatin	Mouse model of human carcinoma cell line KB.	The antitumor efficacy of drug-conjugate was superior to that of oxaliplatin. Also, the animals did not develop acute cold hypersensitivity, which is frequently experienced by patients after oxaliplatin administration.	[140]
PEG	Alendronate	Lung mucosal	The drug-conjugate suppressed lung mucosal toxicity after pulmonary delivery, whereas the administration of the free drug-induced significant toxicity.	[141]

Table 3.
Key observations made from other drug conjugates.

6. Effect of covalent drugs conjugation on the pharmacokinetic profile of the drug

The pharmacokinetic profile of drugs is a very crucial aspect that is considered for clinical application. It is interesting to observe that the pharmacokinetic profile of drugs is becoming better due to covalent drug conjugation as demonstrated by drugs encapsulated to nano/micro-delivery systems. The conjugation of drugs to biomaterials has opened opportunities to alter the pharmacokinetics and biodistribution of the drugs within the human body [120]. The alteration of the pharmacokinetics of the drug offers advantages such as prevention of the rapid clearance or metabolism of the drug. In addition, the drugs are carried to the targeted site of pharmacological action. Drug conjugation to nano/micro-delivery system has shown to be a powerful technique that can alter the pharmacokinetic profile of the drug, thus minimize the side effect of various anticancer drugs such as doxorubicin.

One of the studies that reported the enhanced pharmacokinetic properties of anticancer drug encapsulated to a nanoparticle is that conducted by Vandriess et al. [80]. It was observed that the nanoparticles containing the drug enhanced the drug accumulation and a subsequent reduction of tumor growth in an *in vivo* zebrafish model. Also, another study has revealed that self-assembling drug polymer conjugates which allows a covalent attachment of the drug to the hydrophilic part of the polymer can improve the pharmacokinetic profile of drugs. Thus, covalently conjugating drugs to delivery systems improves pharmacokinetic profiles and physicochemical problems associated with certain free drugs [142]. Benefits from covalent conjugations include prevention of rapid renal clearance, and improved drug solubility is derived. It is however important to note that the attachment of a large number of hydrophobic drugs to nanocarriers such as polymers may result in unwanted aggregation and precipitation in some cases [143].

In one of the first studies, research groups such as Kataoka et al. took advantage of the self-aggregation behavior of drug conjugates to develop a micelle forming drug conjugate [144]. In their study, doxorubicin (DOX) was conjugated to a poly (ethylene glycol)-poly(aspartic acid) block copolymer (PEG-b-P(Asp(DOX)), and the pharmacokinetic profile was investigated. It was observed that there was no interaction between the drug and serum albumin, which is known to bind to the DOX. The inability for the drug and the serum albumin to interact indicates the shielding ability of the nano/micro-delivery system which led to a good biodistribution and therapeutic effect of the drug. Other subsequent studies by the same research group aimed to improve the synthesis [145] and pharmacokinetics profile [146, 147] of the same drug-polymer conjugate. The drug conjugate was designed via an amide bond which can only cleave to release the drug by enzymatic action. The results showed that the drug conjugate had a better pharmacokinetic profile when compared to the free DOX. Interestingly, the conjugate was better tolerated despite needing a higher dose to achieve the same effect as free DOX.

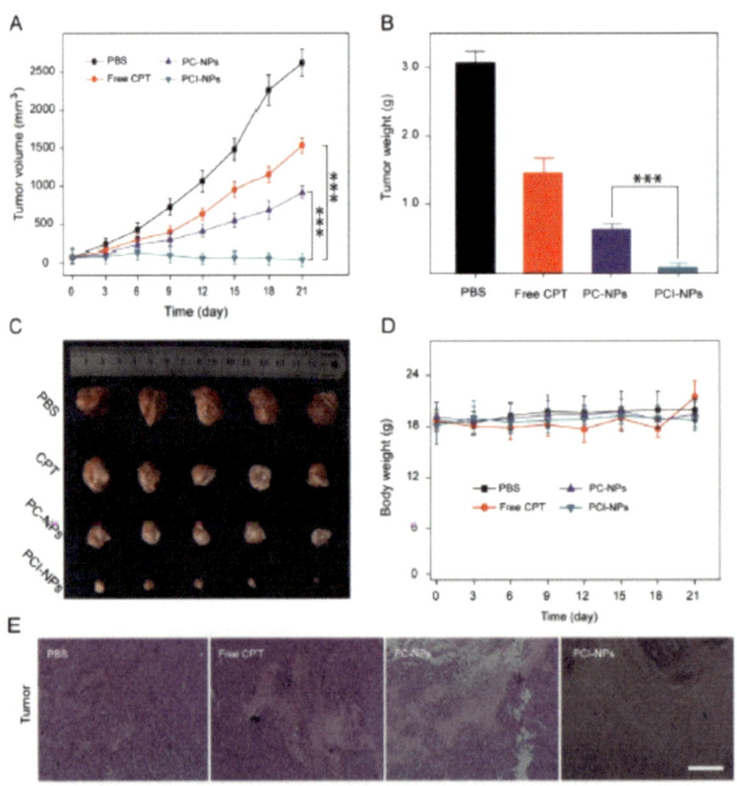

Figure 10.
Control (phosphate buffer system), camptothecin (CPT), and micellar nanoparticles drug conjugates (PC-NPs and PCI-NPs) effectiveness on 22 tumor-bearing BALB/c mice after (A) graphs displaying tumor growth inhibition (B) effect on tumor shrinkage after treatment with PBS, CPT, PC-NPs, and PCI-NPs at 21st day post-treatment of the mice (C) micro-photographs of the harvested tumors. (D) Changes in the bodyweight of the mice during treatment. (E) H&E histological images of different treatment groups. Adapted with permission from [115].

Similarly, more recent studies have further shown that covalent linked prodrugs improve the pharmacokinetics and biodistribution of the conjugated drug as reported by Ibrahim and co-workers. H22 tumor model was induced in BALB/c [115]; the mice were exposed to conjugated drug delivery system and free-drug camptothecin (CPT), respectively. From the results, conjugates had a significantly had better pharmacokinetic profile than the free drug, this also led to increased accumulation of the drug within the tumor tissues and consequently better activity. This observation can be associated with the enhanced permeability and retention (EPR) effect provided by the nano/micro-delivery system. An additional observation which is the biodistribution effect of the drug conjugate is seen in the outstanding inhibition of tumor growth that resulted in better tumor shrinkage when compared to other groups (**Figure 10**). After 21 days of treatment, the drug-conjugated delivery system had a 33-fold less of tumor when compared to the untreated group. It is presumed that the acidity of the tumor contributed to the enhanced anticancer effect by the drug conjugated delivery system after cellular uptake of the nanoparticles, and the drug was released in the cytosol. This might have been the reason for the overall better activity of the conjugated drugs compared to the free drug. This was attributed to the extended blood circulation and better accumulation of conjugates in tumor compared to free CPT. Overall, these studies suggest that by covalently conjugating drugs into nano/micro-delivery systems, and a more enhanced pharmacokinetic profile of drugs can be obtained.

7. Disease site targeting via covalent conjugation

The delivery of drugs to sites of target, where the action of the drug is required, is challenging due to various physicochemical, biopharmaceutical, and pharmacokinetic barriers the drug may face [143]. In order to address these issues, new approaches such as drug covalently conjugated to nano/micro-delivery systems are being explored which alters the pharmacokinetic properties of the drug. This is achieved by using drug various carriers such as polymers [148, 149] liposomes [150], and dendrimers [151] that are capable of protecting the payload drug and delivering it to the disease site. The nano/micro-delivery systems help in accumulating the drug in the tumor site and prolong the circulation time [80]. This consequently leads to a successful drug target to the specific disease site. Drug conjugates have been widely utilized in the field of cancer therapy because they can passively target cancer disease sites by permeating and retain the drug via tumor's leaky vasculature [152]. Apart from the ability of the nano/micro-delivery system to protect the drug from degradative processes such as hydrolysis and metabolism before arriving at the target site, the drug is able to accumulate in the targeted site. This ability is a major advantage that drug conjugates proffers, which enhances their antitumor activity. Additionally, the ability of the drug conjugate to disassemble provides the opportunity to tune the drug release rate at the target site. More so, the tuning or decorating the surface of the nanostructure (drug conjugate) can lead to enhanced tumor targeting compared to drugs in their free form [143]. The enhanced drug efficacy reported in the studies discussed earlier is closely associated with the ability of the drug conjugate to target the specific disease site.

The advantages of covalently conjugating drugs to nano/micro-delivery systems to target disease sites or site of infections has shown effective by results obtained by various researchers who employed different therapeutic agents and nano/micro-delivery systems in targeting specific disease sites as highlighted in **Table 3**. In all the reported study on drug targeting using drug conjugates, a superior targeting of drugs to disease site was displayed by the drug encapsulated to nano/micro-delivery systems via covalent conjugation compared to the free drug. Thus, it implies that covalently conjugated drug-nano/micro-delivery systems have the potential to specifically target disease site; hence, it can be used to treat and manage diseases that appear to be challenging to combat.

8. Conclusions and future perspectives

Drug encapsulation to nano/micro-delivery systems is a field in nanotechnology that has been growing substantially over the last two decades. Specifically, the covalent conjugation of drugs to different nano/micro-delivery systems is one of the drug encapsulation techniques that is gaining increasing attention. Various nanocarriers are currently developed and explored for the delivery of a wide range of therapeutic agents such as peptides, small molecules, and drugs. The several advantages offered by covalently conjugating this therapeutics into nanocarriers have made them gradually more attractive. These advantages include prolonged circulation, controlled release, improved solubility, reduced immunogenicity, specific site targeting, enhanced biosafety pharmacokinetics and biodistribution, and combination or concurrent integration of therapeutics in a single carrier. Due to the great strides that have been achieved in the development of effective drug delivery systems via covalent conjugation and their immense potential, some of these conjugates are gaining entrance into the market. Therefore, it is anticipated that covalent conjugation will continue to advance to facilitate the translation of current research findings into innovative treatments for a broad range of diseases. However, it is still very important to have a comprehensive knowledge of the ideal physiochemical properties, safety, drug release rates and efficacy, pharmacokinetic behavior, and clearance kinetics of these systems before preclinical development and clinical translation. Hence, more efforts and focused research are required to address the knowledge gaps and provide desired information that can accelerate their clinical translation and application in diverse fields of biomedicine. The computational and theoretical modeling approach can also be employed to correlate and answer certain outcomes by providing concrete design parameters.

Author details

Victoria Fasiku[1], Edith K. Amuhaya[2*], Kingo M. Rajab[3] and Calvin A. Omolo[2*]

1 Discipline of Pharmaceutical Sciences, College of Health Sciences, University of KwaZulu-Natal, Durban, South Africa

2 Department of Pharmaceutics, School of Pharmacy and Health Sciences, United States International University-Africa, Nairobi, Kenya

3 Department of Biomedical Sciences, College of Health Sciences, University of Dodoma, Dodoma, Tanzania

*Address all correspondence to: eamuhaya@usiu.ac.ke; comolo@usiu.ac.ke

IntechOpen

© 2020 The Author(s). Licensee IntechOpen. This chapter is distributed under the terms of the Creative Commons Attribution License (http://creativecommons.org/licenses/by/3.0), which permits unrestricted use, distribution, and reproduction in any medium, provided the original work is properly cited. (cc) BY

References

[1] Petros RA, DeSimone JM. Strategies in the design of nanoparticles for therapeutic applications. Nature Reviews Drug Discovery. 2010;**9**: 615-627

[2] Omolo CA, Kalhapure RS, Agrawal N, Jadhav M, Rambharose S, Mocktar C, et al. A hybrid of mPEG-b-PCL and G1-PEA dendrimer for enhancing delivery of antibiotics. Journal of Controlled Release. 2018;**290**: 112-128

[3] Hassan D, Omolo CA, Gannimani R, Waddad AY, Mocktar C, Rambharose S, et al. Delivery of novel vancomycin nanoplexes for combating methicillin resistant Staphylococcus aureus (MRSA) infections. International Journal of Pharmaceutics. 2019;**558**: 143-156

[4] Omolo CA, Megrab NA, Kalhapure RS, Agrawal N, Jadhav M, Mocktar C, et al. Liposomes with pH responsive 'on and off' switches for targeted and intracellular delivery of antibiotics. Journal of Liposome Research. 2019:1-19

[5] Ulbrich K, Hola K, Subr V, Bakandritsos A, Tucek J, Zboril R. Targeted drug delivery with polymers and magnetic nanoparticles: Covalent and noncovalent approaches, release control, and clinical studies. Chemical Reviews. 2016;**116**:5338-5431

[6] Omolo CA, Kalhapure RS, Agrawal N, Rambharose S, Mocktar C, Govender T. Formulation and molecular dynamics simulations of a fusidic acid nanosuspension for simultaneously enhancing solubility and antibacterial activity. Molecular Pharmaceutics. 2018;**15**:3512-3526

[7] das Neves J, Araújo F, Andrade F, Amiji M, Bahia MF, Sarmento B. Biodistribution and pharmacokinetics of dapivirine-loaded nanoparticles after vaginal delivery in mice. Pharmaceutical Research. 2014;**31**:1834-1845

[8] Maji R, Omolo CA, Agrawal N, Maduray K, Hassan D, Mokhtar C, et al. pH-responsive lipid–dendrimer hybrid nanoparticles: An approach to target and eliminate intracellular pathogens. Molecular Pharmaceutics. 2019;**16**: 4594-4609

[9] Lee JH, Yeo Y. Controlled drug release from pharmaceutical nanocarriers. Chemical Engineering Science. 2015;**125**:75-84

[10] Weinbreck F, de Vries R, Schrooyen P, de Kruif CG. Complex coacervation of whey proteins and gum arabic. Biomacromolecules. 2003;**4**: 293-303

[11] Chiappetta DA, Sosnik A. Poly (ethylene oxide)–poly (propylene oxide) block copolymer micelles as drug delivery agents: Improved hydrosolubility, stability and bioavailability of drugs. European Journal of Pharmaceutics and Biopharmaceutics. 2007;**66**:303-317

[12] Vrignaud S, Benoit J-P, Saulnier P. Strategies for the nanoencapsulation of hydrophilic molecules in polymer-based nanoparticles. Biomaterials. 2011;**32**: 8593-8604

[13] Elvira C, Gallardo A, San Roman J, Cifuentes A. Covalent polymer-drug conjugates. Molecules. 2005;**10**:114-125

[14] D'Emanuele A, Attwood D. Dendrimer-drug interactions. Advanced Drug Delivery Reviews. 2005;**57**: 2147-2162

[15] Kim S-W, Lee YK, Kim S-H, Park J-Y, Lee DU, Hong JH, et al. Covalent, non-covalent, encapsulated nanodrug regulate the fate of intra- and extracellular

trafficking : Impact on cancer and normal cells. Scientific Reports. 2017;7:1-17. Article id: 6454

[16] Kaminskas LM, McLeod VM, Porter CJH, Boyd BJ. Association of chemotherapeutic drugs with dendrimer nanocarriers: An assessment of the merits of covalent conjugation compared to noncovalent encapsulation. Molecular Pharmaceutics. 2012;**9**:355-373

[17] Kaminskas LM, Boyd BJ, Karellas P, Krippner GY, Lessene R, Kelly B, et al. The impact of molecular weight and PEG chain length on the systemic pharmacokinetics of pegylated poly L-lysine dendrimers. Molecular Pharmaceutics. 2008;**5**:449-463

[18] Saito G, Swanson JA, Lee KD. Drug delivery strategy utilizing conjugation via reversible disulfide linkages: Role and site of cellular reducing activities. Advanced Drug Delivery Reviews. 2003;**55**:199-215

[19] Lele B, Hoffman A. Mucoadhesive drug carriers based on complexes of poly (acrylic acid) and PEGylated drugs having hydrolysable PEG–anhydride–drug linkages. Journal of Controlled Release. 2000;**69**:237-248

[20] Khandare J, Minko T. Polymer–drug conjugates: Progress in polymeric prodrugs. Progress in Polymer Science. 2006;**31**:359-397

[21] Agarwal HK, Chhikara BS, Hanley MJ, Ye G, Doncel GF, Parang K. Synthesis and biological evaluation of fatty acyl ester derivatives of (−)-2′,3′-dideoxy-3′-thiacytidine. Journal of Medicinal Chemistry. 2012;**55**: 4861-4871

[22] Debart F, Abes S, Deglane G, Moulton HM, Clair P, Gait MJ, et al. Chemical modifications to improve the cellular uptake of oligonucleotides. Current Topics in Medicinal Chemistry. 2007;7:727-737

[23] Agarwal HK, Chhikara BS, Bhavaraju S, Mandal D, Doncel GF, Parang K. Emtricitabine prodrugs with improved anti-HIV activity and cellular uptake. Molecular Pharmaceutics. 2013; **10**:467-476

[24] Takalani F, Kumar P, Kondiah PP, Choonara YE, Pillay V. Lipid–drug conjugates and associated carrier strategies for enhanced antiretroviral drug delivery. Pharmaceutical Development and Technology. 2020;**25**: 267-280

[25] Adhikari P, Pal P, Das AK, Ray S, Bhattacharjee A, Mazumder B. Nano lipid-drug conjugate: An integrated review. International Journal of Pharmaceutics. 2017;**529**:629-641

[26] Nobs L, Buchegger F, Gurny R, Allémann E. Current methods for attaching targeting ligands to liposomes and nanoparticles. Journal of Pharmaceutical Sciences. 2004;**93**: 1980-1992

[27] Hoare DG, Koshland DE. A method for the quantitative modification and estimation of carboxylic acid groups in proteins. Journal of Biological Chemistry. 1967;**242**:2447-2453

[28] Werengowska-Ciećwierz K, Wiśniewski M, Terzyk AP, Furmaniak S. The chemistry of bioconjugation in nanoparticles-based drug delivery system. Advances in Condensed Matter Physics. 2015;**2015** (2015):198175-198202

[29] Yousefpour P, Atyabi F, Vasheghani-Farahani E, Movahedi A-AM, Dinarvand R. Targeted delivery of doxorubicin-utilizing chitosan nanoparticles surface-functionalized with anti-Her2 trastuzumab. International Journal of Nanomedicine. 2011;**6**:1977-1990

[30] Kurtoglu YE, Mishra MK, Kannan S, Kannan RM. Drug release characteristics

of PAMAM dendrimer–drug conjugates with different linkers. International Journal of Pharmaceutics. 2010;**384**: 189-194

[31] Duhem N, Danhier F, Pourcelle V, Schumers J-M, Bertrand O, LeDuff CS, et al. Self-assembling doxorubicin–tocopherol succinate prodrug as a new drug delivery system: Synthesis, characterization, and in vitro and in vivo anticancer activity. Bioconjugate Chemistry. 2014;**25**:72-81

[32] Yokoyama M, Miyauchi M, Yamada N, Okano T, Sakurai Y, Kataoka K, et al. Characterization and anticancer activity of the micelle-forming polymeric anticancer drug adriamycin-conjugated poly(ethylene glycol)-poly (aspartic acid) block copolymer. Cancer Research. 1990;**50**:1693

[33] Nathan A, Zalipsky S, Ertel SI, Agathos SN, Yarmush ML, Kohn J. Copolymers of lysine and polyethylene glycol: A new family of functionalized drug carriers. Bioconjugate Chemistry. 1993;**4**:54-62

[34] Gupta A, Asthana S, Konwar R, Chourasia M. An insight into potential of nanoparticles-assisted chemotherapy of cancer using gemcitabine and its fatty acid prodrug: A comparative study. Journal of Biomedical Nanotechnology. 2013;**9**:915-925

[35] Kizhedath A, Wilkinson S, Glassey J. Applicability of predictive toxicology methods for monoclonal antibody therapeutics: Status quo and scope. Archives of Toxicology. 2017;**91**: 1595-1612

[36] Maruyama K, Takizawa T, Yuda T, Kennel SJ, Huang L, Iwatsuru M. Targetability of novel immunoliposomes modified with amphipathic poly(ethylene glycol)s conjugated at their distal terminals to monoclonal antibodies. Biochimica et Biophysica Acta. 1995;**1234**:74-80

[37] Dvir T, Bauer M, Schroeder A, Tsui JH, Anderson DG, Langer R, et al. Nanoparticles targeting the infarcted heart. Nano Letters. 2011;**11**:4411-4414

[38] Sonawane SJ, Kalhapure RS, Govender T. Hydrazone linkages in pH responsive drug delivery systems. European Journal of Pharmaceutical Sciences. 2017;**99**:45-65

[39] Matson JB, Stupp SI. Drug release from hydrazone-containing peptide amphiphiles. Chemical Communications. 2011;**47**:7962-7964

[40] Vijayakameswara Rao N, Mane S, Kishore A, Sarma JD, Shunmugam R, et al. Norbornene derived doxorubicin copolymers as drug carriers with pH responsive hydrazone linker. Biomacromolecules. 2012;**13**:221-230

[41] Gu Y-J, Cheng J, Jin J, Cheng SH, Wong W-T. Development and evaluation of pH-responsive single-walled carbon nanotube-doxorubicin complexes in cancer cells. International Journal of Nanomedicine. 2011;**6**:2889

[42] Christie RJ, Fleming R, Bezabeh B, Woods R, Mao S, Harper J, et al. Stabilization of cysteine-linked antibody drug conjugates with N-aryl maleimides. Journal of Controlled Release. 2015;**220**:660-670

[43] Anhorn MG, Wagner S, Kreuter J, Langer K, von Briesen H. Specific targeting of HER2 overexpressing breast cancer cells with doxorubicin-loaded trastuzumab-modified human serum albumin nanoparticles. Bioconjugate Chemistry. 2008;**19**(12):2321-2331

[44] Park JW, Hong K, Carter P, Asgari H, Guo LY, Keller GA, et al. Development of anti-p185(HER2) immunoliposomes for cancer therapy. Proceedings of the National Academy of Sciences of the United States of America. 1995;**92**:1327-1331

[45] Kirpotin D, Park JW, Hong K, Zalipsky S, Li WL, Carter P, et al. Sterically stabilized anti-HER2 immunoliposomes: Design and targeting to human breast cancer cells in vitro. Biochemistry. 1997;**36**:66-75

[46] Lu YJ, Wei KC, Ma CCM, Yang SY, Chen JP. Dual targeted delivery of doxorubicin to cancer cells using folate-conjugated magnetic multi-walled carbon nanotubes. Colloids and Surfaces B: Biointerfaces. 2012;**89**:1-9

[47] West K, Otto S. Reversible covalent chemistry in drug delivery. Current Drug Discovery Technologies. 2005;**2**: 123-160

[48] Chari RV. Expanding the Reach of Antibody-Drug Conjugates. ACS Medicinal Chemistry Letters. 2016:7 (11):974-976

[49] Rau H, Baron J, Hersel U, Krusch M. Prodrugs Containing an Aromatic Amine Connected by an Amido Bond to a Linker, in Google Patents. 2015

[50] Gawali SL, Barick KC, Shetake NG, Rajan V, Pandey BN, Kumar NN, et al. pH-labile magnetic nanocarriers for intracellular drug delivery to tumor cells. ACS Omega. 2019;**4**:11728-11736

[51] Ghosh AK, Brindisi M. Organic carbamates in drug design and medicinal chemistry. Journal of Medicinal Chemistry. 2015;**58**: 2895-2940

[52] Kölmel DK, Kool ET. Oximes and hydrazones in bioconjugation: Mechanism and catalysis. Chemical Reviews. 2017;**117**:10358-10376

[53] Fancui M, Quanxin W, Zhuangzhuang Q, Yan Y. Micelles prepared with cinnamaldehyde and vancomycin by Schiff base reaction. International Journal of New Technology and Research. 2018;**4**

[54] Xiao N, Liang H, Lu J. Degradable and biocompatible aldehyde-functionalized glycopolymer conjugated with doxorubicin via acid-labile Schiff base linkage for pH-triggered drug release. Soft Matter. 2011;**7**: 10834-10840

[55] Bhakay A, Rahman M, Dave RN, Bilgili EJP. Bioavailability enhancement of poorly water-soluble drugs via nanocomposites: Formulation–processing aspects and challenges. 2018; **10**:86

[56] Benedetto Tiz D, Kikelj D, Zidar N. Overcoming problems of poor drug penetration into bacteria: Challenges and strategies for medicinal chemists. Expert Opinion on Drug Discovery. 2018;**13**:497-507

[57] Lock LL, LaComb M, Schwarz K, Cheetham AG, Lin Y-A, Zhang P, et al. Self-assembly of natural and synthetic drug amphiphiles into discrete supramolecular nanostructures. Faraday Discussions. 2013;**166**:285-301

[58] Omolo CA, Kalhapure RS, Jadhav M, Rambharose S, Mocktar C, Ndesendo VM, et al. Pegylated oleic acid: A promising amphiphilic polymer for nano-antibiotic delivery. 2017;**112**: 96-108

[59] Su H, Zhang P, Cheetham AG, Koo JM, Lin R, Masood A, et al. Supramolecular crafting of self-assembling camptothecin prodrugs with enhanced efficacy against primary cancer cells. Theranostics. 2016;**6**:1065

[60] Cheetham AG, Zhang P, Lin YA, Lock LL, Cui H. Supramolecular nanostructures formed by anticancer drug assembly. Journal of the American Chemical Society. 2013;**135**:2907-2910

[61] Ma X, Bai S, Zhang X, Ma X, Jia D, Shi X, et al. Enhanced tumor penetration and chemotherapy efficiency by covalent self-assembled

nanomicelle responsive to tumor microenvironment. Biomacromolecules. 2019;**20**:2637-2648

[62] Wang Y, Cheetham AG, Angacian G, Su H, Xie L, Cui H. Peptide–drug conjugates as effective prodrug strategies for targeted delivery. Advanced Drug Delivery Reviews. 2017;**110**:112-126

[63] Lu Y, Lin J, Wang L, Zhang L, Cai C. Self-assembly of copolymer micelles: Higher-level assembly for constructing hierarchical structure. Chemical Reviews. 2020

[64] Amitay Y, Shmeeda H, Patil Y, Gorin J, Tzemach D, Mak L, et al. Pharmacologic studies of a prodrug of mitomycin C in pegylated liposomes (Promitil®): High stability in plasma and rapid thiolytic prodrug activation in tissues. Pharmaceutical Research. 2016; **33**:686-700

[65] Karaman R. Prodrugs design based on inter- and intramolecular chemical processes. Chemical Biology & Drug Design. 2013;**82**:643-668

[66] Scicluna MC, Vella-Zarb L. Evolution of nanocarrier drug-delivery systems and recent advancements in covalent organic framework–drug systems. ACS Applied Nano Materials. 2020;**3**:3097-3115

[67] Taresco V, Alexander C, Singh N, Pearce AK. Stimuli-responsive prodrug chemistries for drug delivery. Advanced Therapeutics. 2018;**1**:1800030

[68] Tian L, Yang Y, Wysocki LM, Arnold AC, Hu A, Ravichandran B, et al. Selective esterase–ester pair for targeting small molecules with cellular specificity. Proceedings of the National Academy of Sciences. 2012;**109**:4756-4761

[69] Ding C, Li Z. A review of drug release mechanisms from nanocarrier systems. Materials Science and Engineering: C. 2017;**76**:1440-1453

[70] Wang Z, Deng X, Ding J, Zhou W, Zheng X, Tang G. Mechanisms of drug release in pH-sensitive micelles for tumour targeted drug delivery system: A review. International Journal of Pharmaceutics. 2018;**535**:253-260

[71] Dillon KM, Powell CR, Matson JB. Self-immolative prodrugs: Effective tools for the controlled release of sulfur signaling species. Synlett. 2019;**30**: 525-531

[72] Meng X, Gao M, Deng J, Lu D, Fan A, Ding D, et al. Self-immolative micellar drug delivery: The linker matters. Nano Research. 2018;**11**: 6177-6189

[73] Senevirathne SA, Washington KE, Biewer MC, Stefan MC. PEG based anti-cancer drug conjugated prodrug micelles for the delivery of anti-cancer agents. Journal of Materials Chemistry B. 2016;**4**:360-370

[74] Lee E, Kim H, Lee I-H, Jon S. In vivo antitumor effects of chitosan-conjugated docetaxel after oral administration. Journal of Controlled Release. 2009;**140**:79-85

[75] Duncan R, Vicent MJ. Do HPMA copolymer conjugates have a future as clinically useful nanomedicines? A critical overview of current status and future opportunities. Advanced Drug Delivery Reviews. 2010;**62**:272-282

[76] Jung B, Jeong Y-C, Min J-H, Kim J-E, Song Y-J, Park J-K, et al. Tumor-binding prodrug micelles of polymer–drug conjugates for anticancer therapy in HeLa cells. Journal of Materials Chemistry. 2012;**22**:9385-9394

[77] Konkle BA, Stasyshyn O, Chowdary P, Bevan DH, Mant T, Shima M, et al. Pegylated, full-length, recombinant factor VIII for prophylactic and on-demand treatment of severe hemophilia A. Blood, The Journal of the

American Society of Hematology. 2015; **126**:1078-1085

[78] Coyle T, Reding MT, Lin J, Michaels L, Shah A, Powell J. Phase I study of BAY 94-9027, a PEG ylated B-domain-deleted recombinant factor VIII with an extended half-life, in subjects with hemophilia A. Journal of Thrombosis and Haemostasis. 2014;**12**: 488-496

[79] Devarajan PV, Dawre SM, Dutta R. Infectious diseases: Need for targeted drug delivery. In: Targeted Drug Delivery: Concepts and Design. Springer; 2015. pp. 113-148

[80] Van Driessche A, Kocere A, Everaert H, Nuhn L, Van Herck S, Griffiths G, et al. pH-sensitive hydrazone-linked doxorubicin nanogels via polymeric-activated Ester scaffolds: Synthesis, assembly, and in vitro and in vivo evaluation in tumor-bearing zebrafish. Chemistry of Materials. 2018; **30**:8587-8596

[81] Cao X, Le C, Lim K, Thi H, Kim G, Gal Y. Redox-responsive core cross-linked prodrug micelles prepared by click chemistry for pH-triggered doxorubicin delivery. Express Polymer Letters. 2017;**11**:832-845

[82] Kamaly N, Xiao Z, Valencia PM, Radovic-Moreno AF, Farokhzad OC. Targeted polymeric therapeutic nanoparticles: Design, development and clinical translation. Chemical Society Reviews. 2012;**41**:2971-3010

[83] Augustijns P, Annaert P, Heylen P, Van den Mooter G, Kinget R. Drug absorption studies of prodrug esters using the Caco-2 model: Evaluation of ester hydrolysis and transepithelial transport. International Journal of Pharmaceutics. 1998;**166**:45-53

[84] Amsberry KL, Gerstenberger AE, Borchardt RT. Amine prodrugs which utilize hydroxy amide lactonization. II. A potential esterase-sensitive amide prodrug. Pharmaceutical Research. 1991;**8**:455-461

[85] Meinig JM, Ferrara SJ, Banerji T, Banerji T, Sanford-Crane HS, Bourdette D, et al. Targeting fatty-acid amide hydrolase with prodrugs for CNS-selective therapy. ACS Chemical Neuroscience. 2017;**8**:2468-2476

[86] Kraut J. Serine proteases: Structure and mechanism of catalysis. Annual Review of Biochemistry. 1977;**46**: 331-358

[87] Otto HH, Schirmeister T. Cysteine proteases and their inhibitors. Chemical Reviews. 1997;**97**:133-172

[88] Häse C, Finkelstein RA. Bacterial extracellular zinc-containing metalloproteases. Microbiology and Molecular Biology Reviews. 1993;**57**: 823-837

[89] Martin MT, Angeles TS, Sugasawara R, Aman NI, Napper AD, Darsley MJ, et al. Antibody-catalyzed hydrolysis of an unsubstituted amide. Journal of the American Chemical Society. 1994;**116**:6508-6512

[90] Dai X, De Mesmaeker A, Joyce GF. Cleavage of an amide bond by a ribozyme. Science. 1995;**267**:237-240

[91] Kalia J, Raines RT. Hydrolytic stability of hydrazones and oximes. Angewandte Chemie (International Ed. in English). 2008;**47**:7523-7526

[92] Ross PL, Wolfe JL. Physical and chemical stability of antibody drug conjugates: Current status. Journal of Pharmaceutical Sciences. 2016;**105**: 391-397

[93] Fontaine SD, Reid R, Robinson L, Ashley GW, Santi DV. Long-term stabilization of Maleimide–Thiol conjugates. Bioconjugate Chemistry. 2015;**26**:145-152

[94] Modarresi-Saryazdi SM, Haddadi-Asl V, Salami-Kalajahi M. N, N'-methylenebis (acrylamide)-crosslinked poly (acrylic acid) particles as doxorubicin carriers: A comparison between release behavior of physically loaded drug and conjugated drug via acid-labile hydrazone linkage. Journal of Biomedical Materials Research Part A. 2018;**106**:342-348

[95] Dong C, Zhou Q, Xiang J, Liu F, Zhou Z, Shen Y. Self-assembly of oxidation-responsive polyethylene glycol-paclitaxel prodrug for cancer chemotherapy. Journal of Controlled Release. 2020;**321**:529-539

[96] Stirland DL, Nichols JW, Miura S, Bae YH. Mind the gap: A survey of how cancer drug carriers are susceptible to the gap between research and practice. Journal of Controlled Release. 2013;**172**: 1045-1064

[97] Sun Q, Zhou Z, Qiu N, Shen Y. Rational design of cancer nanomedicine: Nanoproperty integration and synchronization. Advanced Materials. 2017;**29**:1606628

[98] Rao KSVK, Zhong Q, Bielski ER, da Rocha SRP. Nanoparticles of pH-responsive, PEG–doxorubicin conjugates: Interaction with an in vitro model of lung adenocarcinoma and their direct formulation in propellant-based portable inhalers. Molecular Pharmaceutics. 2017;**14**: 3866-3878

[99] Chakroun RW, Wang F, Lin R, Wang Y, Su H, Pompa D, et al. Fine-tuning the linear release rate of paclitaxel-bearing supramolecular filament hydrogels through molecular engineering. ACS Nano. 2019;**13**: 7780-7790

[100] Mura S, Nicolas J, Couvreur P. Stimuli-responsive nanocarriers for drug delivery. Nature Materials. 2013; **12**:991-1003

[101] Zhou Z, Ma X, Murphy CJ, Jin E, Sun Q, Shen Y, et al. Molecularly precise dendrimer–drug conjugates with tunable drug release for cancer therapy. Angewandte Chemie International Edition. 2014;**53**:10949-10955

[102] Zhou Q, Shao S, Wang J, Xu C, Xiang J, Piao Y, et al. Enzyme-activatable polymer–drug conjugate augments tumour penetration and treatment efficacy. Nature Nanotechnology. 2019;**14**:799-809

[103] Bhattacharyya J, Bellucci JJ, Weitzhandler I, McDaniel JR, Spasojevic I, Li X, et al. A paclitaxel-loaded recombinant polypeptide nanoparticle outperforms Abraxane in multiple murine cancer models. Nature Communications. 2015;**6**:1-12

[104] Wang J, Sun X, Mao W, Sun W, Tang J, Sui M, et al. Tumor redox heterogeneity-responsive prodrug nanocapsules for cancer chemotherapy. Advanced Materials. 2013;**25**:3670-3676

[105] Wang J, Hu S, Mao W, Xiang J, Zhou Z, Liu X, et al. Assemblies of peptide-Cytotoxin conjugates for tumor-homing chemotherapy. Advanced Functional Materials. 2019; **29**:1807446

[106] Shen Y, Jin E, Zhang B, Murphy CJ, Sui M, Zhao J, et al. Prodrugs forming high drug loading multifunctional nanocapsules for intracellular cancer drug delivery. Journal of the American Chemical Society. 2010;**132**:4259-4265

[107] Li J, Hu Z-E, Yang X-L, Wu W-X, Xing X, Gu B, et al. GSH/pH dual-responsive biodegradable camptothecin polymeric prodrugs combined with doxorubicin for synergistic anticancer efficiency. Biomaterials Science. 2019;7: 3277-3286

[108] Tang J, Zeng Z, Yan J, Chen C, Liu J, Feng X. Quantitative and high

drug loading of self-assembled prodrug with defined molecular structures for effective cancer therapy. Journal of Controlled Release. 2019;**307**:90-97

[109] Danial M, Telwatte S, Tyssen D, Cosson S, Tachedjian G, Moad G, et al. Combination anti-HIV therapy via tandem release of prodrugs from macromolecular carriers. Polymer Chemistry. 2016;7:7477-7487

[110] Danial M, Andersen AH, Zuwala K, Cosson S, Riber CF, Smith AA, et al. Triple activity of lamivudine releasing sulfonated polymers against HIV-1. Molecular Pharmaceutics. 2016;**13**: 2397-2410

[111] Shibata A, McMullen E, Pham A, Belshan M, Sanford B, Zhou Y, et al. Polymeric nanoparticles containing combination antiretroviral drugs for HIV type 1 treatment. AIDS Research and Human Retroviruses. 2013;**29**: 746-754

[112] Jiang Y, Cao S, Bright DK, Bever AM, Blakney AK, Suydam IT, et al. Nanoparticle-based ARV drug combinations for synergistic inhibition of cell-free and cell–cell HIV transmission. Molecular Pharmaceutics. 2015;**12**:4363-4374

[113] Xiao Y, Liu J, Guo M, Zhou H, Jin J, Liu J, et al. Synergistic combination chemotherapy using carrier-free celastrol and doxorubicin nanocrystals for overcoming drug resistance. Nanoscale. 2018;**10**:12639-12649

[114] Zhao C-Y, Cheng R, Yang Z, Tian Z-M. Nanotechnology for cancer therapy based on chemotherapy. Molecules. 2018;**23**:826

[115] Ibrahim A, Twizeyimana E, Lu N, Ke W, Mukerabigwi JF, Mohammed F, et al. Reduction-responsive polymer prodrug micelles with enhanced endosomal escape capability for efficient intracellular translocation and drug release. ACS Applied Bio Materials. 2019;**2**:5099-5109

[116] Lu D, Wen X, Liang J, Gu Z, Zhang X, Fan Y. A pH-sensitive nano drug delivery system derived from pullulan/doxorubicin conjugate. Journal of Biomedical Materials Research Part B: Applied Biomaterials: An Official Journal of The Society for Biomaterials, The Japanese Society for Biomaterials, and The Australian Society for Biomaterials and the Korean Society for Biomaterials. 2009;**89**:177-183

[117] Yoo HS, Lee KH, Oh JE, Park TG. In vitro and in vivo anti-tumor activities of nanoparticles based on doxorubicin–PLGA conjugates. Journal of Controlled Release. 2000;**68**:419-431

[118] Shuai X, Ai H, Nasongkla N, Kim S, Gao J. Micellar carriers based on block copolymers of poly (ε-caprolactone) and poly (ethylene glycol) for doxorubicin delivery. Journal of Controlled Release. 2004;**98**:415-426

[119] Ma L, Lin X, Li C, Xu Z, Chan C-Y, Tse M-K, et al. A cancer cell-selective and low-toxic bifunctional heterodinuclear Pt(IV)–Ru(II) anticancer prodrug. Inorganic Chemistry. 2018;**57**:2917-2924

[120] Larson N, Ghandehari H. Polymeric conjugates for drug delivery. Chemistry of Materials. 2012;**24**:840-853

[121] Du J-Z, Du X-J, Mao C-Q, Wang J. Tailor-made dual pH-sensitive polymer–doxorubicin nanoparticles for efficient anticancer drug delivery. Journal of the American Chemical Society. 2011;**133**:17560-17563

[122] Cai K, He X, Song Z, Yin Q, Zhang Y, Uckun FM, et al. Dimeric drug polymeric nanoparticles with exceptionally high drug loading and quantitative loading efficiency. Journal of the American Chemical Society. 2015; **137**:3458-3461

[123] Su L, Li R, Khan S, Clanton R, Zhang F, Lin Y-N, et al. Chemical design of both a glutathione-sensitive dimeric drug guest and a glucose-derived nanocarrier host to achieve enhanced osteosarcoma lung metastatic anticancer selectivity. Journal of the American Chemical Society. 2018;**140**:1438-1446

[124] Miller K, Erez R, Segal E, Shabat D, Satchi-Fainaro R. Targeting bone metastases with a bispecific anticancer and antiangiogenic polymer–alendronate–taxane conjugate. Angewandte Chemie International Edition. 2009;**48**:2949-2954

[125] Paz-Ares L, Ross H, O'brien M, Riviere A, Gatzemeier U, Von Pawel J, et al. Phase III trial comparing paclitaxel poliglumex vs docetaxel in the second-line treatment of non-small-cell lung cancer. British Journal of Cancer. 2008; **98**:1608-1613

[126] Chitkara D, Mittal A, Behrman SW, Kumar N, Mahato RI. Self-assembling, amphiphilic polymer–gemcitabine conjugate shows enhanced antitumor efficacy against human pancreatic adenocarcinoma. Bioconjugate Chemistry. 2013;**24**:1161-1173

[127] Ishiguro S, Cai S, Uppalapati D, Turner K, Zhang T, Forrest WC, et al. Intratracheal administration of hyaluronan-cisplatin conjugate nanoparticles significantly attenuates lung cancer growth in mice. Pharmaceutical Research. 2016;**33**:2517-2529

[128] Tsuchiya K, Uchida T, Kobayashi M, Maeda H, Konno T, Yamanaka H. Tumor-targeted chemotherapy with SMANCS in lipiodol for renal cell carcinoma: Longer survival with larger size tumors. Urology. 2000;**55**:495-500

[129] Wang W, Li C, Zhang J, Dong A, Kong D. Tailor-made gemcitabine prodrug nanoparticles from well-defined drug–polymer amphiphiles prepared by controlled living radical polymerization for cancer chemotherapy. Journal of Materials Chemistry B. 2014;**2**:1891-1901

[130] Chen X, Chen X, Chen W, Ma X, Huang J, Chen R. Extended peginterferon alfa-2a (Pegasys) therapy in Chinese patients with HBeAg-negative chronic hepatitis B. Journal of Medical Virology. 2014;**86**:1705-1713

[131] Trapani A, Di Gioia S, Ditaranto N, Cioffi N, Goycoolea FM, Carbone A, et al. Systemic heparin delivery by the pulmonary route using chitosan and glycol chitosan nanoparticles. International Journal of Pharmaceutics. 2013;**447**:115-123

[132] Mastria EM, Chen M, McDaniel JR, Li X, Hyun J, Dewhirst MW, et al. Doxorubicin-conjugated polypeptide nanoparticles inhibit metastasis in two murine models of carcinoma. Journal of Controlled Release. 2015;**208**:52-58

[133] Zhong Q, Bielski ER, Rodrigues LS, Brown MR, Reineke JJ, da Rocha SR. Conjugation to poly (amidoamine) dendrimers and pulmonary delivery reduce cardiac accumulation and enhance antitumor activity of doxorubicin in lung metastasis. Molecular Pharmaceutics. 2016;**13**:2363-2375

[134] Eskow Jaunarajs KL, Standaert DG, Viegas TX, Bentley MD, Fang Z, Dizman B, et al. Rotigotine polyoxazoline conjugate SER-214 provides robust and sustained antiparkinsonian benefit. Movement Disorders. 2013;**28**:1675-1682

[135] Park JH, Kwon S, Lee M, Chung H, Kim J-H, Kim Y-S, et al. Self-assembled nanoparticles based on glycol chitosan bearing hydrophobic moieties as carriers for doxorubicin: in vivo biodistribution and anti-tumor activity. Biomaterials. 2006;**27**:119-126

[136] Murata M, Yonamine T, Tanaka S, Tahara K, Tozuka Y, Takeuchi H. Surface modification of liposomes using polymer-wheat germ agglutinin conjugates to improve the absorption of peptide drugs

by pulmonary administration. Journal of Pharmaceutical Sciences. 2013;**102**: 1281-1289

[137] Ernsting MJ, Tang W-L, MacCallum NW, Li S-D. Preclinical pharmacokinetic, biodistribution, and anti-cancer efficacy studies of a docetaxel-carboxymethylcellulose nanoparticle in mouse models. Biomaterials. 2012;**33**:1445-1454

[138] Wang H, Wei J, Yang C, Zhao H, Li D, Yin Z, et al. The inhibition of tumor growth and metastasis by self-assembled nanofibers of taxol. Biomaterials. 2012;**33**:5848-5853

[139] Yang C, Bian M, Yang Z. A polymer additive boosts the anti-cancer efficacy of supramolecular nanofibers of taxol. Biomaterials Science. 2014;**2**:651-654

[140] Ueno T, Endo K, Hori K, Ozaki N, Tsuji A, Kondo S, et al. Assessment of antitumor activity and acute peripheral neuropathy of 1, 2-diaminocyclohexane platinum (II)-incorporating micelles (NC-4016). International Journal of Nanomedicine. 2014;**9**:3005

[141] Katsumi H, Takashima M, Sano J-I, Nishiyama K, Kitamura N, Sakane T, et al. Development of polyethylene glycol-conjugated alendronate, a novel nitrogen-containing bisphosphonate derivative: Evaluation of absorption, safety, and effects after intrapulmonary administration in rats. Journal of Pharmaceutical Sciences. 2011;**100**: 3783-3792

[142] Duncan R. Polymer conjugates as anticancer nanomedicines. Nature Reviews Cancer. 2006;**6**:688-701

[143] Cheetham AG, Chakroun RW, Ma W, Cui H. Self-assembling prodrugs. Chemical Society Reviews. 2017;**46**: 6638-6663

[144] Yokoyama M, Miyauchi M, Yamada N, Okano T, Sakurai Y, Kataoka K, et al. Characterization and anticancer activity of the micelle-forming polymeric anticancer drug adriamycin-conjugated poly (ethylene glycol)-poly (aspartic acid) block copolymer. Cancer Research. 1990;**50**:1693-1700

[145] Yokoyama M, Okano T, Sakurai Y, Kataoka K. Improved synthesis of adriamycin-conjugated poly (ethylene oxide)-poly (aspartic acid) block copolymer and formation of unimodal micellar structure with controlled amount of physically entrapped adriamycin. Journal of Controlled Release. 1994;**32**:269-277

[146] Kwon GS, Yokoyama M, Okano T, Sakurai Y, Kataoka K. Biodistribution of micelle-forming polymer–drug conjugates. Pharmaceutical Research. 1993;**10**:970-974

[147] Kwon G, Suwa S, Yokoyama M, Okano T, Sakurai Y, Kataoka K. Enhanced tumor accumulation and prolonged circulation times of micelle-forming poly (ethylene oxide-aspartate) block copolymer-adriamycin conjugates. Journal of Controlled Release. 1994;**29**:17-23

[148] Croy S, Kwon G. Polymeric micelles for drug delivery. Current Pharmaceutical Design. 2006;**12**: 4669-4684

[149] Ahmad Z, Shah A, Siddiq M, Kraatz H. Polymeric micelles as drug delivery vehicles. RSC Advances. 2014; **4**:17028-17038. Go to original source

[150] Pattni BS, Chupin VV, Torchilin VP. New developments in liposomal drug delivery. Chemical Reviews. 2015;**115**:10938-10966

[151] Medina SH, El-Sayed ME. Dendrimers as carriers for delivery of chemotherapeutic agents. Chemical Reviews. 2009;**109**:3141-3157

[152] Torchilin V. Tumor delivery of macromolecular drugs based on the EPR effect. Advanced Drug Delivery Reviews. 2011;**63**:131-135

Chapter 5

Microencapsulation for Clinical Applications and Transplantation by Using Different Alginates

Beyza Goncu and Emrah Yucesan

Abstract

Microencapsulation has been the most frequently used technique for several different disciplines such as cell-based therapies and/or transplantation. Technology is based on the idea of combining and coating a material or isolating from an external source. Microencapsulation may be performed with different materials and, among natural biocompatible materials, alginate-based microencapsulation technique is the most appropriate material for microencapsulation. The structural components of alginate materials are the derivatives of alginic acid, which is found in brown algae as an intercellular gel matrix. This alginate is preferred for clinical applications due to its safety in human studies. Therefore, the choice and the combined system need to be carefully optimized to achieve biocompatible application through cell microencapsulation especially for long term. Specifications of alginate such as primary source, isolation process, viscosity, and purity contribute to improve its biocompatibility. Clinically, cell microencapsulation is the major contribution to the field of transplantation by its technique and additionally provides local immune isolation. This chapter discusses the potential benefits of clinically suitable alginates and their applications. This promising technology may highlight its considerable potential for patients that require transplantation and/or replacement therapy in the future.

Keywords: microencaspulation, alginate, cell therapy, drug delivery, transplantation

1. Introduction

Cell encapsulation is a process that involves immune protection of the living cell by using different polymers. The polymers can be distinguished into two main groups: natural origin (i.e., polysaccharides, polynucleotides, polypeptides) [1] and synthetic polymers (i.e., polyethylene glycol, polyvinyl alcohol, polyurethane, etc.). Several attempts have been made by scientists to use natural, synthetic, and semi-synthetic polymers in the field of encapsulation. The first approach was made in 1933 by Bisceglie et al. and used enveloped membrane to demonstrate tumor cell survival in the abdominal cavity of guinea pigs [2]. In his report, the cells survived for 12 days by diffusion of the nutrients. However, at that time immunoisolation technology was not known or understood [3]. Later, in 1943 Algire et al. reported a transparent chamber for atherapeutic approach *in vivo* [4]. Since this report, therapeutic demands enhanced this encapsulation technology in a way that combines the polymer source (produced synthetically or isolated from natural sources) and their functionality by using its characterization.

Several advantages and disadvantages have been reported about synthetic polymers [5]. Mechanical specifications can be more easily engineered or modified with the desired characteristics and particularly can be produced with larger amounts [6–8]. The main deficit of synthetic polymers is that they require toxic substances during the capsulation process; therefore, cell viability is a true obstacle after encapsulation [8, 9]. In this regard, synthetic polymers are frequently used in combination with different devices such as macrocapsules. Before accommodation of the encapsules, first, synthetic polymers are manufactured in the absence of living tissue/cells, and second, tissue/cells are combined with the device to preserve direct contact of the toxic solvents [1]. The most common synthetic polymers are poly(ethylene glycol) [10], polyvinyl alcohol [11], polyurethane [12], poly(ether sulfone) [13], polypropylene [14], sodium polystyrene sulfate [15], polyacrylate [16], polyphosphazene [17], AN69 [18], and lastly polytetrafluoroethylene [19].

Natural polymers have been proposed for immunoisolation based on two distinct features. First, there is no interference with the functionality of cells/tissues and second, the stability of the structure they provide during encapsulation [1, 20]. Conventionally, the most frequently used polymers from natural sources are cellulose [21], chitosan [22], collagen [23], agarose [24], and alginate [25]. The experimental success mainly depends on the application and mimicry potential of the natural polymers. Among these, in this chapter, we mainly focused on the alginate-based encapsulation and its clinical application.

2. Alginates

The most versatile biomaterials among natural polymers are alginates, which are used in a wide range of applications including diffusion systems, drug delivery, as a wound dressing, and for encapsulation when the transplantation has to be a substitute [25–27]. Alginates are hydrophilic compounds that are naturally found in the cell wall, extracellular matrix of brown algae and some species of bacteria, for example, *Pseudomonas aeruginosa* and *Azotobacter vinelandii* [26, 27]. The most common algae source is brown seaweed. During alginate extraction, alginic acid is generally obtained and converted to a form of salt [26]. Several forms of alginates are currently approved by the Food and Drug Administration (FDA) for use, particularly in the replacement of missing/nonfunctioning endocrine-related diseases [28].

2.1 Gelling and ionic cross-linking of alginates

Alginates are linear copolymers that include two hexuronic acid residues that become dimeric blocks, which are composed of β-D-mannuronic (M) and α-L-guluronic (G) acids for building the entire molecule [29]. These blocks are known as the building blocks of alginates. Mainly, the ratio of G and M blocks depends on the source of the algae type [9]. The important feature of these building blocks is the sensitivity to binding of multivalent cations. This is the starting point of this water-soluble polysaccharide, which allows alginate to form as hydrogels. This characteristic of the hydrogel equilibrates between the environment and the relatively physiologic internal environment [29]. The divalent cations and hydrogel feature depends on the divalent ion's affinity to alginate. Several studies reported high-rate ion affinity results in a stronger gel structure. In order to decrease the ion binding strength, divalent cations should be chosen from the following order: $Pb^{2+}>Cu^{2+}>Cd^{2+}>Ba^{2+}>Sr^{2+}>Ca^{2+}>Co^{2+}>Ni^{2+}>Zn^{2+}>Mn^{2+}$ [1, 29, 30] (**Figure 1**). Controlling cation addition to maintain a porous alginate structure is a critical step.

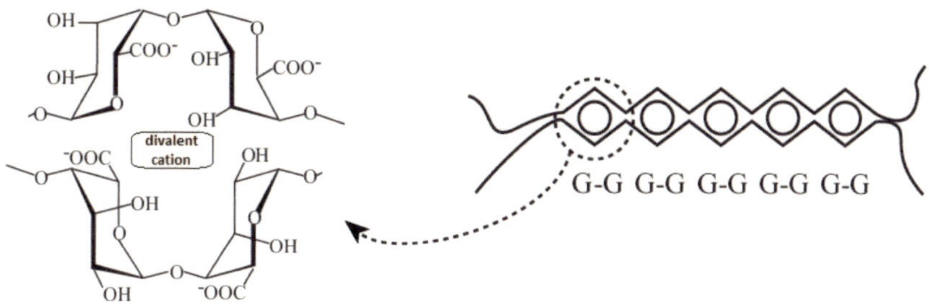

Figure 1.
Representative image for the formation of egg-box ionic cross-links between guluronic acid-rich monomer units (box) and the divalent cations (eggs). Reprinted from Baumberger and Ronsin (2009) [31], an open access article distributed under the terms of the creative commons by attribution 4.0 (CC-BY 4.0).

Successful formation of alginate spheres for delivery purposes requires suitable and selective methods. In 2006, Darrabie et al. identified gelling-cation stability by determining swelling, which contributes to colloid osmotic pressure. They suggested that Ca^{2+} is more hygroscopic and less prominent swelling occurs when compared with Ba^{2+} [32]. Protecting the conformational polymer blocks during preparation of the alginate gels for microencapsulation has been reported using different methods including conjugation of long alkyl chains [33] or dodecylamine [34], temperature (up to 60°C ± 1°C) [35, 36], emulsification by cationic agent [37], and ionotropic gelation of alginate layers [38], etc. Slow gelation utilizes the alginate solution in a more uniform structure in a gradual manner [35].

In the latter case, Lee et al. reported a degree of cross-linking of the alginate can influence a low dose of drug entrapment and unsuitable pore sizes for transplantation. In addition, the efficiency of the microcapsule size or content was found irrelevant, although the preparation step of the water-soluble alginate itself appears to be responsible for the arrangement of the polymer blocks [37]. Cross-linking capacity of the alginates can be modifiable and flexible (**Figure 2**). There are more than 200 types of biocompatible alginates manufactured so far [25, 26]. Moreover, due to the different cross-linking degree of various alginate types, switch in homogenous distribution of the graft/drug during the encapsulation process may occur [36].

Both features of alginates promote several advantages over other polymers such as the stability of the building blocks (-G and/or/both -M repetitively); elasticity of the alginate hydrogel; surface roughness, which is related to elasticity as well, approximately 1% of the alginate can entrap a hundred times more water than its weight; and lastly permitting the ability of oxygen and nutrient permeation inside the spheres.

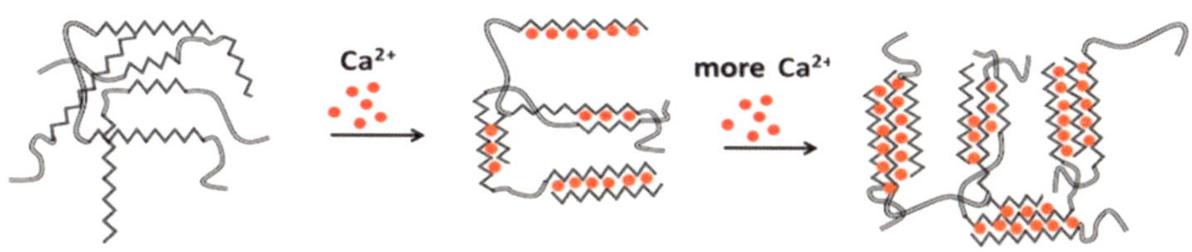

Figure 2.
Representative image of alginate gelation process by continued calcium cations. Reprinted from Dumitru et al. [39], an open access article distributed under the terms of the creative commons by attribution 4.0 (CC-BY 4.0).

2.2 Biotolerability over biocompatibility

Source-dependent impurities may have detrimental effects. Safe and effective delivery of the therapeutic graft/drug with the alginate carrier is frequently mentioned as biocompatible. This naturally derived product provides immunoprotection and most of the studies reported purity of its building block structure preventing a host response when transplanted. Therefore, this makes alginate the most common material for microencapsulation. Higher water-carrying capability of alginates has been shown to directly maintain diffusion and this shows immune-safe characteristics [3]. A decade ago, Kendall et al. focused on the various components of alginate blocks and compared their purity and sphere sizes depending on the cationic agent. They reported that higher purification of alginate prevents imperfections and size/shape properties would affect immunogenicity [40]. Several other reports also demonstrated that -G and -M blocks of the alginate gel need a balance whereas the distribution of these proportions indicates the biocompatibility of the purified alginate is influenced by its viscosity [41–43]. One of the most obvious results from the studies that explains the difference between the building block's balance in alginate gels is higher -M blocks mainly stimulate and induce an immune response [41, 44–46].

There are many immunogenic substances such as endotoxins, proteins, and polyphenols in natural polymers including alginates. Those molecules may diffuse the outer surface from the capsules and then induce an unwanted immune response against the capsules [3]. There are highly conserved molecular motifs that are present in nature and pathogens known as pathogen-associated molecular patterns (PAMPs). PAMPs provoke pattern recognition receptors (PRRs) to enhance inflammatory response [47]. The presence of PAMPs in natural products and alginate as well is not a direct threat; however, complement activation has been reported for encapsulated islets [48]. Therefore, complement activation has a more destructive effect than the inflammatory response; it may activate and produce large quantities of cytokines to induce a stronger response.

Immunoprotective properties still require the exact characterization and preparation of the material to be used as a delivery agent. Despite giving most of the efforts to optimize the encapsulation process, the applicability of this technology has still resulted in an insufficient investigation of graft/drug delivery. In 2014, Rokstad et al. described the duration and the type of host responses and divided the whole process into three categories: acute inflammation, chronic inflammation, and the long-lasting granulation tissue phase [48]. Based on the publications from islet transplantation studies, it was reported that the granulation phase mainly refers to the "vascularized fibrous tissue containing a moderate epithelial histiocytic response" [49–52]. Solely, it is important to observe these responses and that leads to the question: Why do alginate microencapsules contribute to these chain of events even when their purity, stability, and biocompatibility are comparable to most other polymers? Immunocompatibility of the alginate microencapsules should not be determined only by the features of alginate and its preparation process, but should also be evaluated for its protein absorption capability as well.

A profound impact might be introduced with the biotolerability term. Biotolerability is a term for a strategy of making biocompatible encapsulations to induce none/minimal host response. A seemingly minimal cellular overgrowth for graft provides the free diffusion of nutrients, oxygen, and some therapeutic proteins, and controlled drug release from the microcapsules. We should emphasize that the alginate microspheres are not meant to prevent an immune response yet to protect the carrier against an immune response. Therefore, the biocompatibility term not clear enough to explain the biotolerability of the carrier system.

2.3 Vascularization

The vascularization process of the microencapsules is another requirement to increase the survival of the transplanted graft. Sufficient vascularization may be achieved by improving the physical features of the spheres such as the size of the spheres or micropores and the amount/density of the graft/cells. The main argument against vascularization is hypoxia and oxidative stress whereby it develops inside the microspheres [53]. Insufficient oxygenation and nutrition occur particularly in the absence of ideal vascularization. A prerequisite is that the functional performance of the microencapsules often depends on the surface-to-volume ratio. This implies that free diffusion of nutrients and oxygen is necessary and this directly interferes with vascularization.

The majority of researchers developed different strategies to allow a fast exchange of nutrition and demonstrated several boundaries to ensure a low or no inflammatory response while supplying oxygen-nutrients inside [29, 53]. Currently, the accepted limitations of the islet transplantation are defined with three main strategies: first, the cell-to-volume ratio should not exceed 10% even if a large number of cells are required to reach curative treatment. Second, microencapsules should be kept <1 mm, once they reach the spheres they do not maintain their biphasic effect (releasing insulin after a glucose challenge) and also an immune response may be triggered. Third, direct vascular access of the microencapsules to the optimal transplantation site, for instance, glucose must pass and be observed in the transplantation site and then islets release insulin to diffuse through circulation. The whole process requires time and larger amounts to reach an effective dose to lower glucose [1, 53, 54].

3. Clinical applications

A broad range of clinical applications of the microencapsulation process have shown promising results despite encountering some biotolerability issues. Multiple disciplines have been using this alginate encapsulation technology including chemistry, protein science, and cell therapy (mostly transplantation and immunology field). The most studied and reported diseases include Type 1 diabetic patients (T1DM) [55], permanent hypoparathyroidism patients [56], scaffold systems for tissue engineering [57], bone regeneration [58, 59], leukemia (an *in vivo* study that uses alginate to encapsulate specialized hybridoma cells) [60], and even neurodegenerative diseases [61]. Some of the clinical studies about cell therapy are compiled in **Table 1**.

Based on the current experience with alginate, most of the studies have already performed transplantation of beta-cells (islets). The first and well-known clinical trial with islet transplantation was performed in 1994 by Soon-Shiong et al. They reported 9 months of survival of the microencapsules, which were prepared with high guluronic acid containing alginate [49]. Another case reported how islet transplantation was prepared with alginate- poly-l-ornithine and that the patient's need for insulin decreased after transplantation [62]. Following two case reports, Tuch et al. used barium alginate to encapsulate islets and transplanted these into four recipients. In their report, grafts showed various survival rates and did not restore insulin requirements [51]. Considering the last case reports, several companies took the stage and initiated clinical trials to overcome T1DM by using macro- and micro-encapsulation with alginate and other polymers. In 2014, Scharp and Marchetti evaluated the outcomes of islet encapsulation from companies with larger clinical studies, respectively. The increased interest in islet transplantation reached its most

Alginate type	Graft survival	Graft	Year	Reference
Alginate high in guluronic acid	9 months	Beta-cells (Islets)	1994	[49]
Ultrapure alginate (68% glucuronic acid)	3 months	Beta-cells (Islets)	2013	[50]
Barium alginate	Various duration for four recipients	Beta-cells (Islets)	2009	[51]
poly-l-ornithine-sodium alginate	<1 year	Beta-cells (Islets)	2006	[62]
Ultra-purified sodium alginate	3 years	Beta-cells (Islets)	2011	[63]
Alginate-Poly-L-Ornithine	<8 months	Beta-cells (Islets)	2010	[64]
Collagen/Alginate	n/a	Beta-cells (Islets)	2010	[65]
Sodium alginate	3 months	Parathyroid cells	1997	[66]
Amitogenic alginate	<3 months	Parathyroid cells	2001	[43]
n/a	1 year	Parathyroid tissue particles	2001	[67]
n/a	n/a	Parathyroid cells	2004	[68]
Sodium alginate	<20 months	Parathyroid cells	2009	[69]
Ultrapure-low viscosity high guluronic acid-rich alginate	>1 year	Parathyroid cells	2019	[56]

Table 1.
Some of the examples of alginate derivates used in microencapsulation studies.

popular level between 2010 and 2012 [54]. For the last 2 years, researchers provided detailed *in vivo* experiments and defined an alginate encapsulation strategy in a more enhanced way [52, 60, 70, 71] . The vast majority of attempts have been made to treat T1DM and the critical requirements remain to be elucidated in the future.

Another endocrine replacement therapy performed for hypoparathyroidism by encapsulated parathyroid tissue/cell transplantation (PTX) was described only in seven case reports for 12 recipients [43, 56, 67–69, 72, 73] between 1997 and 2019. Six of these case studies used alginate for encapsulation. In 1997, Hasse et al. performed the first microencapsulated PTX for two recipients and reported 3 months of graft survival [72]. The second one, performed by Zimmerman et al. in 2001 for one recipient showed no trace of parathyroid tissue particles nor microcapsules, after 3 months, from histological samples from the implantation site of the recipient [43]. The third transplantation case reported up to 1 year graft survival by Tibell et al. and they had macroencapsulated the parathyroid tissue particles and transplanted into four recipients [67]. Another case by Ulrich et al. reported two PTX recipients had elevations in PTH levels and reduced the supplementation requirement into half dose [68]. In 2009, Cabane et al. microencapsulated the enzymatically isolated parathyroid cells in one recipient and reported the longest follow-up data with 20 months of graft survival [69]. The last and seventh case performed by Yucesan et al. in 2019 microencapsulated parathyroid cell transplantation for one recipient reported and the results followed for a year with success [56]. Despite these achievements, the necessity of immunoisolation for parathyroid allotransplantation requires more case studies with long-term follow-up data.

A different therapy for using microencapsulation is cell therapy for neurodegenerative diseases. The development of a delivery strategy is limited due to the blood–brain barrier; however, principle studies in animal models may offer new approaches including gene delivery, cell-based delivery, and also biomaterial drug delivery [61]. In the past year, several *in vivo* studies have been reported for neurodegenerative diseases [71, 74–76]. Galli et al. used alginate-poly-L-lysine-alginate (APA) microcapsules and cross-linked the spheres with both Ca^{2+} and Ba^{2+}. They have used this system as a transporter to carry a specialized cell clone for codon optimization of the cerebral dopamine neurotrophic factor gene. According to their recent data, this system has the potential to deliver polymer-encapsulated-drug conjugates for the treatment of Parkinson's and Alzheimer's diseases [76].

4. Conclusion

Immunoisolating construct tuning may be achieved by defining the mechanical properties, molecular weight, cross-linking density of the polymer, and the concentration balance between the therapeutic graft/drug and the biomaterial. These proportions still require optimal decisions even with the known performances of encapsulated cells.

Significant efforts have been made so far by ongoing studies from research laboratories and biotechnology companies, which continue to encounter microencapsulation strategies at every step. The future perspective is strong enough to overcome the current limitations. Nevertheless, alginate is the best natural product to be used by many different disciplines at the same time.

Conflict of interest

The authors declare no conflict of interest.

Author details

Beyza Goncu[1]* and Emrah Yucesan[2]

1 Experimental Research Center, Bezmialem Vakif University, Istanbul, Turkey

2 Department of Medical Biology, Faculty of Medicine, Bezmialem Vakif University, Istanbul, Turkey

*Address all correspondence to: bsgoncu@gmail.com; bgoncu@bezmialem.edu.tr

IntechOpen

© 2020 The Author(s). Licensee IntechOpen. This chapter is distributed under the terms of the Creative Commons Attribution License (http://creativecommons.org/licenses/by/3.0), which permits unrestricted use, distribution, and reproduction in any medium, provided the original work is properly cited.

References

[1] de Vos P, Lazarjani HA, Poncelet D, Faas MM. Polymers in cell encapsulation from an enveloped cell perspective. Advanced Drug Delivery Reviews. 2014;**67-68**:15-34

[2] Bisceglie V. Über die antineoplastische Immunität. Zeitschrift für Krebsforschung. 1934;**40**(1):141-158

[3] David A, Day J, Shikanov A. Immunoisolation to prevent tissue graft rejection: Current knowledge and future use. Experimental Biology and Medicine (Maywood, N.J.). 2016;**241**(9):955-961

[4] Algire GH. An Adaptation of the Transparent-Chamber Technique to the Mouse. JNCI: Journal of the National Cancer Institute. 1943;**4**(1):1-11

[5] Song R, Murphy M, Li C, Ting K, Soo C, Zheng Z. Current development of biodegradable polymeric materials for biomedical applications. Drug Design, Development and Therapy. 2018;**12**:3117-3145

[6] Piskin E. Biodegradable polymers as biomaterials. Journal of Biomaterials Science. Polymer Edition. 1995;**6**(9):775-795

[7] Gill I, Ballesteros A. Bioencapsulation within synthetic polymers (Part 1): sol-gel encapsulated biologicals. Trends in Biotechnology. 2000;**18**(7):282-296

[8] Gill I, Ballesteros A. Bioencapsulation within synthetic polymers (Part 2): non-sol-gel protein-polymer biocomposites. Trends in Biotechnology. 2000;**18**(11):469-479

[9] de Vos P, van Schilfgaarde R. Biocompatibility Issues. In: Kühtreiber WM, Lanza RP, Chick WL, editors. Cell Encapsulation Technology and Therapeutics. Boston, MA: Birkhäuser Boston; 1999. pp. 63-75

[10] Zalipsky S, Mullah N, Harding JA, Gittelman J, Guo L, DeFrees SA. Poly(ethylene glycol)-grafted liposomes with oligopeptide or oligosaccharide ligands appended to the termini of the polymer chains. Bioconjugate Chemistry. 1997;**8**(2):111-118

[11] Emerich DF, Hammang JP, Baetge EE, Winn SR. Implantation of polymer-encapsulated human nerve growth factor-secreting fibroblasts attenuates the behavioral and neuropathological consequences of quinolinic acid injections into rodent striatum. Experimental Neurology. 1994;**130**(1):141-150

[12] Seymour RB, Kauffman GB. Polyurethanes: A class of modern versatile materials. Journal of Chemical Education. 1992;**69**(11):909

[13] Abe T, Kato K, Fujioka T, Akizawa T. The blood compatibilities of blood purification membranes and other materials developed in Japan. International Journal of Biomaterials. 2011;**2011**:375390

[14] Coates GW, Waymouth RM. Oscillating stereocontrol: A strategy for the synthesis of thermoplastic elastomeric polypropylene. Science. 1995;**267**(5195):217-219

[15] Brown LF, Detmar M, Claffey K, Nagy JA, Feng D, Dvorak AM, et al. Vascular permeability factor/vascular endothelial growth factor: A multifunctional angiogenic cytokine. EXS. 1997;**79**:233-269

[16] Young TH, Yao NK, Chang RF, Chen LW. Evaluation of asymmetric poly(vinyl alcohol) membranes for use in artificial islets. Biomaterials. 1996;**17**(22):2139-2145

[17] Teasdale I, Bruggemann O. Polyphosphazenes: Multifunctional,

biodegradable vehicles for drug and gene delivery. Polymers (Basel). 2013;**5**(1):161-187

[18] Prevost P, Flori S, Collier C, Muscat E, Rolland E. Application of AN69 hydrogel to islet encapsulation. Evaluation in streptozotocin-induced diabetic rat model. Annals of the New York Academy of Sciences. 1997;**831**:344-349

[19] Buder B, Alexander M, Krishnan R, Chapman DW, Lakey JR. Encapsulated islet transplantation: Strategies and clinical trials. Immune Netw. 2013;**13**(6):235-239

[20] Paredes Juarez GA, Spasojevic M, Faas MM, de Vos P. Immunological and technical considerations in application of alginate-based microencapsulation systems. Frontiers in Bioengineering and Biotechnology. 2014;**2**:26

[21] Miyamoto T, Takahashi S, Ito H, Inagaki H, Noishiki Y. Tissue biocompatibility of cellulose and its derivatives. Journal of Biomedical Materials Research. 1989;**23**(1):125-133

[22] Chandy T, Mooradian DL, Rao GH. Evaluation of modified alginate-chitosan-polyethylene glycol microcapsules for cell encapsulation. Artificial Organs. 1999;**23**(10):894-903

[23] Lee CH, Singla A, Lee Y. Biomedical applications of collagen. International Journal of Pharmaceutics. 2001;**221**(1-2):1-22

[24] Iwata H, Amemiya H, Matsuda T, Takano H, Hayashi R, Akutsu T. Evaluation of microencapsulated islets in agarose gel as bioartificial pancreas by studies of hormone secretion in culture and by xenotransplantation. Diabetes. 1989;**38**(Suppl 1):224-225

[25] Tonnesen HH, Karlsen J. Alginate in drug delivery systems. Drug Development and Industrial Pharmacy. 2002;**28**(6):621-630

[26] Jost A, Sapra A. Alginate. Treasure Island (FL): StatPearls; 2019

[27] Sánchez P, Hernández RM, Pedraz JL, Orive G. Encapsulation of cells in alginate gels. In: Guisan JM, editor. Immobilization of Enzymes and Cells. Third ed. Totowa, NJ: Humana Press; 2013. pp. 313-325

[28] Montanucci P, Terenzi S, Santi C, Pennoni I, Bini V, Pescara T, et al. Insights in behavior of variably formulated alginate-based microcapsules for cell transplantation. BioMed Research International. 2015;**2015**:965804

[29] Lopes M, Abrahim B, Veiga F, Seica R, Cabral LM, Arnaud P, et al. Preparation methods and applications behind alginate-based particles. Expert Opinion on Drug Delivery. 2017;**14**(6):769-782

[30] Poojari R, Srivastava R. Composite alginate microspheres as the next-generation egg-box carriers for biomacromolecules delivery. Expert Opinion on Drug Delivery. 2013;**10**(8):1061-1076

[31] Baumberger T, Ronsin O. From thermally activated to viscosity controlled fracture of biopolymer hydrogels. The Journal of Chemical Physics. 2009;**130**(6):061102

[32] Darrabie MD, Kendall WF, Opara EC. Effect of alginate composition and gelling cation on microbead swelling. Journal of Microencapsulation. 2006;**23**(6):613-621

[33] Pelletier S, Hubert P, Payan E, Marchal P, Choplin L, Dellacherie E. Amphiphilic derivatives of sodium alginate and hyaluronate for cartilage repair: Rheological properties. Journal of Biomedical Materials Research. 2001;**54**(1):102-108

[34] Leonard M, De Boisseson MR, Hubert P, Dalencon F, Dellacherie E. Hydrophobically modified alginate hydrogels as protein carriers with specific controlled release properties. Journal of Controlled Release. 2004;**98**(3):395-405

[35] Lee KY, Mooney DJ. Alginate: Properties and biomedical applications. Progress in Polymer Science. 2012;**37**(1):106-126

[36] Whelehan M, Marison IW. Microencapsulation using vibrating technology. Journal of Microencapsulation. 2011;**28**(8): 669-688

[37] Lee HY, Chan LW, Heng PW. Influence of partially cross-linked alginate used in the production of alginate microspheres by emulsification. Journal of Microencapsulation. 2005;**22**(3):275-280

[38] Ehrhart F, Mettler E, Bose T, Weber MM, Vasquez JA, Zimmermann H. Biocompatible coating of encapsulated cells using ionotropic gelation. PLoS One. 2013;**8**(9):e73498

[39] Dumitru LM, Manoli K, Magliulo M, Ligonzo T, Palazzo G, Torsi L. A hydrogel capsule as gate dielectric in flexible organic field-effect transistors. APL Materials. 2014;**3**(1):014904

[40] Kendall WF Jr, Darrabie MD, El-Shewy HM, Opara EC. Effect of alginate composition and purity on alginate microspheres. Journal of Microencapsulation. 2004;**21**(8):821-828

[41] Tam SK, Dusseault J, Bilodeau S, Langlois G, Halle JP, Yahia L. Factors influencing alginate gel bio-compatibility. Journal of Biomedical Materials Research. Part A. 2011;**98**(1):40-52

[42] Klock G, Pfeffermann A, Ryser C, Grohn P, Kuttler B, Hahn HJ, et al. Biocompatibility of mannuronic acid-rich alginates. Biomaterials. 1997;**18**(10):707-713

[43] Zimmermann U, Cramer H, Jork A, Thürmer F, Zimmermann H, Fuhr G, et al. Microencapsulation-based cell therapy. Biotechnology. 2001:547-571

[44] Otterlei M, Ostgaard K, Skjak-Braek G, Smidsrod O, Soon-Shiong P, Espevik T. Induction of cytokine production from human monocytes stimulated with alginate. Journal of Immunotherapy. 1991;**10**(4):286-291

[45] Espevik T, Otterlei M, Skjak-Braek G, Ryan L, Wright SD, Sundan A. The involvement of CD14 in stimulation of cytokine production by uronic acid polymers. European Journal of Immunology. 1993;**23**(1):255-261

[46] Kulseng B, Skjak-Braek G, Ryan L, Andersson A, King A, Faxvaag A, et al. Transplantation of alginate microcapsules: Generation of antibodies against alginates and encapsulated porcine islet-like cell clusters. Transplantation. 1999;**67**(7):978-984

[47] Mogensen TH. Pathogen recognition and inflammatory signaling in innate immune defenses. Clinical Microbiology Reviews. 2009;**22**(2):240-273

[48] Rokstad AM, Lacik I, de Vos P, Strand BL. Advances in biocompatibility and physico-chemical characterization of microspheres for cell encapsulation. Advanced Drug Delivery Reviews. 2014;**67-68**:111-130

[49] Soon-Shiong P, Heintz RE, Merideth N, Yao QX, Yao Z, Zheng T, et al. Insulin independence in a type 1 diabetic patient after encapsulated islet transplantation. Lancet. 1994;**343**(8903):950-951

[50] Jacobs-Tulleneers-Thevissen D, Chintinne M, Ling Z, Gillard P,

Schoonjans L, Delvaux G, et al. Sustained function of alginate-encapsulated human islet cell implants in the peritoneal cavity of mice leading to a pilot study in a type 1 diabetic patient. Diabetologia. 2013;**56**(7):1605-1614

[51] Tuch BE, Keogh GW, Williams LJ, Wu W, Foster JL, Vaithilingam V, et al. Safety and viability of microencapsulated human islets transplanted into diabetic humans. Diabetes Care. 2009;**32**(10):1887

[52] Bochenek MA, Veiseh O, Vegas AJ, McGarrigle JJ, Qi M, Marchese E, et al. Alginate encapsulation as long-term immune protection of allogeneic pancreatic islet cells transplanted into the omental bursa of macaques. Nature Biomedical Engineering. 2018;**2**(11):810-821

[53] Colton CK. Oxygen supply to encapsulated therapeutic cells. Advanced Drug Delivery Reviews. 2014;**67-68**:93-110

[54] Scharp DW, Marchetti P. Encapsulated islets for diabetes therapy: history, current progress, and critical issues requiring solution. Advanced Drug Delivery Reviews. 2014;**67-68**:35-73

[55] Vaithilingam V, Bal S, Tuch BE. Encapsulated islet transplantation: Where do we stand? The Review of Diabetic Studies. 2017;**14**(1):51-78

[56] Yucesan E, Basoglu H, Goncu B, Akbas F, Ersoy YE, Aysan E. Microencapsulated parathyroid allotransplantation in the omental tissue. Artificial Organs. 2019;**43**(10):1022-1027

[57] Reakasame S, Boccaccini AR. Oxidized alginate-based hydrogels for tissue engineering applications: A review. Biomacromolecules. 2018;**19**(1):3-21

[58] Nabavinia M, Khoshfetrat AB, Naderi-Meshkin H. Nano-hydroxyapatite-alginate-gelatin microcapsule as a potential osteogenic building block for modular bone tissue engineering. Materials Science & Engineering. C, Materials for Biological Applications. 2019;**97**:67-77

[59] Zhou X, Liu P, Nie W, Peng C, Li T, Qiang L, et al. Incorporation of dexamethasone-loaded mesoporous silica nanoparticles into mineralized porous biocomposite scaffolds for improving osteogenic activity. International Journal of Biological Macromolecules. 2020;**149**:116-126

[60] Lang MS, Hovenkamp E, Savelkoul HF, Knegt P, Van Ewijk W. Immunotherapy with monoclonal antibodies directed against the immunosuppressive domain of p15E inhibits tumour growth. Clinical and Experimental Immunology. 1995;**102**(3):468-475

[61] Emerich DF, Orive G, Thanos C, Tornoe J, Wahlberg LU. Encapsulated cell therapy for neurodegenerative diseases: From promise to product. Advanced Drug Delivery Reviews. 2014;**67-68**:131-141

[62] Calafiore R, Basta G, Luca G, Lemmi A, Montanucci MP, Calabrese G, et al. Microencapsulated pancreatic islet allografts into nonimmunosuppressed patients with type 1 diabetes: First two cases. Diabetes Care. 2006;**29**(1):137-138

[63] Basta G, Montanucci P, Luca G, Boselli C, Noya G, Barbaro B, et al. Long-term metabolic and immunological follow-up of nonimmunosuppressed patients with type 1 diabetes treated with microencapsulated islet allografts: Four cases. Diabetes Care. 2011;**34**(11):2406-2409

[64] Tan PL. Company profile: Tissue regeneration for diabetes and

neurological diseases at living cell technologies. Regenerative Medicine. 2010;**5**(2):181-187

[65] Dufrane D, Goebbels RM, Gianello P. Alginate macroencapsulation of pig islets allows correction of streptozotocin-induced diabetes in primates up to 6 months without immunosuppression. Transplantation. 2010;**90**(10):1054-1062

[66] An D, Wang LH, Ernst AU, Chiu A, Lu YC, Flanders JA, et al. An atmosphere-breathing refillable biphasic device for cell replacement therapy. Advanced Materials. 2019;**31**(52):e1905135

[67] Tibell A, Rafael E, Wennberg L, Nordenstrom J, Bergstrom M, Geller RL, et al. Survival of macroencapsulated allogeneic parathyroid tissue one year after transplantation in nonimmunosuppressed humans. Cell Transplantation. 2001;**10**(7):591-599

[68] Ulrich F, Klupp J, Thürmer F, Rayes N, Seehofer D, Tullius S, et al. Allotransplantation of encapsulated human parathyroid tissue in patients with permanent hypoparathyroidism. Transplantation. 2004;**78**:79

[69] Cabane P, Gac P, Amat J, Pineda P, Rossi R, Caviedes R, et al. Allotransplant of microencapsulated parathyroid tissue in severe postsurgical hypoparathyroidism: A case report. Transplantation Proceedings. 2009;**41**(9):3879-3883

[70] Safley SA, Kenyon NS, Berman DM, Barber GF, Willman M, Duncanson S, et al. Microencapsulated adult porcine islets transplanted intraperitoneally in streptozotocin-diabetic non-human primates. Xenotransplantation. 2018;**25**(6):e12450

[71] Liu Q, Chiu A, Wang LH, An D, Zhong M, Smink AM, et al. Zwitterionically modified alginates mitigate cellular overgrowth for cell encapsulation. Nature Communications. 2019;**10**(1):5262

[72] Hasse C, Klock G, Schlosser A, Zimmermann U, Rothmund M. Parathyroid allotransplantation without immunosuppression. Lancet. 1997;**350**(9087):1296-1297

[73] Khryshchanovich V, Ghoussein Y. Allotransplantation of macroencapsulated parathyroid cells as a treatment of severe postsurgical hypoparathyroidism: Case report. Annals of Saudi Medicine. 2016;**36**(2):143-147

[74] Emerich DF, Kordower JH, Chu Y, Thanos C, Bintz B, Paolone G, et al. Widespread striatal delivery of GDNF from encapsulated cells prevents the anatomical and functional consequences of excitotoxicity. Neural Plasticity. 2019;**2019**:6286197

[75] Paolone G, Falcicchia C, Lovisari F, Kokaia M, Bell WJ, Fradet T, et al. Long-term, targeted delivery of GDNF from encapsulated cells is neuroprotective and reduces seizures in the pilocarpine model of epilepsy. The Journal of Neuroscience. 2019;**39**(11):2144-2156

[76] Galli E, Lindholm P, Kontturi LS, Saarma M, Urtti A, Yliperttula M. Characterization of CDNF-secreting ARPE-19 cell clones for encapsulated cell therapy. Cell Transplantation. 2019;**28**(4):413-424

Chapter 6

Coconut Phospholipid Species: Isolation, Characterization and Application as Drug Delivery System

Dwi Hudiyanti, Nur Kamila, Febriani Kusuma Wardani and Khairul Anam

Abstract

The purpose of this study was to isolate the ethanolamine species of coconut phospholipid and to investigate their potency as drug delivery system by using it to encapsulate vitamin C. The study consisted of two stages: the first stage was isolation and characterization of coconut phosphatidylethanolamine species; and the second stage was utilization of coconut phosphatidylethanolamine liposomes to encapsulate vitamin C. A dark brown gel of coconut phosphatidylethanolamine species (CocoPEs) was isolated from dried coconut meat (9.3×10^{-3}%, w/w). At least 15 species were found in coconut phosphatidylethanolamine. The fatty acyl chains of the species were capric, linoleic, oleic, stearic and arachidic acyl chains. At least four different phases were identified on CocoPEs i.e. planar-shape gel phase, rippling phase, liquid crystal phase and hexagonal phase. The temperature (T_p) was at 25.29°C for changing from planar-shaped gel to rippling phase, 32.62°C (T_m) for major transition from gel to liquid crystal, and 65.53°C (T_h) from liquid crystal to hexagonal phase. All of CocoPEs liposomes encapsulation efficiency with cholesterol concentration up to 30% were above 80%. CocoPEs showed great potency as encapsulation material. It had high encapsulation efficiency and addition of cholesterol to the liposome membrane only slightly reduced the efficiency.

Keywords: cholesterol, *Cocos nucifera* L., coconut phosphatidylethanolamine, drug delivery, encapsulation, fatty acyl chain, liposome, phase behavior, phospholipid

1. Introduction

Phospholipids are major constituent of cellular membrane hence they have excellent biocompability. They are amphiphilic molecules which usually built by glycerol backbone with two different polarity groups attached to it. On the one hand is the hydrophilic group renowned as the head group which then becomes the basis of species classification of phospholipids, such as phosphatidylcholine (PC), phosphatidyletanolamine (PE), and phosphatidylserine (PS). On the other hand is the hydrophobic fatty acyl chains distinguished as the tails. The variation of the length and the saturation, the bonding position of fatty acyl chains to glycerol backbone as well as the head group type become a crucial part of their application, for instance in drug delivery systems.

The development of phospholipids based drug delivery systems have been proven prominent by the emergence of many phospholipid-related drug formulation. Among of them are doxorubicin in stealth liposomes for cancer treatment, which has been on the market since 1995 [1, 2]; Verteporfin in cationic liposomes for molecular degeneration [3] and vincristine in conventional liposome for Non-Hodgkin lymphoma [2]. They have been used in clinic, and achieve good results. Many more phospholipids based liposomal preparation have been developed to find better therapeutic results [4–6]. Furthermore various sources, synthetic and natural, have been explored [2, 7].

The isolation of phospholipids from natural sources cost lower than synthesizing them hence the preference is the isolation of natural phospholipids. For natural origin, the more pure they are, the greater the value is [8]. Phospholipids from natural origin can be refined into diverse levels, comprising food and pharmaceutical grade [2, 9]. In term of natural phospholipids, different source enhance the species variety of phospholipids [7]. Egg yolk and soybean phospholipids mainly consist of phosphatidylcholine species but they have differences in the tail portions which influence their physical, chemical properties and their applications. Other natural phospholipids that currently are being explored extensively are sunflower [10–12], candlenut [13], jack bean [14], sesame [13, 15–17] and coconut [13, 15, 16, 18–22].

Coconut is one of the native plantations in tropical countries and produces mainly copra and coconut oil. Exploration of coconut by-products such as coconut phospholipids needs to be done to increase the added value of these coconut plantations. Previous studies have found that dried coconut contain phospholipids from cephaline species with their fatty acyl chains are dodecanoic and octanoic acyl chains [15]. Purification with eluent chloroform: methanol (9:1) follows by identification using thin layer chromatography (TLC) also detects the presence of phosphatidylcholine (PC), phosphatidyletanolamine (PE), and phosphatidylserine (PS) species in coconut phospholipids (CocoPLs) [20, 21].

In the matter of its application, coconut liposomes (CocoPLs liposomes) have been used in the encapsulation of hydrophilic agent namely carboxyfluoresence and vitamin C and resulted in that CocoPLs liposomes has high efficiency of encapsulation [16, 19, 22]. The addition of cholesterol improves the encapsulation efficiency and low storage temperature reduces CocoPLs liposomes leakage. The results advocated the CocoPLs potency as drug delivery material. Moreover since we have established that CocoPLs consist of many phospholipid species therefore it would be valuable to study the component of the species and their capability as drug delivery system. In this study we explore the isolation and purification of coconut phospholipid species specifically coconut phosphatidylethanolamine (CocoPEs) and utilization of their liposomes (CocoPEs liposomes) for vitamin C encapsulation with various cholesterol concentrations. To our knowledge this is the first study of such.

2. Materials and methods

2.1 Materials

Materials used in this study were ripe coconut meat purchased from local market, TLC silica gel 60 F_{254} plate, silica gel powder 60 G for thin layer chromatography, various solvents and regents for analytical grade.

2.2 Coconut phospholipid (CocoPLs) isolation

Isolation technique was carried out based on the previous method used [20, 21]. Briefly coconut meat powder was macerated in a chloroform: methanol (2:1, v/v) mixture. The filtrate obtained was washed using 0.9% NaCl. The lipid was evaporated until thick coconut lipid extract were obtained. The extract was then subjected to solvent partition using n-hexane and ethanol 87%. The lower phase was evaporated to yield brownish yellow extract of CocoPLs.

2.3 Coconut phosphatidyletanolamines (CocoPEs) separation using vacuum liquid chromatography

About 5 g of CocoPLs was mixed with 5 g of silica gel in a small amount of chloroform: methanol (9:1, v/v) solution to form a silica slurry. The slurry was then stirred until the mixture was dried and formed fine powder of CocoPLs-SG.

A total of 80 mg of silica gel was poured into a chromatography column and compressed by vacuum. The column was rinsed using chloroform:methanol (9:1, v/v) eluent and vacuumed until all the eluent was eluted. The CocoPLs-SG powder was poured onto the column. Then the column was subjected to compression. Elution was performed using 10 ml of chloroform:methanol (9:1, v/v) solution. Fraction eluted from the column was collected into clean vials. The fraction was analyzed using TLC plate. The spot on the TLC plate was identified with 10% H_2SO_4 and ninhydrin. Elution was repeated every 10 ml of the eluent until the TLC plate did not show any spot when subjected to identification. The CocoPLs fractions contained ethanolamine species were gathered into an evaporating flask and evaporated at 40°C to obtain dark brownish gel of CocoPEs.

2.4 Characterization of CocoPLs and CocoPEs

Both CocoPLs and CocoPEs obtained were characterized using FT-IR (Prestige 21 Shimadzu), GC-MS (Shimadzu QP2010S), and LCMSMS (Waters Xevo TQD) and DSC (Shimadzu DSC-60A). The FTIR was employed to probe the phospholipids functional groups. The GC-MS was used to determine the phospholipids fatty acyl chains. The LC-MS/MS was for identifying the chemical component of CocoPEs and the DSC analysis was carried out to explore the CocoPEs phase behavior.

2.5 Vitamin C encapsulation in coconut liposomes

In this research, vitamin C (VC) was used as a model for hydrophilic drug to be encapsulated in coconut liposome [13, 16, 17, 22]. Stock solution of 500 ppm CocoPEs with cholesterol concentration (0%, 10%, 20%, 30%, 40% w/w) were made. A total of 2 mL of each stock solution was diluted with chloroform to 10 mL and poured into a test tube. The liquid solution was evaporated using N_2 gas flow to form a thin layer. After that hydration process was carried out. Around 10 mL of phosphate buffer solution was added to the thin film. The mixture was subjected to freeze-thawing process until the thin film was dispersed completely. The dispersions contained empty coconut liposome and was used as control. Other set of dispersions were prepared by adding 8 ppm (C_0) VC solution in phosphate buffer pH 7.4 to each 2 mL stock solution and followed by similar process to obtained encapsulated VC in coconut liposome dispersion. The VC concentration in the filtrates obtained after all coconut liposome dispersions were centrifuged were analyzed using UV-Vis spectrophotometer at 265 nm. The concentration of VC was calculated from the filtrate absorbance and represented as $C_{liposome+VC}$ and $C_{empty\ liposome}$ in equation 2.

In addition we used CocoPLs as comparison. The encapsulation efficiency of VC in coconut liposome was determined based on Eqs. (1) and (2):

$$EE = \frac{C_0 - C_t}{C_0} \times 100\% \qquad (1)$$

$$C_t = C_{liposome+VC} - C_{empty\ liposome} \qquad (2)$$

where *EE* is the encapsulation efficiency; C_0 is the initial concentration of VC; and C_t is the unencapsulated VC concentration.

3. Result and discussion

3.1 Isolation and separation

A brownish yellow gel of CocoPLs was obtained from dried coconut meat ($6.86 \times 10^{-2}\%$, w/w) (**Figure 1**). The result was confirmed by the appearance similarity of the CocoPLs from the previous research [20, 21]. The CocoPLs was then subjected to separation to obtain CocoPEs.

In the separation process using vacuum column chromatography, CocoPLs was eluted continuously using chloroform:methanol (9:1, v/v). Each fraction of 10 mL eluent was collected and subjected to identification. As much as 520 fractions were obtained to elute CocoPEs from the CocoPLs samples completely. Identification by

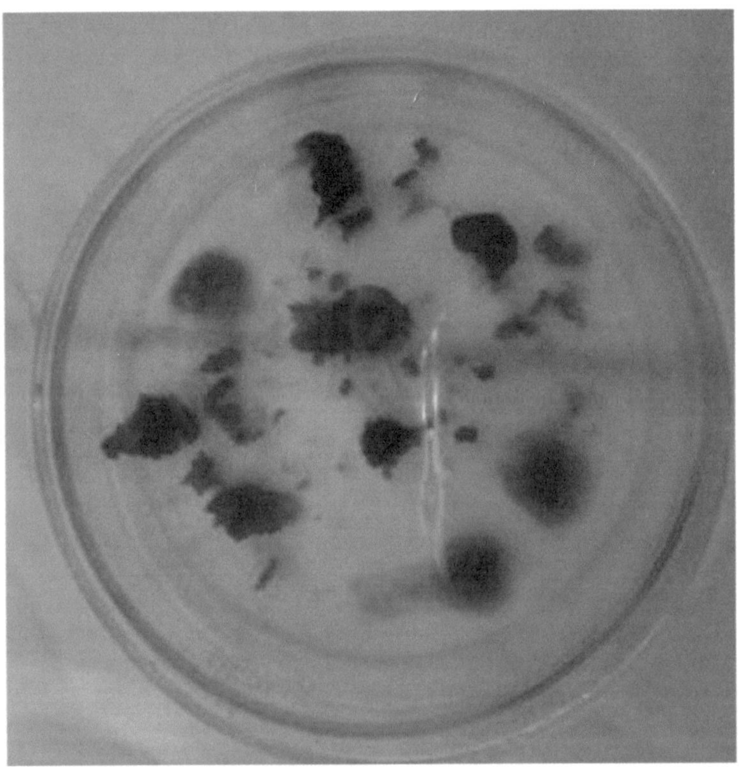

Figure 1.
CocoPLs.

TLC using 10% H_2SO_4 and ninhydrin spotting agent [23] resulted in that CocoPEs were present in the 105th to the 520th fraction.

The fraction contained CocoPEs were then combined and evaporated to remove the eluent that resulted in dark brown CocoPEs gel (9.8×10^{-3}%, w/w of dried coconut meat) (**Figure 2**).

3.2 Functional groups identification

The functional groups identification of CocoPLs and CocoPEs was conducted by FTIR spectra analysis. The FTIR spectra of both CocoPLs and CocoPEs were displayed on **Figure 3**. To analyze further the spectra were scrutinized using a deconvolution program [21, 24], at wavenumbers 3500–2800 cm^{-1} and 1800–700 cm^{-1} as presented in **Figure 4**.

The absorption data obtained from both FTIR spectra and deconvolution analysis were compared (see **Table 1**) to the specific infrared absorption area for phospholipids proposed by Stuart [25] and Hudiyanti et al. [20, 21]. The presence of a typical spectrum of phospholipids was clearly revealed. Significant differences between CocoPLs and CocoPEs spectra was disclosed by the typical absorption of choline and ethanolamine groups on both spectra of CocoPLs and CocoPEs. The choline group absorptions; $(CH_3)_3N^+$ asymmetric bending and $(CH_3)_3N^+$ asymmetry stretching; were not present on the CocoPEs spectra. The typical absorption that indicate the presence of ethanolamine species by N-H vibration absorptions was displayed on CocoPLs and CocoPEs spectra. This evident indicated that CocoPLs contained choline and ethanolamine species while CocoPEs did not contain choline

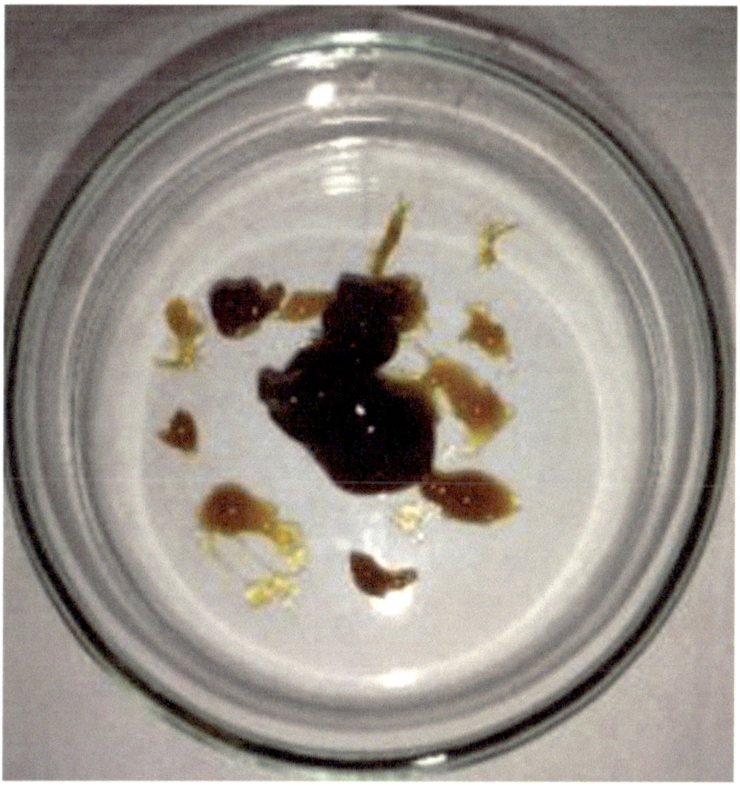

Figure 2.
CocoPEs.

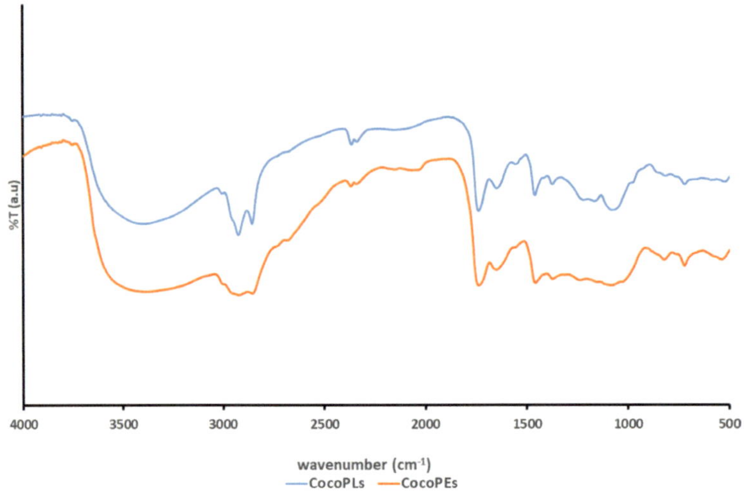

Figure 3.
CocoPLs and CocoPEs absorption spectra.

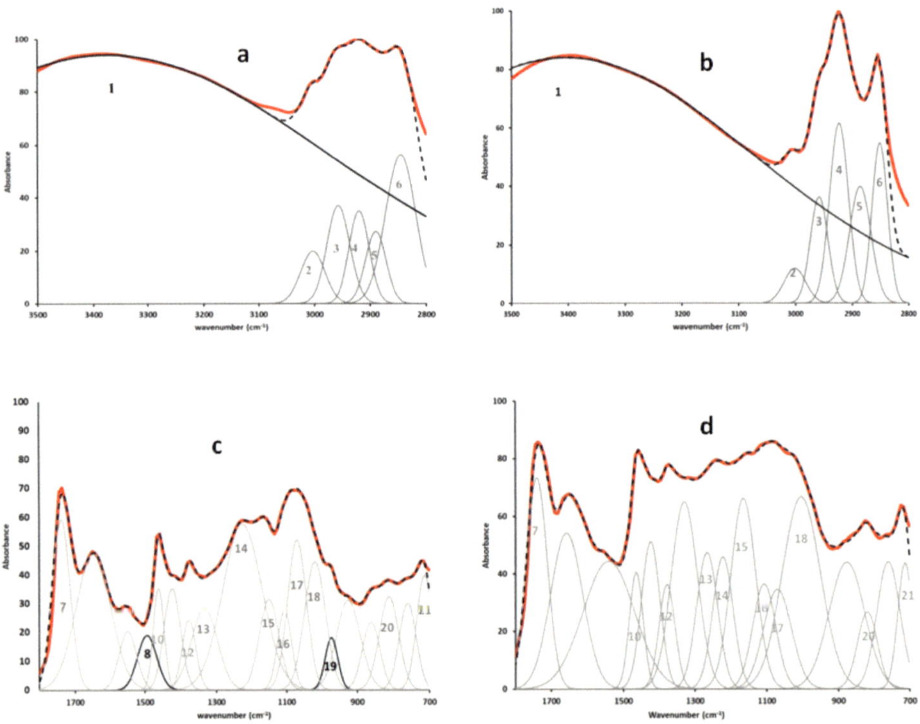

Figure 4.
Deconvolution results: (a) CocoPLs at wavenumbers 1800–700 cm^{-1}; (b) CocoPLs at wavenumbers 3500–2800 cm^{-1}; (c) CocoPEs at wavenumbers 1800–700 cm^{-1}; (d) CocoPEs at wavenumbers 3500–2800 cm^{-1}.

species. From The FTIR spectra point of view this data disclosed that the CocoPEs separation from CocoPLs was successful.

3.3 Characterization of fatty acyl chains

The fatty acyl chains content of CocoPLs and CocoPEs was analyzed by GC-MS. The CocoPLs chromatogram was presented on **Figure 5**. A total of nine

No.	Absorption type	References [15, 20, 21, 25] (cm^{-1})	CocoPLs (cm^{-1})	CocoPEs (cm^{-1})	CocoPLs Deconvolution (cm^{-1})	CocoPEs Deconvolution (cm^{-1})
1.	**N-H vibration**	**3471**	**3394**	**3379**	**3403**	**3373**
2.	=C-H stretching	3010	—	—	3001	3002
3.	CH_3 asymmetric stretching	2956	—	—	2958	2956
4.	CH_2 asymmetric stretching	2920	2924	2924	2923	2919
5.	CH_3 symmetric stretching	2870	—	—	2885	2890
6.	CH_2 symmetric stretching	2850	2854	2854	2850	2848
7.	C=O stretching, sn-1 chain trans-conformation	1730	1735	1735	1738	1739
8.	**(CH3)3N+ asymmetric bending**	**1485**	—	—	**1493**	—
9.	CH_2 scissoring	1473, 1472, 1468, 1463	—	—	—	—
10.	CH_3 asymmetric bending	1460	1458	1458	1461	1464
11.	$(CH_3)_3N_+$ symmetric bending	1405	—	—	—	—
12.	CH_3 symmetric bending	1378	1373	1373	1376	1378
13.	CH_3 rocking ribbon progression	1400–1200	—	—	1333	1266
14.	PO_2^-asymmetric stretching	1228	1226	1242	1225	1222
15.	CO-O-C asymmetric stretching	1170	1165	—	1150	1165
16.	PO_2^- symmetric stretching	1085	—	1080	1106	1107
17.	CO-O-C symmetric stretching	1070	1072	—	1071	1070
18.	C-O-P stretching	1047	—	—	1020	1003
19.	**(CH3)3N+ asymmetric stretching**	**972**	—	—	**973**	—
20.	P-O asymmetric stretching	820	817	—	813	819
21.	CH_2 rocking	730, 720, 718	717	725	714	713

Bold entries represented the typical absorption of choline and ethanolamine groups on both spectra of CocoPLs and CocoPEs.

Table 1.
Typical Absorption of CocoPLs and CocoPEs functional groups.

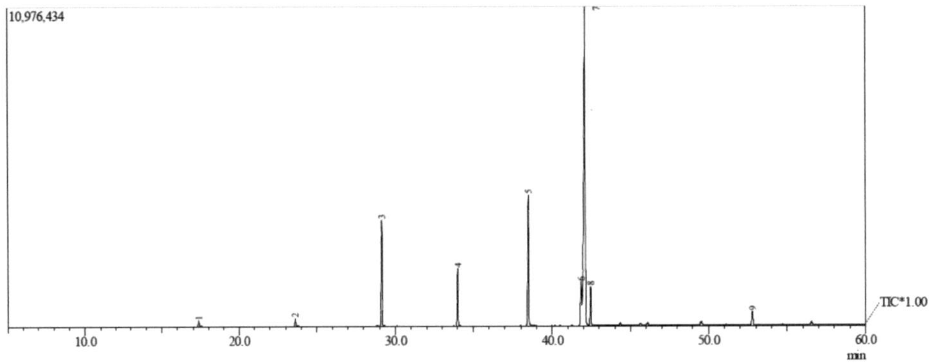

Figure 5.
CocoPLs chromatogram.

Peak number	t_R (min)	Fatty acyl chains	Area (%)
3.	29.164	Lauric acid, C12:0 (dodecanoic acid)	11.31
4.	34.037	Myristic acid, C14:0 (tetradecanoic acid)	5.71
5.	38.497	Palmitic acid, C16:0 (hexadecanoic acid)	15.26
6.	41.872	Linoleic acid, C18:2 (9(Z),12(Z)-octadecadienoic acid)	6.00
7.	42.117	Oleic acid, C18:1 (9(Z)-octadecenoic acid)	55.18
8.	42.482	Stearic acid, C18:0 (octadecanoic acid)	3.97
9.	52.794	Lignoceric acid, C24:0 (tetracosanoic acid)	1.49

Table 2.
The fatty acyl chains of CocoPLs.

peaks was recognized. Seven peaks were with abundance above 1%. The chromatogram suggested that there were at least 9 types of fatty acyl chains present on the CocoPLs. The MS reading revealed the identity of these fatty acyl chains. Three fatty acyl chains worth mentioning with the abundance more than 10%, i.e., lauric acid, palmitic acid and oleic acid which were indicated by peak number 3 (abundance of 11.31%); peak number 5 (15.26%); and peak number 7 (55.18%). The result was in agreement with previous research [15, 20, 21]. The seven fatty acyl chains recognized in CocoPLs was displayed on **Table 2**.

The chromatogram of CocoPEs was disclosed on **Figure 6**. The resulting chro matogram exposed the presence of five peaks with abundance above 1% which suggested the presence of five types of fatty acyl chains in the CocoPEs. Three of them had great abundance i.e. capric, linoleic and oleic acids as indicated by peak number 2, 3 and 4 and with abundance of 17.09%, 43.17% and 31.88% respectively. The MS reading of fatty acyl chains content in the CocoPEs was tabulated on **Table 3**.

Tables 2 and **3** revealed differences to some extent in fatty acyl chains composition between CocoPLs and CocoPEs. CocoPLs had more variation in fatty acyl chains type compared to CocoPEs. This fact plausible considering that CocoPEs was obtained from the separation of CocoPLs. The separation was mainly based on the common head group namely ethanolamine that reflected on the polarity of the separated CocoPEs molecules hence the choice of the separation eluent. More over fatty acyl chains profile were closely related to the position of phospholipid species in the bio-membrane bilayer [26–28]. Phosphatidylethanolamine (PE) species

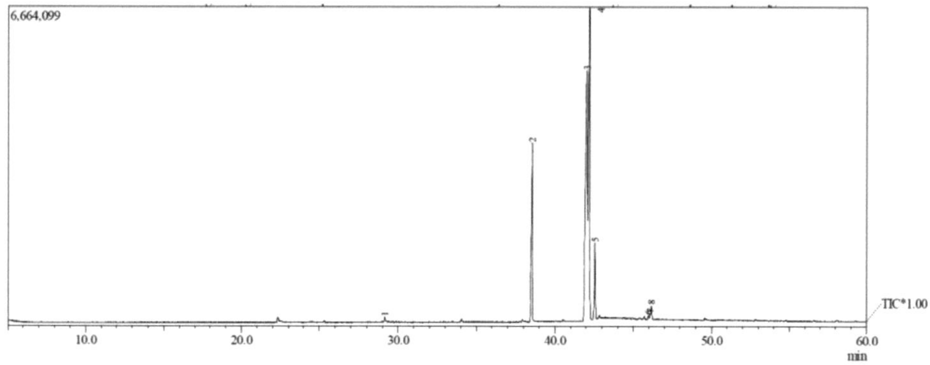

Figure 6.
CocoPEs chromatogram.

Peak number	t_R (min)	Fatty acyl chains	Area (%)
2.	38.566	Capric acid, C10:0 (decanoic acid)	17.09
3.	42.041	Linoleic acid, C18:2 (9(Z),12(Z)-octadecadienoic acid)	43.17
4.	42.198	Oleic acid, C18:1 (9(Z)-octadecenoic acid)	31.88
5.	42.555	Stearic acid, C18: 0 (octadecanoic acid)	5.93
8.	46.186	Arachidic acid, C20:0 (eicosanoic acid)	1.04

Table 3.
The Fatty acyl chains of CocoPEs.

generally would be positioned in the inner leaflet of bilayer due to their molecular geometry, i.e. cylinder [2]. The PE species molecular shape was supported by more abundance composition of unsaturated fatty acyl chains in the CocoPEs extract, **Table 3**.

3.4 Parent ion screening

Based on the fatty acyl chains of the CocoPEs we conducted parent ion screening using LCMSMS. The CocoPEs parent ion spectrogram was presented on **Figure 7**. The spectrogram gave us a representation of the molecular species composing CocoPEs extract. At least 11 molecular species of CocoPEs were found. The CocoPEs molecular species was tabulated on **Table 4**. The molecular species was predicted based on the head group and combination of two fatty acyl chains for the nonpolar part of CocoPEs species. These similar species would govern the CocoPEs phase behavior and other properties as well.

3.5 Phase behavior

Every phospholipid species has unique phase behavior that related to their molecular structure and phase behavior. The phase behavior of CocoPLs and CocoPEs were investigated by thermal analysis using DSC. The thermogram for CocoPLs, **Figure 8**, exhibited a small peak at 28.85°C and larger peak at 83.95°C. These peaks indicated that CocoPLs underwent phase changes as temperature changes. A pre-transition process from planar-shaped gel (L_b') to the rippling phase (P_b') was at a temperature of 28.85°C (T_p), then proceed with the

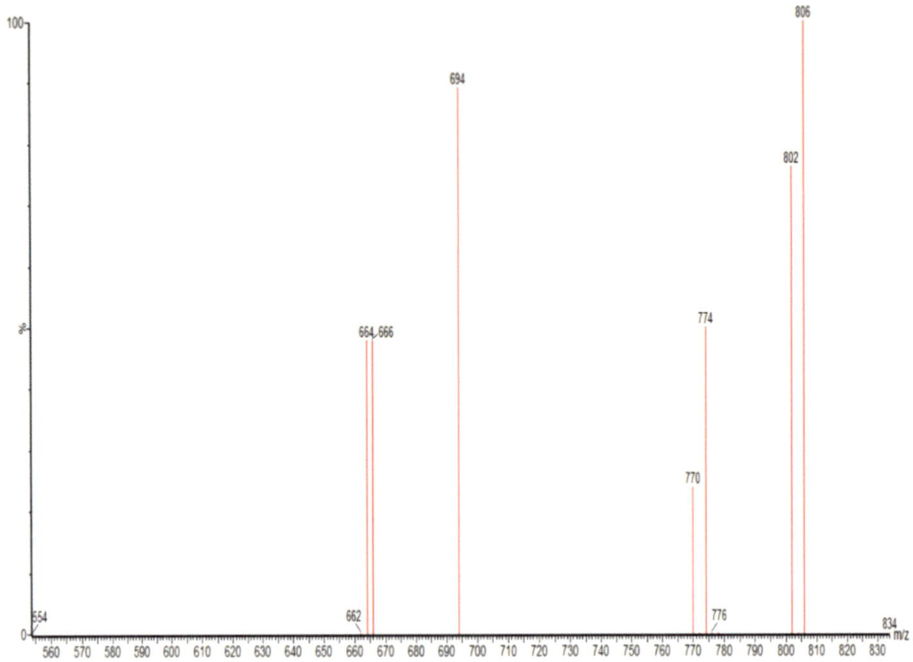

Figure 7.
CocoPEs spectrogram.

No.	m/z (M-H)	Molecular weight	CocoPEs molecular species	
			Head group	Fatty acyl chains
1.	554	555	Ethanolamine	Capric acid Capric acid
2.	662	663	Ethanolamine	Capric acid Linoleic acid
3.	664	665	Ethanolamine	Capric acid Oleic acid
4.	666	667	Ethanolamine	Capric acid Stearic acid
5.	694	695	Ethanolamine	Capric acid Arachidic acid
6.	770	771	Ethanolamine	Linoleic acid Linoleic acid
7.	774	775	Ethanolamine	Oleic acid Oleic acid
8.	776	777	Ethanolamine	Oleic acid Stearic acid
9.	802	803	Ethanolamine	Linoleic acid Arachidic acid
10.	806	807	Ethanolamine	Stearic acid Arachidic acid
11.	834	835	Ethanolamine	Arachidic acid Arachidic acid

Table 4.
CocoPEs molecular species prediction.

main transition from gel (L_b') to the liquid crystal phase (L_a) at a temperature of 83.95°C (T_m) [29–31]. T_p and T_m were the pre-transition and melting temperature correspondingly.

Different phase behavior of CocoPEs was exhibited in **Figure 9**. The thermogram for CocoPEs was more complex than CocoPLs indicated that CocoPEs had more complex phase transition than CocoPLs. CocoPEs displayed pre-transition process from planar-shaped gel (L_b') to a rippling phase (P_b') at a temperature of 25.29°C (T_p), followed by a major transition from gel (L_b') to liquid crystal phase (L_a) at a temperature of 32.62°C (T_m), and then a transition from the liquid crystal phase (L_a) to hexagonal phase (H) at a temperature of 65.53°C (T_h) [32]. The

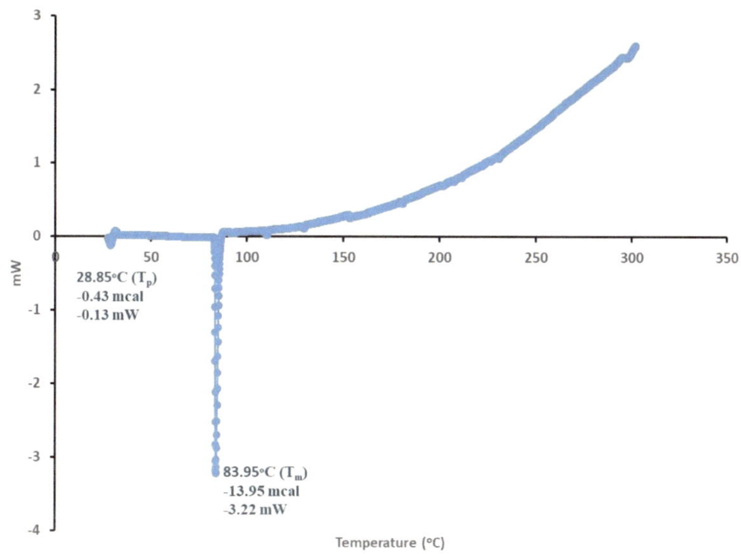

Figure 8.
Thermal analysis of CocoPLs.

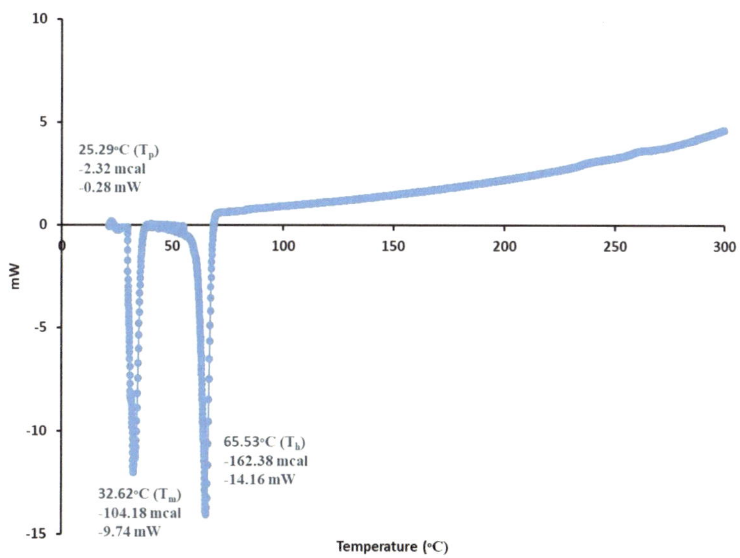

Figure 9.
Thermal analysis of CocoPEs.

hexagonal phase formation was consistent to cylindrical molecular shape attributed to CocoPEs. The CocoPEs gradual change of phase was estimated because of the similar molecular species composing CocoPEs.

The phase behavior of CocoPEs dan CocoPLs above indicated that they were both had complex self-assembly structures which would be beneficial for future applications [2].

3.6 Encapsulation of vitamin C in coconut (CocoPLs and CocoPEs) liposomes

Phospholipids has long been known as drug delivery substance due to their liposome forming ability. Liposome was a spherical aggregation structure with bilayer phospholipid as its shell surrounding aqueous core. This unique structure was especially a perfect vehicle for delivering hydrophilic and hydrophobic drugs with storage and controlled release purposes. In this paper as a preliminary study for further application of coconut phospholipid as drug delivery material we used vitamin C as a hydrophilic drug model to be encapsulated in coconut liposomes. Vitamin C was a hydrophilic drug and would be encapsulated inside the aqueous core of liposome. The study lead to that encapsulation efficiency of vitamin C in CocoPEs were higher than CocoPLs i.e. 94.44% and 92.40% respectively, **Figure 10**.

In relation to their application as drug delivery, liposomes were usually made from phospholipid and a small amount of cholesterol. Cholesterol was added to the liposome membrane to control liposome rigidity and penetrability [33]. Therefore to explore the effect of cholesterol on the encapsulation efficiency of coconut liposomes we also prepared coconut liposomes with several different concentration of cholesterol namely 10%, 20%, 30% and 40%. The encapsulation efficiency of the liposomes were presented on **Figure 10**. The results suggested that addition of cholesterol up to 40% in the liposome's membrane reduced the encapsulation efficiency of CocoPEs and CocoPLs liposomes. Furthermore CocoPEs liposomes demonstrated slighter reduction than CocoPLs liposomes. The encapsulation efficiency of CocoPEs diminished gradually as the cholesterol concentration increased while for CocoPLs liposomes the decline was arbitrary. Addition up to 30% of cholesterol only reduced the CocoPEs encapsulation efficiency to around 80% while CocoPLs was as low as 52%. Cholesterol effect on the encapsulation efficiency of CocoPEs

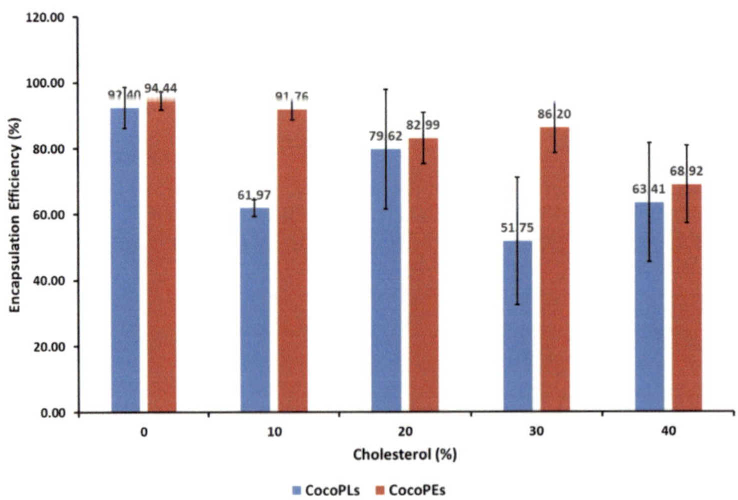

Figure 10.
Encapsulation efficiency of CocoPLs and CocoPEs liposomes with cholesterol composition variation.

liposomes more consistent than CocoPLs. We suspected it was due to the molecular composition of the phospholipid in the membrane. The molecular composition was represented by the composition of functional group and fatty acyl chains in the CocoPEs and CocoPLs, **Tables 1–3**. In the liposome membrane cholesterol interacted with CocoPEs and CocoPLs through their functional groups and fatty acyl chains. Cholesterol with small hydrophilic head group i.e., –OH and big and rigid hydrophobic steroid ring would interact better with small head group phospholipid species like CocoPEs than CocoPLs which had big spherical choline group and possibly other head groups as well. The composition of fatty acyl with double bonds also suspected would give more room for cholesterol hydrophobic moiety. The fatty acyl chains would assume "kink" structure at the double bond position [34, 35] and allocate more space hence more comfortable for cholesterol to integrate. With smaller number of fatty acyl chains type and higher concentration of double bond made cholesterol effect became more systematic in the CocoPEs liposome membrane. The data gave an insight about the application of CocoPEs as encapsulation material. CocoPEs was a good candidate for encapsulation hydrophilic material.

4. Conclusion

A total of (9.8×10^{-3}%, w/w) of coconut phosphatidylethanolamine species (CocoPEs) was isolated from dried coconut meat. The CocoPEs were obtained in the form of a dark brownish gel. Parent ion screening by LCMSMS revealed that 15 species were found in CocoPEs. Characterization of fatty acyl chains by GCMS resulted in that the hydrophobic part of the species were comprised of capric, linoleic, oleic, stearic and arachidic acyl chains. Phase behavior analysis using DSC obtained at least four different phases on CocoPEs i.e. planar-shape gel phase, rippling phase, liquid crystal phase and hexagonal phase. Each phase change occurred at a particular temperature. The pre-transition temperature (T_p) was from planar-shaped gel to rippling phase at 25.29°C, the melting temperature (T_m) for major transition from gel to liquid crystal at 32.62°C, and the hexagonal phase formation from liquid crystal (T_h) at 65.53°C. CocoPEs liposome had high encapsulation efficiency. The presence of cholesterol in the membrane liposome up to 30% did not change much of their encapsulation efficiency. The encapsulation efficiencies were above 80%. Meanwhile coconut phospholipids (CocoPLs) had them above 90% but then decrease irregularly to 52% at 0% and 30% cholesterol respectively.

Acknowledgements

DH and KA would like to express their gratitude of financial support by DIPA Selain APBN FSM UNDIP Riset Madya, 2018.

Conflict of interest

The authors declare that there is no conflict of interests regarding the publication of this chapter.

Author details

Dwi Hudiyanti[1*], Nur Kamila[2], Febriani Kusuma Wardani[2] and Khairul Anam[1]

1 Chemistry Department, Faculty of Science and Mathematics, Diponegoro University, Semarang, Indonesia

2 Chemistry Program, Chemistry Department Faculty of Science and Mathematics, Diponegoro University, Semarang, Indonesia

*Address all correspondence to: dwi.hudiyanti@live.undip.ac.id

IntechOpen

© 2019 The Author(s). Licensee IntechOpen. This chapter is distributed under the terms of the Creative Commons Attribution License (http://creativecommons.org/licenses/by/3.0), which permits unrestricted use, distribution, and reproduction in any medium, provided the original work is properly cited.

References

[1] Sahu AN. Nanotechnology in herbal medicines and cosmetics. International Journal of Research in Ayurveda and Pharmacy. 2013;**4**:472-474. DOI: 10.7897/2277-4343.04334

[2] Li J, Wang X, Zhang T, Wang C, Huang Z, Luo X, et al. A review on phospholipids and their main applications in drug delivery systems. Asian Journal of Pharmaceutical Sciences. 2015;**10**:81-98. DOI: 10.1016/J.AJPS.2014.09.004

[3] Bozzuto G, Molinari A. Liposomes as nanomedical devices. International Journal of Nanomedicine. 2015;**10**:975-999. DOI: 10.2147/IJN.S68861

[4] Sercombe L, Veerati T, Moheimani F, Wu SY, Sood AK, Hua S. Advances and challenges of liposome assisted drug delivery. Frontiers in Pharmacology. 2015;**6**:286. DOI: 10.3389/fphar.2015.00286

[5] Zylberberg C, Matosevic S. Pharmaceutical liposomal drug delivery: A review of new delivery systems and a look at the regulatory landscape. Drug Delivery. 2016;**23**:3319-3329. DOI: 10.1080/10717544.2016.1177136

[6] Abu Lila AS, Ishida T. Liposomal delivery systems: Design optimization and current applications. Biological & Pharmaceutical Bulletin. 2017;**40**:1-10. DOI: 10.1248/bpb.b16-00624

[7] van Hoogevest P, Wendel A. The use of natural and synthetic phospholipids as pharmaceutical excipients. European Journal of Lipid Science and Technology. 2014;**116**:1088-1107. DOI: 10.1002/ejlt.201400219

[8] Paltauf F, Hermetter A. Phospholipids — Natural, semisynthetic, synthetic. In: Phospholipids. Boston, MA: Springer US; 1990. pp. 1-12. DOI: 10.1007/978-1-4757-1364-0_1

[9] Liu D, Ma F. Soybean phospholipids. In: Krezhova D, editor. Recent Trends for Enhancing the Diversity and Quality of Soybean Products. London: IntechOpen; 2011. pp. 483-500. DOI: 10.5772/20986

[10] Komaiko J, Sastrosubroto A, McClements DJ. Encapsulation of ω-3 fatty acids in nanoemulsion-based delivery systems fabricated from natural emulsifiers: Sunflower phospholipids. Food Chemistry. 2016;**203**:331-339. DOI: 10.1016/J.FOODCHEM.2016.02.080

[11] Cabezas DM, Guiotto EN, Diehl BWK, Tomás MC. Antioxidant and Emulsifying Properties of Modified Sunflower Lecithin by Fractionation with Ethanol-Water Mixtures. In: Muzzalupo I, editor. Food Industry. London: InTechOpen; 2013. pp. 589-602. DOI: 10.5772/53165

[12] Meng X, Pan Q, Ding Y, Jiang L. Rapid determination of phospholipid content of vegetable oils by FTIR spectroscopy combined with partial least-square regression. Food Chemistry. 2014;**147**:272-278. DOI: 10.1016/J.FOODCHEM.2013.09.143

[13] Hudiyanti D, Raharjo TJ, Narsito NS. Investigation on the morphology and properties of aggregate structures of natural phospholipids in aqueous system using cryo-tem. Indonesian Journal of Chemistry. 2012;**12**:54-61. DOI: 10.22146/ijc.21372

[14] Hudiyanti D, Arya AP, Siahaan P, Suyati L. Chemical composition and phospholipids content of Indonesian Jack Bean (*Canavalia ensiformis* L.). Oriental Journal of Chemistry. 2015;**31**:2043-2046. DOI: 10.13005/ojc/310423

[15] Hudiyanti D, Raharjo TJTJ, Narsito N, Noegrohati S. Isolasi Dan Karakterisasi Lesitin Kelapa Dan Wijen. agriTECH. 2012;**32**:23-26. DOI: 10.22146/agritech.9652

[16] Hudiyanti D, Raharjo TJ, Narsito N, Noegrohati S. Study on leakage of sesame (*Sesamum indicum* L.) and coconut (*Cocos nucifera* L.) liposomes. Oriental Journal of Chemistry. 2015;**31**:435-439. DOI: 10.13005/ojc/310152

[17] Hudiyanti D, Fawrin H, Siahaan P. Simultant encapsulation of vitamin C and beta-carotene in sesame (*Sesamum indicum* L.) liposomes. IOP Conference Series: Materials Science and Engineering. 2018;**349**:012014. DOI: 10.1088/1757-899X/349/1/012014

[18] Hudiyanti D, Supardi A, Nugroho S. The characteristics of coconut phospholipids as biosurfactants. Jurnal Sains Dan Matematika. 2012;**20**:93-97

[19] Hudiyanti D, Triana D, Siahaan P. Studi Pendahuluan tentang Enkapsulasi Vitamin C dalam Liposom Kelapa (*Cocos nucifera* L.). Jurnal Kimia Sains dan Aplikasi. 2017;**20**:5. DOI: 10.14710/jksa.20.1.5-8

[20] Hudiyanti D, Al Khafiz MF, Anam K. Coconut (*Cocos nucifera* L.) lipids: Extraction and characterization. Oriental Journal of Chemistry. 2018;**34**:1136-1140. DOI: 10.13005/ojc/340268

[21] Hudiyanti D, Jayanti M, Fuad Al-Khafiz M, Anam K. A study of coconut (*Cocos nucifera* L.) phosphatidylcholine species. Oriental Journal of Chemistry. 2018;**34**:2963-2968. DOI: 10.13005/ojc/340636

[22] Hudiyanti D, Aminah S, Hikmahwati Y, Siahaan P. Cholesterol implications on coconut liposomes encapsulation of beta-carotene and vitamin C. IOP Conference Series: Materials Science and Engineering. 2019;**509**:012037. DOI: 10.1088/1757-899X/509/1/012037

[23] Friedman M. Applications of the ninhydrin reaction for analysis of amino acids, peptides, and proteins to agricultural and biomedical sciences. Journal of Agricultural and Food Chemistry. 2004;**52**:385-406. DOI: 10.1021/jf030490p

[24] Wojdyr M. *Fityk*: A general-purpose peak fitting program. Journal of Applied Crystallography. 2010;**43**:1126-1128. DOI: 10.1107/S0021889810030499

[25] Stuart BH. Infrared Spectroscopy: Fundamentals and Applications. Chichester: John Wiley & Sons; 2004

[26] De Kruyff B, Van Den Besselaar AMHP, Van Deenen LM. Outside-inside distribution and translocation of lysophosphatidylcholine in phosphatidylcholine vesicles as determined by 13C-NMR using (N-13CH3)-enriched lipids. Biochimica et Biophysica Acta - Biomembranes. 1977;**465**:443-453. DOI: 10.1016/0005-2736(77)90263-2

[27] Parisio G, Ferrarini A, Sperotto MM. Model studies of lipid flip-flop in membranes. International Journal of Advances in Engineering Sciences and Applied Mathematics. 2016;**8**:134-146. DOI: 10.1007/s12572-015-0155-9

[28] Marquardt D, Geier B, Pabst G. Asymmetric lipid membranes: Towards more realistic model systems. Membranes (Basel). 2015;**5**:180-196. DOI: 10.3390/membranes5020180

[29] Garidel P, Johann C, Blume A. Non-ideal mixing and fluid–fluid immiscibility in phosphatidic acid–phosphatidylethanolamine mixed

bilayers. European Biophysics Journal. 2011;**40**:891-905. DOI: 10.1007/s00249-011-0707-2

[30] Gennis RB. The Structures and Properties of Membrane Lipids. In: Biomembranes. New York: Springer; 1989. pp. 36-84. DOI: 10.1007/978-1-4757-2065-5_2

[31] Lewis RN, Mantsch HH, McElhaney RN. Thermotropic phase behavior of phosphatidylcholines with omega-tertiary-butyl fatty acyl chains. Biophysical Journal. 1989;**56**:183-193. DOI: 10.1016/S0006-3495(89)82663-3

[32] Jouhet J. Importance of the hexagonal lipid phase in biological membrane organization. Frontiers in Plant Science. 2013;**4**:494. DOI: 10.3389/fpls.2013.00494

[33] Kaddah S, Khreich N, Kaddah F, Charcosset C, Greige-Gerges H. Cholesterol modulates the liposome membrane fluidity and permeability for a hydrophilic molecule. Food and Chemical Toxicology. 2018;**113**:40-48

[34] Róg T, Murzyn K, Gurbiel R, Takaoka Y, Kusumi A, Pasenkiewicz-Gierula M. Effects of phospholipid unsaturation on the bilayer nonpolar region. Journal of Lipid Research. 2004;**45**:326-336. DOI: 10.1194/JLR.M300187-JLR200

[35] Yesylevskyy SO, Demchenko AP, Kraszewski S, Ramseyer C. Cholesterol induces uneven curvature of asymmetric lipid bilayers. The Scientific World Journal. 2013;**2013**:965230. DOI: 10.1155/2013/965230

Section 2

Rheology of Micro-Emulsions

Chapter 7

Rheology of Structured Oil Emulsion

Gudret Isfandiyar Kelbaliyev, Dilgam Babir Tagiyev and Manaf Rizvan Manafov

Abstract

This study is devoted to the rheology of oil emulsions, accompanied by both the formation and destruction of the structure. The presence of particles of a dispersed phase in an oil emulsion, including asphaltenes and resins, determines the formation of coagulation structures as a result of interaction and collision of particles. In this regard, to study the formation of coagulation structures, analytical solutions to the mass transfer equations are proposed, based on which the coalescence and fragmentation frequencies of the droplets are determined. Models and analytical solutions of the equation for the thinning of an interfacial film between droplets with their coalescence in the volume of an oil emulsion are proposed taking into account the Marangoni effect and the effect of asphaltene content. The thickness of the adsorbed layer on the droplet surface was estimated. Many empirical and semi-empirical formulas have been proposed for determining the dependence of viscosity on the content of water and asphalt-resinous substances in oil. Based on the solution of the Fokker-Planck equation, the evolution of the distribution function of droplets in time and size in an oil emulsion is studied.

Keywords: oil emulsion, rheology, coalescence, deformation, breaking, asphaltenes, drop, viscosity, Marangoni effect, distribution function

1. Introduction

The separation processes of oil emulsions are an important stage for the preparation and purification of crude oil from water, mineral salts and various related impurities, asphalt-resinous substances, and paraffins contained in oil. The processes of separation of oil emulsions, the purpose of which is to completely reduce their aggregative and kinetic stability, are carried out in various ways: in gravitational (settling systems and other modifications); in centrifugal, electric, and magnetic fields [1–4]; as well as using filtering through solid and liquid layers, using microwave and membrane technology [5, 6].

Oil emulsions contain water droplets of a sufficiently large size, in connection with which, in most practical applications, high-capacity separation processes use settling systems, and at small sizes and droplet concentrations, using a constant electric field and membrane technologies or combined methods to achieve high degree of purification.

Experimental and theoretical studies indicate a very complex, in disperse composition (separation) and in the flowing physical phenomena (coalescence, deformation, crushing), the structure of the intermediate layer. Many works have been devoted to theoretical and experimental studies of the mechanism of the formation of stabilization and destruction of oil emulsions as heterogeneous media [2, 4]; although many problems associated with the phenomena occur at the oil–water interface, the coalescence and fragmentation of water droplets, separation, and deposition have not been resolved correctly. Oil emulsions are polydisperse media with droplet sizes of 1–150 microns, although coarse (150–1000 microns) and colloidal (0.001–1 microns) particles are found in them. Such a size dispersion has a significant effect on the mechanism of structure formation, structural destruction, separation, and precipitation of droplets in oil emulsions. The mechanism of destruction and coalescence of droplets in oil emulsions can be divided into the following stages [7, 8]:

a. Convergence and collision of droplets of different sizes with the formation of an interfacial film. It should be noted that droplet transfer in a polydisperse medium is determined mainly by hydrodynamic conditions and flow turbulence. Under conditions of isotropic turbulence, the collision frequency of droplets depends on the specific dissipation of the energy of the turbulent flow and the properties of the medium and the dispersed phase [9–12]. As a result of the collision and fixation of two drops with sizes a_1 and a_2, an interfacial film of circular cross section is formed, the radius of which can be determined in the form [13]

$$R_K = \left[\frac{3\pi}{4} P_m (k_1 + k_2) a_r\right]^{1/3} \quad (1)$$

where P_m is the maximum compressive pressure, k_1, k_2 are the elastic coefficients of two drops, $a_r = {a_1 a_2}/{(a_1+a_2)}$ is the average size of the drops, and a_1, a_2 are the diameters of two drops. In [14], the expression for the hydrodynamic compression pressure in a turbulent flow is defined as

$$P_m = \pi a_r^2 \rho_C \vec{U}^2 \quad (2)$$

b. The deformation and destruction of adsorption shells at the oil–water interface in the flow volume at certain temperatures (60–70^{0}C) and pressures.

c. Thinning and rupture of the interfacial film, followed by coalescence and coarsening of the droplets. The rupture of the interfacial film contributes to the coalescence of smaller droplets into larger ones. It is important to note that as a result of the transport of the oil emulsion in the pipes, the droplet crushing rate is much higher than the coalescence rate, as a result of which the oil emulsion is characterized by a large dispersion of droplet size and polydispersity of the medium.

d. Precipitation of droplets and separation of the dispersed phase as a continuous phase (separation).

An equally important factor affecting the efficiency of separation of oil emulsions is the conditions of thinning, tearing of the interfacial film [7], and the coalescence rate associated with the destruction of the adsorbed film on the surface of the droplets with the participation of demulsifiers.

The rheology of oil emulsions is associated with the presence of coagulation phenomena of dispersed particles in the presence of asphalt-resinous substances, accompanied in most cases by structure formation. The rheological properties of oil emulsions largely depend on the state of aggregation (solid phase, droplets, gas bubbles) and the properties of the dispersion medium. However, the presence of a dispersed phase can significantly change these properties under the influence of adhesion forces between particles of a dispersed phase and their interaction with a dispersion medium. In free-dispersed systems, particles of a dispersed phase are not interconnected and are able to independently move in a dispersion medium. In connected dispersed systems, particles of the dispersed phase form continuous spatial networks (structures); they lose their ability to transitional movement, maintaining only oscillatory movements. Unstable disperse systems provide structure formation in the system, up to the formation of aggregates and a skeleton, which can negatively affect the structural state (viscosity, fluidity), changing rheological properties, as well as to obtain precipitation during phase separation, treatment of industrial emissions, wastewater, etc. Aggregate stability characterizes the ability of a dispersed system to maintain a uniform distribution of particles of a dispersed phase over the volume of a dispersed medium without their interaction, providing conditions for the stability of the medium to phase separation. The loss of aggregative stability in concentrated emulsions is associated with coagulation of particles and their enlargement and can manifest itself in the formation of a bulk structure in which the dispersion medium is evenly distributed, thereby changing the rheological properties of the medium. The aggregate stability of dispersed systems with respect to coagulation is determined by the coagulation rate, which, in addition to the intensity of Brownian and hydrodynamic motion and the number of collisions, depends on the properties of the surface layers surrounding the particles. A deeper coagulation process leads to the destruction of the interlayers of the medium and direct contact of the particles, resulting in the formation of rigid coagulation structures and aggregates of particles, or their complete merging in the case of a liquid and gaseous dispersed phase (coalescence) (**Figure 1**).

The formation of coagulation structures and aggregates in the flow volume significantly affects the physical properties of oil emulsions associated with a sharp increase in the structural viscosity of the medium.

Based on this, the aim of this work is to study (a) the phenomena of coalescence, deformation, and crushing of droplets in a turbulent flow and the formation of coagulation structures associated with this; (b) the effect of asphalt-resinous substances on the formation of adsorption films and the structural viscosity of emulsions; (c) issues related to thinning and tearing of an interfacial film; and (d) the evolution of the droplet size and time distribution functions, taking into account coalescence and fragmentation of the droplets.

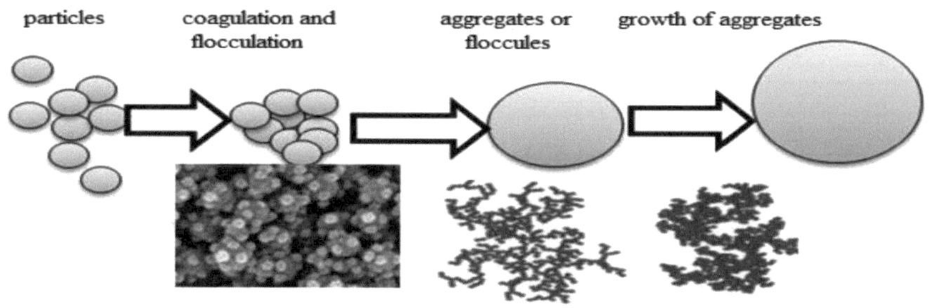

Figure 1.
Scheme of coagulation and formation of aggregates of particles of various structures.

2. Coalescence, deformation, and crushing of droplets in an oil emulsion

The structural and mechanical stability of emulsion systems is associated with the formation of adsorption layers at the oil–water interface, the composition of which consists of asphaltenes, resins, paraffins, mineral salts, and solid particles, i.e., natural surfactants [1–4]. It has been established that metal-paraffin complexes lead to the formation of the shell itself and solid particles (sand, clay, limestone, etc.) contribute to increasing the strength of the shells [3, 4]. An analysis of the composition of these shells on the surface of water droplets of crude oil of various fields shows that the main stabilizers are asphaltenes and resins, which include high-melting paraffins and inorganic mechanical impurities. The structure, composition, and physicochemical properties of asphaltenes, which are very complex compounds, are given in [14–17]. The formation of an adsorption layer on the surface of water droplets with elastic and viscous properties contributes to the stabilization of oil emulsions.

2.1 The influence of asphalt-resinous substances on the separation of oil emulsions

Consequently, the stability of oil emulsions is the result of a physical barrier that prevents tearing of the film when the collision energy between the droplets is insufficient to destroy the adsorption layer. The mechanism of the formation of adsorption films on the surface is determined by the following stages:

a. Diffusive mass transfer of the substance (asphaltenes) from the volume of oil to the surface of water droplets. In [18], the mass flow to the surface of a moving drop per unit time for small numbers $\mathrm{Re} = \frac{Ua_r}{\nu_c} << 1$ is defined as

$$I = \sqrt{\frac{\pi}{6}}\left[\frac{D}{a_r}\frac{\eta_C}{\eta_C + \eta_d}\right]^{1/2} a_r^2 \Delta C \sqrt{U} \tag{3}$$

where $\Delta C = C_0 - C_S$ and C_0, C_S are the contents of asphaltenes and resins in the volume and on the surface. Assuming that the change in the mass of the adsorbed layer is determined by $dm/d\tau = I$, integrating which we obtain $m - m_0 = I\tau$ (τ is the residence time, and m_0 is the initial mass of the adsorbed layer, taken equal to zero). Then, putting $m = \frac{1}{6}\pi\rho_a(a_r + 2\Delta)^3 - \frac{1}{6}\pi\rho_a a_r^3$ and taking into account the insignificance of the expansion terms of the second and third order of smallness ($\frac{\Delta}{a_r} << 1$), we have $m \approx \pi\rho_a a_r^3 \frac{\Delta}{a_r} = I\tau$. Taking into account expression (3), the thickness of the adsorbed layer is defined as

$$\frac{\Delta}{a_r} \approx \frac{1}{\sqrt{6\pi}}\left[\frac{1}{Pe}\frac{1}{1+\gamma}\right]^{1/2}\left(\frac{\Delta C}{\rho_a} St\right) \tag{4}$$

where $\gamma = \eta_d/\eta_C$, $\mathrm{Pe} = \frac{Ua_r}{D}$ is the Peclet number, $\mathrm{St} = \frac{U\tau}{a_r}$ is the modified Strouhal number, and ρ_a is the density of the adsorbed layer. It follows from Eq. (4) that the thickness of the adsorbed layer depends on the diffusion of particles to the surface of the droplet, the size and mobility of the surface of the droplets, and on the concentration of asphaltenes in the flow volume. For the values $Pe = 10^2 - 10^3$ ($D \approx 10^{-10} - 10^{-9} м^2/c$), $\gamma = 0.8$, $\Delta C/\rho_a \approx 10^{-5}$, and $\mathrm{St} = 10^4 - 10^5$, from the equation, we estimate $\Delta/a_r \approx 0.01 - 0.03$. Large values of the number, which are the result of small values of the coefficient of diffusion of particles in a liquid, in some cases determine the prevalence of convective transport of matter over diffusion. Further compaction of the adsorption layer under the influence of external perturbations and chemical transformations contribute to an increase in the density of the layer and the "aging" of emulsions. Despite the insignificant thickness of the adsorption layer compared to the size of the droplet, their strength on the surface of the droplets for various oils ranges from 0.5 to 1.1 $^{N}/_{m^2}$ [3].

b. Adsorption of the substance on the surface of the droplets.

c. Desorption and destruction of the adsorption layer with the participation of surface-active substances (surfactants). If the rate of adsorption and desorption is low compared to the rate of supply of the substance to the surface of the droplet, the process of formation of the adsorption layer is limited by the processes of adsorption and desorption. Assume that the concentration of adsorbed matter in the volume C_0 and on the surface Γ. By analogy with the derivation of the Langmuir equation, if we assume that the adsorption rate of the substance on the surface of the droplet is $W_A = \beta C_0 \left(1 - {}^{\Gamma}/_{\Gamma_\infty}\right)$ and the desorption rate is $W_D = \alpha\Gamma$, then in the equilibrium state $(W_A = W_D)$, we have

$$\Gamma = \frac{KC_0}{1 + K_0 C_0} \tag{5}$$

where α, β are some constants, depending on temperature, $K = {}^{\beta}/_{\alpha}$, $K_0 = {}^{\beta}/_{\alpha\Gamma_\infty}$, and Γ_∞ is the maximum saturation of the droplet surface. Eq. (3) is in good agreement with many experimental data for oils of various fields. **Figure 2** shows the adsorption isotherm of asphaltenes on the surface of water droplets (T = 40°C) [19] for North Caucasian oils and the calculated values according to Eq. (5), where $K = 55, K_0 = 0.5$.

To destroy the adsorption films in the flow volume, various demulsifiers (SAS) are used, which are characterized by high surface activity during adsorption. The mechanism of destruction of adsorption films consists in the diffusion transfer of the demulsifier to the film surface, with further adsorption and penetration of the film into its volume, the formation of defects and cracks in its structure, a change in surface tension, and a decrease in strength properties, which qualitatively changes the rheological properties of the films at the oil-gas interface water. Further separation of oil emulsions is determined by the frequency of droplet collisions, their fixation on the surface, thinning, and rupture of the interfacial film.

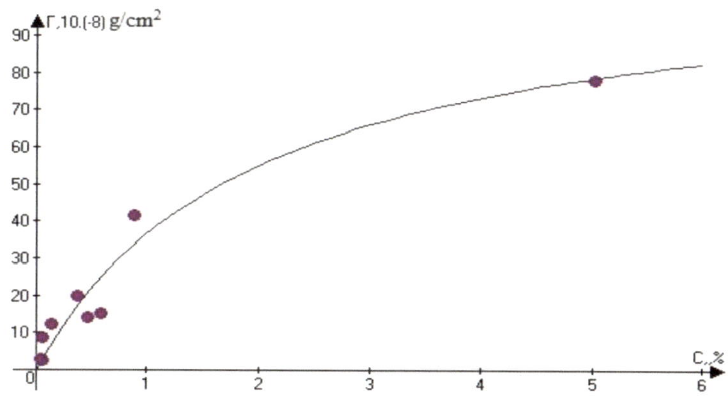

Figure 2.
Dependence of the concentration of adsorbed matter on the surface on the concentration of asphaltenes (points—experiment [19]).

2.2 Thinning and destruction of the interfacial film taking into account the Marangoni effect

When fixing two drops as a result of their collision, the resulting interfacial film under the action of various kinds of forces is thinned to a certain critical thickness and breaks with the further merging of two drops. Assuming that in a flat film of circular cross section the laminar flow, the momentum transfer equation in cylindrical coordinates is written in the form [7, 8].

$$-\frac{\partial P}{\partial r}+\frac{\eta}{gr^2}\frac{\partial^2 V_r}{\partial \theta^2}+\frac{\eta}{g}\frac{\partial^2 V_r}{\partial x^2}=0 \tag{6}$$

$$-\frac{1}{r}\frac{\partial P}{\partial \theta}+\frac{2\eta}{gr^2}\frac{\partial V_r}{\partial \theta}=0 \tag{7}$$

$$\frac{\partial V_x}{\partial x}+\frac{1}{r}\frac{\partial (rV_r)}{\partial r}=0 \tag{8}$$

where P is the pressure in the film, V_r, V_x are the components of the flow velocity in the film, and θ is the polar angle. The boundary conditions for solving these equations are

$$x=\delta,\ -\eta\frac{\partial V_r}{\partial r}=\frac{d\sigma}{dr}+\frac{1}{R_K\sin\theta}\frac{\partial\sigma(\cos\theta)}{\partial\theta} \tag{9}$$

The last condition determines the presence of convective flow in the film according to the Marangoni effect [20–22]. The Marangoni effect can be considered as a thermocapillary flow due to a change in the temperature in the film and a convective flow due to a change in the concentration of the demulsifier and surface tension. Then differentiating (7) with respect to θ

$$\frac{\partial^2 V_r}{\partial \theta^2}=\frac{r}{2\eta g}\frac{\partial^2 P}{\partial \theta^2}$$

and substituting into Eq. (6), we obtain

$$\frac{\eta}{g}\frac{\partial^2 V_r}{\partial x^2}=\frac{\partial P}{\partial r}-\frac{1}{2r}\frac{\partial^2 P}{\partial \theta^2} \tag{10}$$

Integrating Eq. (10) twice and using boundary conditions (9), we obtain

$$V_r=\frac{g}{\eta}\left(\frac{\partial P}{\partial r}-\frac{1}{2r}\frac{\partial^2 P}{\partial \theta^2}\right)\left(\frac{x^2}{2}-\delta x\right)-\frac{x}{\eta}\left(\frac{\partial\sigma}{\partial r}+\frac{1}{R_K\sin\theta}\frac{\partial\sigma(\cos\theta)}{\partial\theta}\right) \tag{11}$$

Solving Eq. (8), taking into account (11), and provided that the value is negligible, we obtain

$$V_x=\frac{d\delta}{dt}=-\frac{1}{r}\frac{\partial}{\partial r}\int_0^\delta rV_r dx=\frac{g\delta^3}{3\eta r}\frac{\partial}{\partial r}\left[r\left(\frac{\partial P}{\partial r}-\frac{1}{2r}\frac{\partial^2 P}{\partial \theta^2}\right)\right]+$$
$$\frac{\delta^2}{2\eta r}\left(\frac{\partial\sigma}{\partial r}+\frac{1}{R_K\sin\theta}\frac{\partial\sigma(\cos\theta)}{\partial\theta}\right) \tag{12}$$

It should be noted that in [19] this equation was proposed in a slightly different form, not taking into account the distribution of pressure and surface tension depending on the angle θ. This wave equation determines the distribution of fluid velocity in the film or the change in film thickness depending on the pressure and distribution of surface tension. Neglecting the second derivatives $\partial^2 P/\partial\theta^2$ and $\partial^2\sigma/\partial r^2$, we obtain

$$\frac{1}{r}\frac{\partial}{\partial r}\left(r\frac{\partial P}{\partial r}\right)=\frac{3\eta}{g\delta^3}V_x-\frac{3}{2g\delta r}\left(\frac{\partial\sigma}{\partial r}+\frac{1}{R_K\sin\theta}\frac{\partial\sigma(\cos\theta)}{\partial\theta}\right) \tag{13}$$

Integrating Eq. (13) twice, provided that $r=R_K$ and $P=P_0(R_K)$, we obtain

$$\begin{aligned}P(r)=P_0(R_K)+\frac{3V_x\eta}{2\delta^3 g}\left(R_K^2-r^2\right)-\\ \frac{3}{2g\delta}\left(\Delta\sigma(r)\ln\frac{r}{R_K}+\frac{r}{R_K\sin\theta}\frac{\partial\sigma(\cos\theta)}{\partial\theta}\right)\end{aligned} \tag{14}$$

where $P_0(R_K)$ is the external pressure at the periphery of the film. The force acting on the interfacial film with a uniform distribution of matter along the radius $(\Delta\sigma(r)\approx 0)$ is

$$F=\int_0^{R_K}P(r)ds\approx P_0\pi R_K^2+\frac{3\pi V_x}{2g}\frac{\eta R_K^4}{\delta^3}-\frac{\pi R_K^2}{g\delta\sin\theta}\frac{\partial\sigma}{\partial\theta} \tag{15}$$

Putting that $\Delta P=F-P_0\pi R_K^2$, we define

$$V_x=\frac{2g\delta^3}{3\pi\eta R_K^4}\Delta P+\frac{2\delta^2}{3\eta R_K^2\sin\theta}\frac{\partial\sigma}{\partial\theta} \tag{16}$$

Putting $d\delta/dt\approx V_x$, we define the equation of thinning of the interfacial film in the form

$$\frac{d\delta}{dt}=\frac{2g\Delta P}{3\pi\eta R_K^4}\delta^3+\frac{2\delta^2}{3\eta R_K^2\sin\theta}\frac{\partial\sigma}{\partial\theta} \tag{17}$$

For ΔP we define the following expression $\Delta P=(P_D+P_K)\pi R_K^2+\Pi$, where P_D, P_K is the dynamic and capillary pressure $\left(P_K=2\sigma/g\delta\right)$ acting in the film; Π is the wedging pressure, defined both for a spherical drop and $\Pi=-\frac{AR_k^2}{6\delta^3}$ for deformable drops; and A is the van der Waals-Hamaker constant $\left(A\sim 10^{-21}J\right)$ [23, 24].

Given the foregoing, the equation of thinning of the interfacial film (17) can be represented as

$$\frac{d\delta}{dt}=b_1\delta^3+b_2\delta^2-b_3\delta, \tag{18}$$

$$t=0,\delta=\delta_0$$

where $b_1=\frac{2gP_D}{3\eta R_K^4}$, $b_2=\frac{2}{3\eta R_K^2}\left(2\sigma+\frac{1}{\sin\theta}\frac{\partial\sigma}{\partial\theta}\right)$, and $b_3=\frac{1}{9}\frac{Aa_rg}{\pi\eta R_K^4}$. The general solution of Eq. (18) will be presented in the form of a transcendental expression:

$$\ln\frac{\delta^2}{\delta_0^2}\frac{b_1\delta_0^2+b_2\delta_0-b_3}{b_1\delta^2+b_2\delta-b_3}-\frac{b_2}{\sqrt{\Delta}}\ln\frac{\left(2b_1\delta+b_2-\sqrt{\Delta}\right)\left(2b_1\delta_0+b_2+\sqrt{\Delta}\right)}{\left(2b_1\delta+b_2+\sqrt{\Delta}\right)\left(2b_1\delta_0+b_2-\sqrt{\Delta}\right)}=-2b_3t \tag{19}$$

where $\Delta=\frac{2}{9\eta^2R_K^2}\left[\frac{g^2P_DAa_r}{\pi R_K^4}+2\left(\frac{\sigma}{3}+\Delta\sigma\right)^2\right]$. Solution (19) is a complex expression for determining the change in the thickness of an interfacial film $\delta(t)$, in connection with which we consider more specific cases:

a. For thin films, we can put that $P_D<<P_K-\Pi/\pi R_K^2$. In this case, the solution of Eq. (18) will be presented as a special case (19):

$$\delta(t)=\frac{\delta_0\exp\left(b_3t\right)}{1+\beta_1\delta_0\left(\exp\left(b_3t\right)-1\right)} \tag{20}$$

where $\beta_1=\frac{b_2}{b_3}=\frac{6\pi R_k^2}{Aa_rg}\left(2\sigma+\frac{1}{\sin\theta}\frac{\partial\sigma}{\partial\theta}\right)$. For very thin films, solution (18) appears as

$$\delta(t)\approx\delta_0\exp\left(-b_3t\right) \tag{21}$$

where $\beta_3=\frac{2}{3}\frac{P_Dg\delta_0}{\eta R_K^2}$. In the case of deformable drops, we have

$$\delta(t)\approx\delta_0-\beta_2t \tag{22}$$

where $\beta_2=\frac{Ag}{9\pi\eta\delta_0R_K^2}$.

b. For thick films, we can put that $(P_D+P_K)>>{}^{\Pi}/_{\pi R_K^2}$. It is important to note that the main forces determining the discontinuity of the interfacial film at its large thicknesses are the forces due to velocity pulsations, i.e., hydrodynamic forces. Provided that $P_D>>P_K$, the decision is presented in the form

$$\delta(t)=\frac{\delta_0}{\sqrt{1+\beta_3t}} \tag{23}$$

If $P_D<<P_K$, then we have

$$\delta(t)=\frac{\delta_0}{1+b_2\delta_0t} \tag{24}$$

The above solutions (20)–(24) can be used in practical calculations of the thickness of the interfacial film for special cases. As follows from Eq. (20), the Marangoni effect is a partial correction to the surface tension coefficient in the coefficient b_2, although it can have a significant effect on the nature of the flow and on the velocity distribution in the interfacial films (12) and (16).

It should be noted that various chemical reagents and demulsifiers significantly reduce the surface tension of the film and significantly increase the rate of thinning of the interfacial film (**Figure 3**).

Figure 4 shows a comparison of experimental and calculated values according to Eq. (17) for thinning the film thickness, and after reaching the critical value thickness $\delta\le\delta_{cr}$, the calculation according to formula (24) is most acceptable.

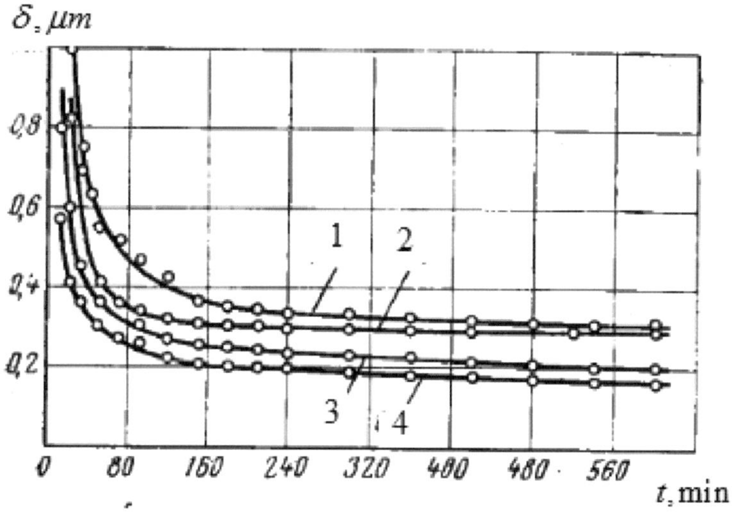

Figure 3.
Change in the thickness of the interfacial film for various concentrations of demulsifier (g/l): 1, 0.02; 2, 0.01; 3, 0.005; 4, 0.002.

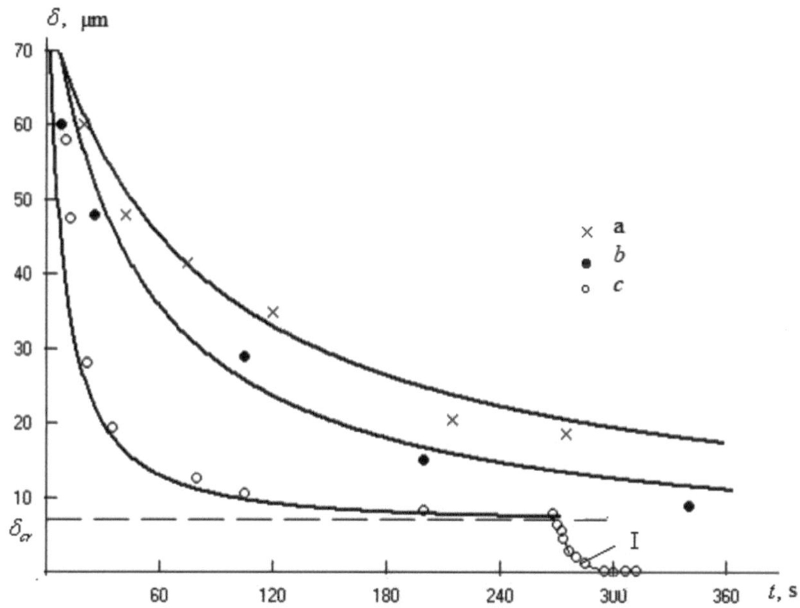

Figure 4.
Comparison of the calculated (17) and experimental values [25] of the thickness of the interfacial film versus time at various concentrations (g/l) of the demulsifier (g/l): a, 0.2; b, 0.5; c, 1.0 *(I, calculation according to Eq. (24)).*

2.3 Coalescence, deformation, and crushing of droplets in an isotropic turbulent flow

The processes of coalescence and fragmentation of droplets are reversible phenomena and can be described by similar equations.

The crushing of droplets and bubbles in an isotropic turbulent flow is an important factor for increasing the interfacial surface and the rate of heat and mass transfer in dispersed systems. The crushing mechanism of deformable particles is determined by many factors, among which it is important to note the following:

a. The effect of turbulent pulsations of a certain frequency on the surface of droplets and bubbles on the change in shape.

b. Boundary instability on the surface of the droplet, determined by the turbulization of the boundary layer or general instability as a result of reaching the droplet size maximum value $a \geq a_{max}$.

c. The influence of the external environment, in which the droplet crushing is defined as the equilibrium between the external forces from the continuous phase (dynamic pressure) and the surface tension forces that resist the destruction of the droplet. It should be noted that this condition can also characterize the deformation of the shape of drops and bubbles.

d. As a result of mutual elastic collision with intensive mixing of the system. It is important to note that not every collision of droplets and bubbles leads to their coalescence and coalescence, and during an elastic collision, a droplet can decay into fragments, thereby changing the size distribution spectrum, although there is no work indicating the number of particles formed as a result of such decay.

A general review of the fragmentation of droplets and bubbles is given in the work [26], where issues related to the frequency of crushing and the nature of the particle size distribution function are considered, although the analysis of the maximum and minimum sizes and the characteristic features of the effect of secondary crushing processes on the change in the function of the multimodal distribution of drops are not considered. Despite the many mechanisms for crushing droplets and bubbles, an important parameter characterizing this process is the frequency of crushing in a turbulent flow, the definition of which has been the subject of many works. It should be noted that the mechanisms of coalescence and fragmentation of droplets are similar and differ only in the dependence of energy dissipation on the number of particles. Based on the analysis of surface energy and kinetic energy of a turbulent flow, the following expression is proposed for the droplet crushing frequency [26]:

$$\omega(a) = C_1 a^{-2/3} \varepsilon_R^{1/3} \exp\left(-\frac{C_2 \sigma}{\rho_c \varepsilon_R^{2/3} a^{5/3}}\right) \tag{25}$$

In an isotropic turbulent flow, coalescence and fragmentation of droplets are determined by their turbulent diffusion, represented as [18, 27].

$$\begin{aligned} D_T &\approx \alpha(\varepsilon_R/\lambda)^{1/3}\lambda, \quad \lambda > \lambda_0 \\ D_T &\approx \alpha(\varepsilon_R/\lambda)^{1/2}\lambda^2, \quad \lambda < \lambda_0 \end{aligned} \tag{26}$$

The process of coalescence and crushing can be considered as a mass transfer process, in connection with which, the change in the number of particles taking into account the diffusion coefficients at $\lambda > \lambda_0$ and Pe < <1 can be written as [7–10].

$$
\begin{aligned}
&\frac{\partial N}{\partial t}=\frac{\alpha}{r^2}\frac{\partial}{\partial r}\left[\mu_P^2\varepsilon_R^{1/2}r^{10/3}\frac{\partial N}{\partial r}\right]\\
&t=0, r>R, N=N_0\\
&t>0, r=R, N=0\\
&r\to\infty, N=N_0
\end{aligned}
\tag{27}
$$

The general solution of this boundary value problem under certain assumptions will be presented as

$$
\begin{aligned}
&N(r,t)=\sum_{n=1}^{\infty}A_nJ_2\left[\mu_n(r/R)^{1/3}\right]\exp\left(-\mu_n^2t\right)\\
&A_n=\frac{2}{R^2}\frac{\int_0^R N_0J_0\left(\mu_n(r/R)^{1/3}\right)rdr}{J_1^2\left(\mu_n^2\right)}
\end{aligned}
\tag{28}
$$

The frequency of coalescence and crushing is defined as

$$
\omega=D_T\frac{\partial N}{\partial r}|_{r=R}\approx C_1\left(\frac{\varepsilon_R}{a^2}\right)^{1/3}\exp\left(-C_2\left(\varepsilon_R/a^2\right)^{1/3}t\right)
\tag{29}
$$

We introduce the relaxation time for the coalescence of droplets in a turbulent flow in the form

$$
\begin{aligned}
&\lambda>\lambda_0,\quad \tau_{PT}=\left(\frac{a^2}{\varepsilon_R}\right)^{1/3}\\
&\lambda<\lambda_0,\quad \tau_{PT}=\left(\frac{\nu_c}{\varepsilon_R}\right)^{1/2}
\end{aligned}
\tag{30}
$$

Then the coalescence frequency is defined as

$$
\omega=D_T\frac{\partial N}{\partial r}|_{r=R}\approx C_1\left(\frac{\varepsilon_R}{a^2}\right)^{1/3}\exp\left(-C_2t/\tau_{PT}\right)
\tag{31}
$$

Thus, if $t< <\tau_{PT}$ rapid coalescence and droplet coalescence occur, as a result of which we have

$$
\omega=C_1\left(\frac{\varepsilon_R}{a^2}\right)^{1/3}
\tag{32}
$$

Similarly, it is possible to determine the frequency of coalescence and crushing at $\lambda<\lambda_0$ using the second Eq. (26); for the diffusion coefficient for a viscous flow, the crushing frequency can be determined by the following expression:

$$
\omega(a)=C_{01}N_0a^3\left(\frac{\varepsilon_R}{\nu_c}\right)^{1/2}\exp\left[\frac{\sigma}{\left(\nu_c\varepsilon_R\right)^{1/2}a\rho_c}\right]
\tag{33}
$$

As follows from this equation, the frequency of fragmentation of droplets and bubbles in a viscous region or in a liquid medium is inversely proportional to the viscosity of the medium $\sim\nu_c^{-1/2}$, and the time for crushing droplets is taken in the form $\tau\sim\sigma/(\rho_c\varepsilon_Ra)$, although in [18] it is defined as $\tau\sim a^{2/3}\varepsilon_R^{-1/3}$. For processes of droplet crushing with the number of particles N_0 in a turbulent flow, the droplet crushing frequency for a high droplet crushing rate, these expressions are simplified to the form $t << (a^2/\varepsilon_{RD})^{1/3}$

$$\omega_D(a) \approx C_1 \mu_p^2 N_0 a^3 \left(\frac{\varepsilon_{RD}}{a^2}\right)^{1/3}, \lambda > \lambda_0 \tag{34}$$

or for a viscous flow $t << (\nu_c/\varepsilon_{RD})^{1/2}$

$$\omega_D(a) \approx C_2 \mu_p^2 N_0 a^3 \left(\frac{\varepsilon_{RD}}{a^2}\right)^{1/2}, \lambda < \lambda_0 \tag{35}$$

With an increase in the concentration of the dispersed phase, particle collisions occur, accompanied by the phenomena of coagulation, crushing, and the formation of coagulation structures in the form of a continuous loose network of interconnected particles. With an increase in particle concentration, the effective viscosity increases linearly if the particles of the dispersed phase are distant from each other at sufficiently large distances that exclude intermolecular interaction and are rigid undeformable balls.

In a number of works, depending on the crushing mechanism, the following formulas are proposed for the crushing frequency [28–32]:

$$\omega(a) = C_3 a^{-2/3} \varepsilon_R^{1/3} \left(\frac{2}{\sqrt{\pi}}\right) \Gamma\left(\frac{3}{2} \frac{C_4 \sigma}{\rho_c \varepsilon_R^{2/3} a^{5/3}}\right),$$

$$\omega(a) = C_5 \varepsilon_R^{1/3} erfc\left(\sqrt{C_6 \frac{\sigma}{\rho_c \varepsilon_R^{2/3} a^{5/3}} + C_7 \frac{\eta_d}{\sqrt{\rho_c \rho_d \varepsilon_R^{1/3} a^{4/3}}}}\right), \tag{36}$$

$$\omega(a) = \frac{a^{5/3} \varepsilon_R^{19/15} \rho_c^{7/5}}{\sigma^{7/5}} exp\left(-\frac{\sqrt{2}\sigma^{9/5}}{a^3 \rho_c^{9/5} \varepsilon_R^{6/5}}\right), ; \omega(a) = C_8 n erfc\left(C_9 \frac{\sigma^{3/2}}{n^3 d_T^3 \rho_c^{3/2} a^{3/2}}\right)^{1/3}, .$$

The last equation determines the frequency of droplet crushing in the mixing devices and depends on the mixing parameters [20, 33]. For multiphase systems with a volume fraction of droplets φ, the crushing frequency can be determined in the form

$$\omega(a) = \frac{\varepsilon_R^{1/3}}{a^{2/3}(1+\varphi)} \exp\left(-C_{11} \frac{(1+\varphi)^2 \sigma}{\rho_d a^{5/3} \varepsilon_R^{2/3}}\right) \tag{37}$$

The crushing rate of droplets in an isotropic turbulent flow is characterized by the crushing rate constant, defined as

$$\mathrm{Re}_d < 1, \; k_R = A_0 \frac{\varepsilon_R^{1/3}}{a^{2/3}} \exp\left(-\frac{A_1 \sigma}{\rho_c \varepsilon_R^{2/3} a^{5/3}}\right) \tag{38}$$

$$\mathrm{Re}_d > 1, \; k_R = A_0 \frac{\rho_c a^{2/3} \varepsilon_R^{1/3}}{\eta_c} \exp\left(-\frac{A_1 \sigma}{\rho_c \varepsilon_R^{2/3} a^{5/3}}\right) \tag{39}$$

In principle, the expression given in brackets characterizes the ratio of surface energy ($E_\sigma \sim \pi a^2 \sigma / a \sim \pi a \sigma$) to turbulent flow energy

$\left(\overline{E}_T \sim \pi a^2(\Delta P), \left(\Delta P_T = C_1 \rho_c (\varepsilon_R a)^{2/3}\right)\right)$ and characterizes the efficiency of the crushing process

$$\frac{E_\sigma}{\overline{E}_T} \sim \frac{\sigma}{\rho_c \varepsilon_R^{2/3} a^{5/3}} \tag{40}$$

Analyzing Eqs. (29)–(31), it can be noted that the crushing frequency in an isotropic turbulent flow for a region $\lambda > \lambda_0$ is mainly determined by turbulence parameters (specific energy dissipation, scale of turbulent pulsations), medium density, surface stress, and for a viscous flow $\lambda < \lambda_0$, in addition, viscosity of the medium. It is important to note that the fragmentation of droplets and bubbles in an isotropic turbulent flow is preceded by a deformation of their shape, and with significant numbers and sufficiently small numbers, they can take on forms that cannot be described. The equilibrium condition between the surface forces and the external forces of the turbulent flow (40) can also characterize the initial conditions of particle deformation. Coalescence of droplets and bubbles plays an important role in the flow of various technological processes of chemical technology and, above all, in reducing the interfacial surface, in the separation of particles of different sizes, accompanied by their deposition or ascent. The mechanism of coalescence of droplets and bubbles is determined by the following steps: (a) mutual collision of particles with a certain frequency in a turbulent flow; (b) the formation of an interfacial film between two drops and its thinning; (c) rupture of the interfacial film and drainage of fluid from one drop to another, merging and the formation of a new drop. Mutual collisions of particles in the flow volume occur for various reasons:

a. Due to convective Brownian diffusion of the finely dispersed component of particles, which is characteristic mainly for laminar flow at low Reynolds numbers.

b. Due to turbulent flow and turbulent diffusion

c. Due to additional external fields (gravitational, electric, electromagnetic, etc.). If the Kolmogorov turbulence scale λ_0 is smaller or comparable with the size of the droplets in the viscous flow region, then the process is accompanied by a turbulent walk, similar to Brownian, which results in the appearance of turbulent diffusion. However, turbulent diffusion may be characteristic of large particle sizes at large distances λ, due to the high intensity of turbulent pulsations and the heterogeneity of the hydrodynamic field.

d. Due to the effect of engagement as a result of convective transfer of small particles in the vicinity of the incident large particle. As a result of the deposition or ascent of large particles, due to the formation of a hydrodynamic wake, the capture of small particles by large particles significantly increases, which leads to gravitational coalescence if they fall along lines close to the center line. For the processes of droplet coalescence, the capture coefficient plays an important role, which determines the deviation of the real particle capture cross section from the geometric

$$\vartheta = \frac{I}{\pi (L+R)^2 N_0 V_\infty} \tag{41}$$

where I is the mass flow to the surface of the selected particle, ϑ is the capture coefficient, L is the characteristic distance scale, and V_∞ is the velocity of the medium unperturbed by the sphere of flow. The relationship between the Sherwood number and the capture coefficient in convective diffusion has the form

$$Sh = \frac{1}{2}Pe\vartheta\left(1+\frac{R}{L}\right)^2$$

The capture coefficient is defined as

$$\begin{aligned}\vartheta &\approx \frac{4}{\text{Pe}}\left(1-\frac{N_L}{N_0}\right)b_*(1+b_0\text{Pe}), \text{Pe} < < 1;\\ \vartheta &\approx \left(1-\frac{N_L}{N_0}\right)\text{Pe}^{-2/3}\left(1+0.73\text{Pe}^{-1/3}\right), \text{Pe} > > 1\end{aligned} \tag{42}$$

Here N_L is the concentration of particles on the surface of a sphere of radius $r = L$, b_i coefficients;

e. Due to the heterogeneity of the temperature and pressure fields, which contribute to the appearance of forces proportional to the temperature and pressure gradients and acting in the direction of decreasing these parameters. As a result of the action of these forces, the finely dispersed component of the dispersed flow is characterized by their migration due to thermal diffusion and barodiffusion, which also contributes to their collision and coalescence.

f. In addition to the indicated phenomena, physical phenomena (droplet evaporation, condensation) contribute to coalescence, accompanied by the emergence of a hydrodynamic repulsive force (Fassi effect) of the evaporating droplets due to evaporation (Stefan flow) or when the droplet condenses by the appearance of a force acting in the opposite direction. For an inviscid flow and a fast droplet coalescence rate $t < < (a^2/\varepsilon_{RK})^{1/3}$, expressions (29) and (31) are transformed

$$\omega_K(a) \approx C_1\mu_p^2N_0a^3\left(\frac{\varepsilon_{RK}}{a^2}\right)^{1/3}, \lambda > \lambda_0 \tag{43}$$

or for a viscous flow $t < < (\nu_c/\varepsilon_{RK})^{1/2}$

$$\omega_K(a) \approx C_2\mu_p^2N_0a^3\left(\frac{\varepsilon_{RK}}{\nu_c}\right)^{1/2}, \lambda < \lambda_0 \tag{44}$$

where $\lambda_0 = \left(\nu_c^3/\varepsilon_R\right)^{1/4}$ is the Kolmogorov scale of turbulence and ε_R is the specific energy dissipation in the fluid flow and dispersed medium in the presence of coalescence (ε_{RK}) or fragmentation of particles (ε_{RD}), depending on the number of particles in the flow and on their size. These expressions for a two-particle collision of the i–th and j–th drops can be transformed to the form

$$\begin{aligned}\omega_K(a) &\approx C_1\mu_p^2N_0\left(\frac{\varepsilon_{RK}}{\alpha^2}\right)^{1/3}\left(a_i^2+a_j^2\right)^{3/2}, \lambda < \lambda_0\\ \omega_K(a) &\approx C_2\mu_p^2N_0\left(\frac{\varepsilon_{RK}}{\nu_c}\right)^{1/2}\left(a_i^2+a_j^2\right)^{3/2}, \lambda < \lambda_0\end{aligned} \tag{45}$$

As follows from this expression, the collision frequency of particles is inversely proportional to their size $\omega \sim a^{-2/3}$ and increases with increasing concentration of particles in the volume. In these equations (43) μ_p^2 there is a degree of entrainment of particles by a pulsating medium, and for drops of small sizes $\mu_p^2 \to 1$, and for large drops – $\mu_p^2 \to 0$. As follows from formula (45), with increasing viscosity of the medium and particle size, the collision frequency of particles in an isotropic turbulent flow decreases, and, naturally, the probability of the formation of coagulation structures is extremely low. For large Peclet numbers Pe> > 1, using stationary solutions of the convective diffusion equation for fast coagulation, the coalescence frequency can be expressed as

$$\omega_k = C_1 N_0 \left[\left(\frac{\varepsilon_r}{\nu_c}\right) aU\right]^{1/2} a^2 \tag{46}$$

where $C_1 = 8\sqrt{\frac{\pi}{3}}\mu_p^2 a$.

By introducing the Peclet number for isotropic turbulence in the form $\mathrm{Pe} = \frac{U_\infty}{a}\left(\frac{\nu_C}{\varepsilon_R}\right)^{1/2}$, this expression can be rewritten in the form

$$\omega_K = C_1 N_0 U a^2 \mathrm{Pe}^{-1/2} \tag{47}$$

Thus, with an increase in the number Pe, the number of particle collisions decreases, which prevents the formation of coagulation structures. For finely dispersed particles, the number Pe can be expressed as $\mathrm{Pe} = \frac{a}{D}\dot{\gamma}$, which, for isotropic turbulence, is transformed to a form $\mathrm{Pe} = a_1\left(\frac{\nu_C}{\varepsilon_R}\right)^{1/2}\dot{\gamma} = a_1\left(\frac{\eta_C}{\varepsilon_R\rho_C}\right)^{1/2}\frac{\tau}{\eta_C}$, i.e., the Pe number is proportional to the shear stress. Therefore, with $\tau \to \tau_P$, the number Pe becomes infinitely large, which creates the conditions for the formation of coagulation structures.

Coalescence of droplets and bubbles is characterized by the following stages: rapprochement and collision of droplets of different sizes in a turbulent flow with the formation of an interfacial film between them. It should be noted that the transfer of droplets in a polydisperse medium is mainly determined by the hydrodynamic conditions and the intensity of the flow turbulence. Under conditions of isotropic turbulence, the collision frequency of droplets depends on the specific dissipation of the energy of the turbulent flow and the properties of the medium and the dispersed phase.

2.4 Deformation of drops and bubbles

The deformation of droplets and bubbles, first of all, is characterized by a violation of the balance of external and surface stresses acting on the droplet in a turbulent flow. In the simplest case, with insignificance of gravitational and resistance forces, such forces are hydrodynamic head and surface tension. The pressure forces are proportional to the velocity head $F_D \sim \frac{\rho_c U}{2}$, and the surface tension force is proportional to capillary pressure $F_\sigma = \frac{2\sigma}{a_e}$. If the Weber number $We \sim \frac{F_D}{F_\sigma} < < 1$, then for small numbers $\mathrm{Re}_d < < 1$, drops and bubbles have a strictly spherical shape. Under the condition of $F_D \geq F_\sigma$ either $We \geq 1$, $\mathrm{Re}_d > 1$ the surface of the droplet loses stability and it deforms, taking the shape of a flattened ellipsoid of revolution at the beginning, and with a further increase in the number Re_d and We, it assumes various configurations up to the stretched filament, which are not amenable to theoretical investigation and description (**Figure 5**). It should be noted that in dispersed systems, there is a certain maximum size a_{max}, above which the droplets are unstable, deform, and instantly collapse, and the minimum size a_{min}, which

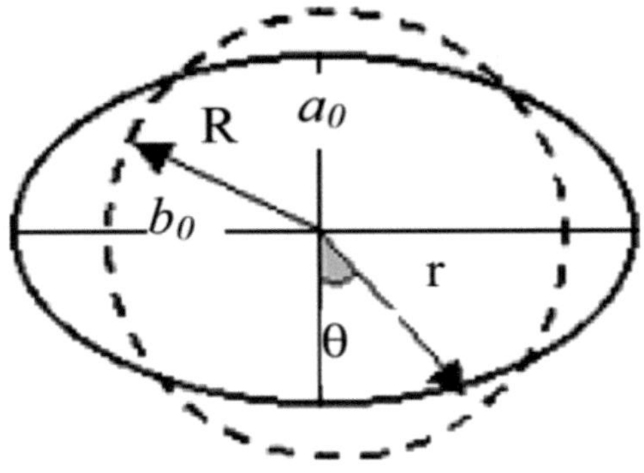

Figure 5.
Schematic representation of the deformation of a drop to an ellipsoidal shape.

determines the lower threshold for the stability of droplets; i.e., under certain conditions, the flows of droplets that have reached these sizes cannot be further fragmented. The maximum particle size characterizes the unstable state of droplets and bubbles, which depend on the hydrodynamic conditions of the dispersed medium flow and, under certain turbulent flow conditions, are prone to shape deformation and fragmentation of a single drop. Usually, deformation of a drop's shape to an ellipsoidal shape is estimated by the ratio of the small axis of the ellipsoid to the large $\chi = a_0/b_0$.

The volumetric deformation of droplets and bubbles is based on a three-dimensional model and results in a change in the shape of a spherical particle to an ellipsoidal one. Moreover, the drop is subjected to simultaneous stretching and compression with a constant volume. In the literature there are a large number of empirical formulas describing the deformation of drops and bubbles. Compared to multidimensional deformation, volumetric deformation is the simplest case with the preservation of a certain shape symmetry (**Figure 6**).

It is important to note that for any deformation of the droplet shape, the surface area of the particle increases with a constant volume of liquid in the droplet, which is an important factor in increasing the interfacial surface.

In [8, 18], the fluctuation frequency of oscillations of the droplet surface using the Rayleigh equation as a result of the influence of turbulent pulsations of a certain frequency on the surface of droplets and bubbles on the shape change is defined as

$$\omega(k) = \left[\left(\frac{2\sigma}{\pi 2\rho_c a^3}\right)\left(\frac{(k+1)(k+2)k(k\text{-}1)}{(k+1)_{\rho d/\rho_c}+1}\right)\right]^{1/2} \tag{48}$$

where is k the wave number. For $k = 2$ using this formula, one can obtain formulas for determining the frequency corresponding to the fragmentation of

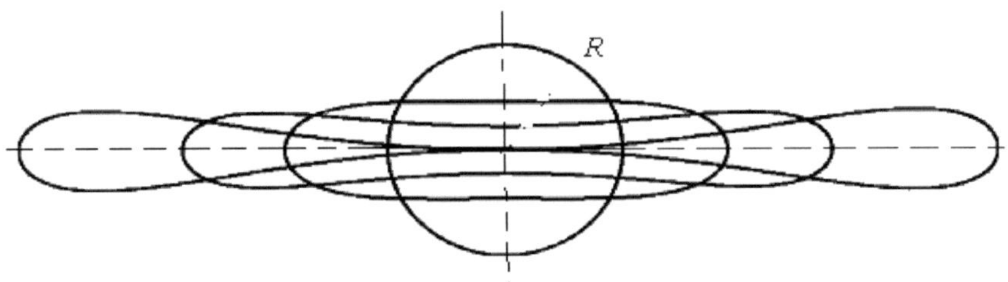

Figure 6.
The characteristic forms of deformation of a spherical drop and bubble.

bubbles $(\rho_d << \rho_c)$ $\omega(a) = \frac{2\sqrt{6}}{\pi}\left(\frac{\sigma}{\rho_c a^3}\right)^{1/2}$ and drops $(\rho_d >> \rho_c)$ $\omega(a) = \frac{4}{\pi}\left(\frac{\sigma}{\rho_d a^3}\right)^{1/2}$. As a result, for minor deformations, the droplet shape is determined by the superposition of linear harmonics

$$r(t,\theta) = R\left[1 + \sum_k A_k \cos(\omega_k t) P_k(\cos\theta)\right] \tag{49}$$

where $P_k(\cos\theta)$ is the Legendre function; Ak are the coefficients of the series, defined as $A_k = A_{k0}\exp(-\beta_k t)$; and β_k is the attenuation coefficient, defined as

$$\beta_k = \frac{(k+1)(k\text{-}1)(2k+1)\eta_d + k(k+2)(2k+2)\eta_c}{[\rho_d(k+1) + \rho_c k]R^2}$$

Expression (49) for small numbers Re_d is represented as

$$r(t,\theta) = R[1 + \xi(\cos\theta)] \tag{50}$$

where $\xi(\cos\theta) = \lambda_m Ac\,\mathrm{Re}_d^2 P_2(\cos\theta) - \frac{3}{70}\lambda_m \frac{11+10\gamma}{1+\gamma} Ac^2\,\mathrm{Re}_d^3 P_3(\cos\theta) + \ldots$, and R is the radius of the spherical particle. Here $\lambda m = \varphi(\gamma)$, and in particular for gas bubbles in an aqueous medium $\lambda_m = 1/4$, for drops of water in air $\lambda_m \to 5/48$, etc. Putting that

$We = Ac\,\mathrm{Re}_d^2$ we get

$$\xi(\cos\theta) = \lambda_m WeP_2(\cos\theta) - \frac{3}{70}\lambda_m \frac{11+10\gamma}{1+\gamma} We^2\,\mathrm{Re}_d^{-1} P_3(\cos\theta) + \ldots. \tag{51}$$

As a parameter characterizing the deformation of droplets and bubbles, we consider the ratio of the minor axis of the ellipsoid a to the major b, i.e., $\chi = a/b$. Having plotted that for $\theta = 90°$, $P_2(\cos 90°) = -0.5$, $P_3(\cos 90°) = 0$, from Eqs. (50) and (51), we can write $a = R(1 + a_0 We)$, and for $\theta = 0°$, $P_2(\cos 0) = 1.0$, $P_3(\cos 0) = -1$ we define $b = R\left(1 + \beta_0 We + \beta_0 We^2\right)$, where $a_0 = 0.5\lambda m$, $\beta_0 = \lambda_m$, $\beta_1 = \frac{3}{70}\lambda_m \frac{11+10\gamma}{1+\gamma}\mathrm{Re}_d^{-1}$.

Then, putting that $\chi = a/b$, we finally obtain the expression for the dependence of the degree of deformation on the number We in the form

$$\chi = \frac{1 + a_0 We}{1 + \beta_0 We + \beta_1 We^2} \tag{52}$$

where We is the Weber number. This expression is characteristic for describing small deformations of droplets. As a result of using experimental studies [33] on the deformation of the shape of bubbles in a liquid medium with different numbers Mo and to expand the field of application of Eq. (51), the following expression is proposed:

$$\chi = \frac{1 + 0.06We}{1 + 0.2We + \beta_1 We^2} \tag{53}$$

where $\beta_1 = 0.005(2 - \ln Mo)$ with a correlation coefficient equal to $r^2 = 0.986$. **Figure** 7 compares the calculated values according to Eq. (53) with experimental data [33].

As follows from **Figure 8**, expression (53) satisfactorily describes the deformation of droplets and bubbles for the region of variation $We < 10$ and $10^{-4} \leq Mo \leq 7$.

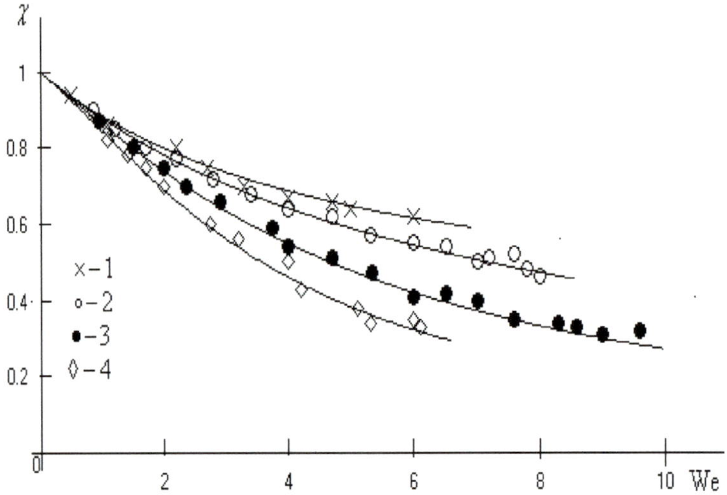

Figure 7.
Dependence of the degree of deformation on the number for various numbers equal to 1, 7; 2, 1.4; 3, 0.023; 4, 0.0001.

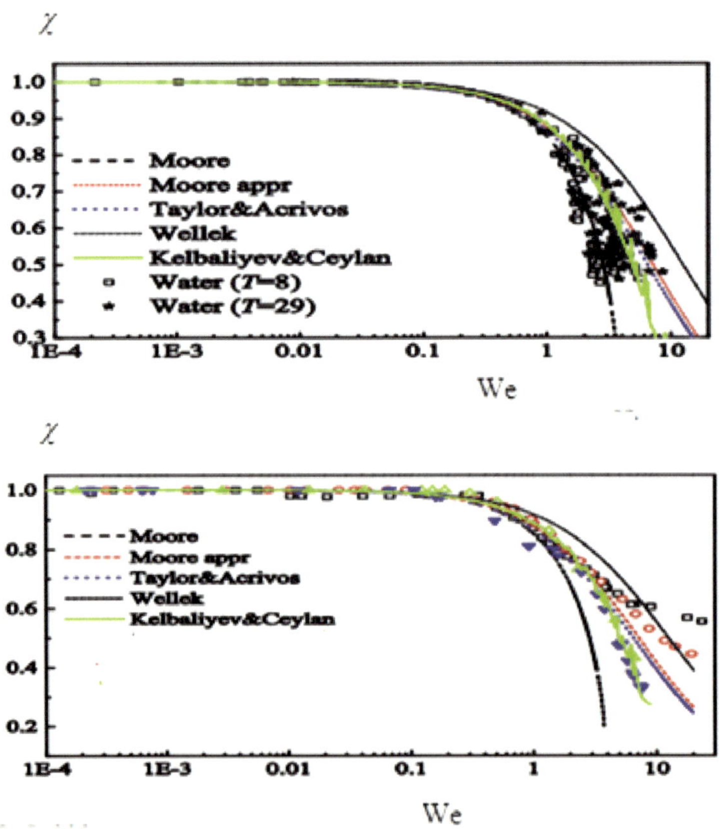

Figure 8.
Comparison of the deformation model (56) of water droplets (pure water in the first graph, glycerol in the second graph) with existing models and experimental data.

Considering only the first term of expression (53) and setting that $P_2(\cos\theta) = 0.5(3\cos^2\theta\text{-}1)$, we obtain

$$r = R\left[1 - \frac{\lambda_0}{2}We(3\cos^2\theta - 1\right] \tag{54}$$

If $\theta = 0$ and $r = a_0$, then expression (54) can be written as

$$a_0 = R(1\text{-}\lambda_0 \mathrm{We}) \tag{55}$$

and if $\theta = \pi/2$ and $r = a_0$, then we have $b_0 = R(1 + \lambda_0/2We)$. Then the relative deformation of the drop is defined as

$$\chi = \frac{a_0}{b_0} = \frac{1 - \lambda_0 We}{1 + (\lambda_0/2)We} \tag{56}$$

Here λ_0, the parameter is determined empirically, using experimental data in the form

$$\lambda_0 = \frac{1}{12}\left(1 - \frac{3}{25}\frac{We}{\mathrm{Re}_d}\right) \tag{57}$$

In [34], this model was used to study the deformation of drops, and a comparison is made with other existing models, the results of which are shown in **Figure 8**.

The authors of [34] note that model (56) is the best compared to existing models.

3. The structural viscosity of oil emulsions

The structural viscosity of a dispersed medium associated with the content of the dispersed phase, as well as with various physical phenomena of interaction between particles, varies from the molecular viscosity of a Newtonian fluid in the absence of dispersed particles ($\varphi = 0$) to shear or bulk viscosity at high particle concentrations ($\varphi \to \varphi_\infty$). Moreover, as experimental studies have shown, the region of the onset of structure formation is clearly distinguished on the curve of viscosity change. The structural viscosity is influenced by the processes of coagulation of particles, accompanied by the formation of coagulation structures in the form of a continuous grid. In most cases, taking these factors into account results in constructing a viscosity model depending on the volume fraction of particles $\eta = f(\varphi)$ or on the fraction of particles and shear stress $\eta = f(\varphi, \tau)$ and shear rate. The rheological oil models of various fields, reflecting the relationship between stress and shear rate through structural viscosity or consistency, obey different laws, exhibiting different properties: visco-plastic, viscoelastic, or having exponential functions. With an increase in the number of particles per unit volume, the effective viscosity of non-Newtonian oil transforms into structural viscosity, which reflects the nature of the formation of this structure. Under certain conditions, rheological models for oil of various fields can be represented by the equations of Bingham ($\tau = \tau_0 + \eta\dot{\gamma}$), Casson ($\tau^{1/2} = \tau_0^{1/2} + k^{1/2}\dot{\gamma}^{1/2}$), Herschel-Bulkley ($\tau = \tau_0 + k\dot{\gamma}^n$), or many other rheological equations. Despite the wide variety of rheological models, in some cases, different models describe the same experimental measurements with equal accuracy. In addition, rheological models differ in the nature of the dependence of the effective viscosity on the content of asphaltenes, resins, and paraffin.

3.1 The dependence of the viscosity of oil emulsions on the water content

One of the important rheological parameters of emulsions is their dynamic viscosity, which depends on the volume fraction, size, and shape of the droplets, on the ratio of the viscosity of the droplets to the viscosity of the medium $\lambda = \eta_d/\eta_c$ (mobility of the surface of the droplets), on the shear stress in concentrated emulsions, etc. Viscosity is the main parameter of structured disperse systems that determines their rheological properties. With an increase in particle concentration, the effective viscosity increases linearly if the particles of the dispersed phase are distant from each other at sufficiently large distances that exclude intermolecular interaction and are rigid undeformable balls (**Table 1**).

A large number of empirical formulas for calculating the viscosity of dispersed media are given in the work [40, 41]. At high concentrations of particles in the volume, taking into account the hydrodynamic interaction of particles, some authors use a modification of the Einstein equation

$$\eta_{ef} = \eta_C(1 + 2,5\varphi + a_0\varphi^2 + a_1\varphi^3 + \dots\dots) \quad (58)$$

where a_i are the coefficients that take into account physical phenomena in a dispersed flow, which in different works take different values.

As a semiempirical expression for calculating the effective viscosity of suspensions, which describes the experimental data well over a wide range of particle concentrations, the Moony formula [7, 8] can be noted

$$\eta_{ef}/\eta_C = \exp\left[\kappa_1\phi/(1-\kappa_2\phi)\right] \quad (59)$$

where κ_1 and κ_2 are coefficients equal to $\kappa_1 = 2,5$ and $0,75 \le \kappa_2 \le 1,5$. This formula for $\varphi \to 0$ provides the limit transition to the Einstein formula.

No.	Formulas for viscosity	Links
1	$\eta_{ef} = \eta_c(1 + 2.5\varphi),\ \varphi < 0.01$	Einstein's formula
2	$\eta_{ef} = \eta_c(1 + 2.5\varphi + 6.2\varphi^2),\ \varphi < 0.1$	[35]
3	$\eta_{ef} = \eta_c\left(1 - \frac{\varphi}{\varphi_\infty}\right)^{-2.5\varphi_\infty},\ \varphi_\infty \approx 0.64$	[36]
4	$\eta_{ef} = \eta_c\left(1 - \frac{\varphi}{\varphi_\infty}\right)^{-2}$	[37]
5	$\eta_{ef} = \eta_c\left(1 - \frac{\varphi}{\varphi_\infty}\right)^{-2.5\varphi_\infty \frac{\eta_d + 0.4\eta_c}{\eta_d + \eta_c}}$	[38]
6	$\eta_{ef} = \eta_c \exp\left[2.5\frac{\eta_d + 0.4\eta_c}{\eta_d + \eta_c}\left(\varphi + \varphi^{5/3} + \varphi^{11/3}\right)\right]$	[38]
7	$\eta_{ef} = \eta_c\left(1 + 2.5\varphi\frac{\eta_d + 0.4\eta_c}{\eta_d + \eta_c}\right)$	[38]
8	$\eta_{ef} = \eta_c \exp\left(\frac{2.5\varphi}{1 + k_1\varphi}\right),\ 0.75 < k_1 < 1.5$	[38]
9	$\eta_{ef} = \eta_c k_1(\varphi/\varphi_\infty)^{1/3}\left[(1 - \varphi/\varphi_\infty)^{1/2} + 1\right]$	[39]
10	$\eta_{ef} = \eta_c k_1\left[1 + 0.75\varphi/\varphi_\infty(1 - \varphi/\varphi_\infty)^{-1}\right]^2$	[39]

Table 1.
Empirical formulas for calculating the effective dynamic viscosity of disperse systems.

Taylor has generalized this equation to the effective viscosity of emulsions

$$\eta_{ef} = \eta_C\left(1 + 2,5\phi\frac{\eta_d + 0,4\eta_C}{\eta_d + \eta_C}\right) \quad (60)$$

where η_d and η_c are the viscosities of the dispersed phase and the medium.

For the effective viscosity of a disperse system, *Ishii and Zuber* offer the following empirical formula

$$\eta_{ef}/\eta_C = \left[1 - \left(\varphi/\varphi_\infty\right)\right]^{-m} \quad (61)$$

where φ_∞ is the volume fraction of particles corresponding to their maximum packing, $\varphi_\infty = 0.5 - 0.74$, and $m = 2.5\varphi_\infty(\eta_d + 0,4\eta_c)/(\eta_d + \eta_c)$. In this formula, the value $\varphi_\infty = 0.62$ is the most suitable for most practical cases. *Kumar et al.* [7, 8] for wide limits changes φ from 0.01 to 0.75 suggested the following formula:

$$\frac{\eta_{ef}}{\eta_C} = \exp\left[2.5\frac{0.4\eta_C + \eta_d}{\eta_C + \eta_d}\left(\phi + \phi^{5/3} + \phi^{11/3}\right)\right] \quad (62)$$

This formula was tested for various liquid–liquid systems and gave the most effective result with a relative error of up to 20%. Many models express the dependence of the viscosity of a disperse system on the limiting concentration of particles φ_p, at which the flow stops on the limiting shear stress. In addition to the above models, there are many empirical and semiempirical expressions in the literature for calculating the viscosity of concentrated systems, although the choice of a model in all cases is based not on the structure formation mechanism, but on the principle of an adequate description of experimental data.

In the literature you can find many other rheological models, using which you can give various dependencies to determine the viscosity of the system [7, 8].

$$\frac{\eta_{ef} - \eta_0}{\eta_0 - \eta_\infty} = f(\dot{\gamma}\theta_w),\ \eta = \eta_\infty + \frac{\eta - \eta_\infty}{1 + (\alpha_0\tau)^m},\ \eta = \eta_\infty + \frac{\eta - \eta_0}{1 + \alpha_0\dot{\gamma}^m + \alpha_1\dot{\gamma}} \quad (63)$$

Here $\gamma = \partial V/\partial y^-$ is the shear rate, τ_0 is the limit value of the shear stress, k^- is the consistency coefficient, and η_∞^- is the viscosity for the suspension in the absence of interaction between the particles.

The empirical models presented are used for specific applications and represent formulas for adequate approximation of experimental data, although we note that attempts to find a general rheological equation for different systems are considered impossible in advance. It is important to note that effective viscosity also depends on particle sizes. However, if we assume that the volume fraction of particles per unit volume is equal to $\varphi = N_0\pi a^3/6$ (N_0 is the number of particles per unit volume), then any expressions that allow us to determine the effective viscosity of a dispersed medium in an indirect order through the volume fraction of particles express the dependence of viscosity on particle size. Effective viscosity does not significantly depend on large particle sizes. **Figure 9** shows the dependence of the effective viscosity on the volume fraction of suspension solid particles for their various sizes, calculated by the formula

$$\eta_{ef} = 1 + 2.5\varphi + 1.5\varphi\exp\left(\frac{0.45\varphi}{(\varphi - \varphi_\infty)^2}\right) \quad (64)$$

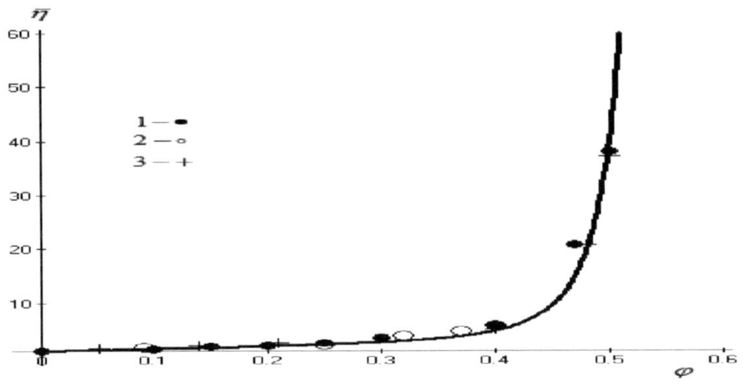

Figure 9.
The dependence of the effective viscosity of suspensions on the fraction of particles and their sizes: 1, 90–105 μm; 2, 45–80 μm; 3, 30–40 μm.

For small particle sizes, the dependence of effective viscosity on particle sizes becomes more noticeable, where the dependence of viscosity on particle sizes is described by the expression

$$\eta_{ef} = 1 + 2,5\varphi + \frac{3}{4}\varphi \exp\left(\frac{m\varphi}{(\varphi - \varphi_\infty)^2}\right), \quad m = 2.2 + 0.03a \tag{65}$$

The correspondence of this dependence to experimental data is shown in **Figure 10**.

As follows from the experimental data and from this formula, the effective viscosity of a dispersed system substantially depends on the volume fraction and particle size. Moreover, with increasing particle size, the effective viscosity also increases. In all likelihood, in this case, coagulation structures and aggregates are not formed, but a simple dense packing of particles is formed.

The effective viscosity of the disperse system grows up to a critical value, which affects the speed and nature of the flow (**Figure 10**). Coagulation structures are formed due to intermolecular bonds between particles, and if liquid interlayers remain between the particles, then the thickness of this interlayer significantly affects the strength of the coagulation structure. The change in the effective viscosity of non-Newtonian oil from the pressure gradient, accompanied by the formation

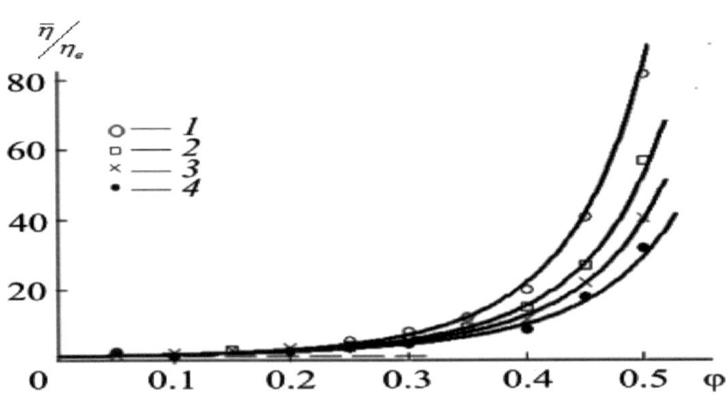

Figure 10.
The calculated (solid curves) experimental (points) of the relative viscosity of the dispersed system from the volume fraction of solid spherical particles and their sizes: 1, a = 0.1 μm; 2, 0.5 μm; 3, 1.0 μm; 4, 1.5 μm.

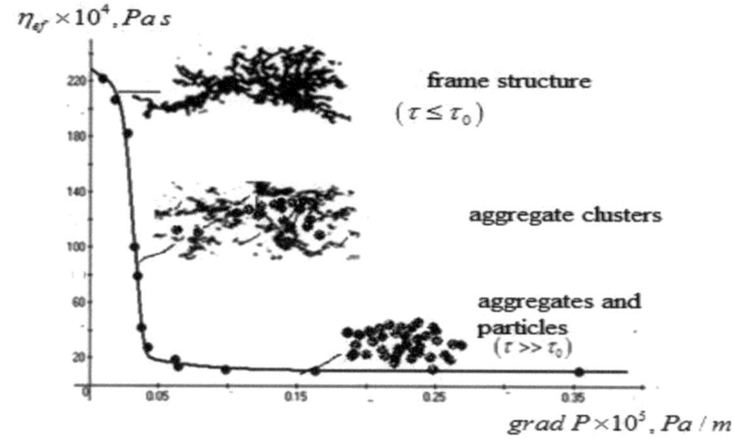

Figure 11.
The dependence of the viscosity of the structured system on the nature of its destruction at various values of the pressure gradient.

and destruction of the structure due to particles of asphaltenes, based on experimental data, is determined by the empirical formula [8, 42].

$$\frac{\eta_{ef} - \eta_\infty}{\eta_0 - \mu_\infty} = \exp\left(-30z^6\right) \tag{66}$$

where η_0, μ_∞ is the initial $(\tau \leq \tau_P)$ and final viscosity of the oil $\tau > > \tau_P, z = grad\ P$. **Figure 11** shows the change in the viscosity of the destroyed structure, although the formation of the same structure also occurs only in the opposite direction; i.e., the system is characterized by thixotropy of the structure.

The viscosity of disperse systems also depends on the size and deformation of the particle shape, and with increasing size, the viscosity increases. Despite the large number and variety of viscosity models of disperse systems, the main studies are devoted to the construction of empirical models without taking into account the mechanism of phenomena that describe experimental data with a certain accuracy. The nature and properties of coagulation structures significantly affect the basic properties of a dispersed medium. It is very difficult to determine the viscosity of composite materials, where the formation of certain structures is an important and necessary problem, where the viscosity depends on the concentration of the components included in this system, molecular weight, temperature, and many other parameters.

The viscosity of free-dispersed systems increases with increasing concentration of the dispersed phase. The presence of particles of the dispersed phase leads to a distortion of the fluid flow near these particles, which affects the viscosity of the dispersed system. If the concentration is negligible, then the collision of the particles is excluded, and the nature of the fluid motion near one of the particles will affect the fluid motion near the others.

The work [43] provides a formula for calculating the viscosity of an oil emulsion for its various types

$$\frac{\eta_{ef}}{\eta_C} = \exp(5\varphi)(1 - 3\varphi + b\varphi) \tag{67}$$

Here η_{ef}, η_C are the dynamic viscosities of the emulsion and oil, φ is the volume fraction of droplets, and b is an emulsion type factor, moreover, b = 7.3 for highly

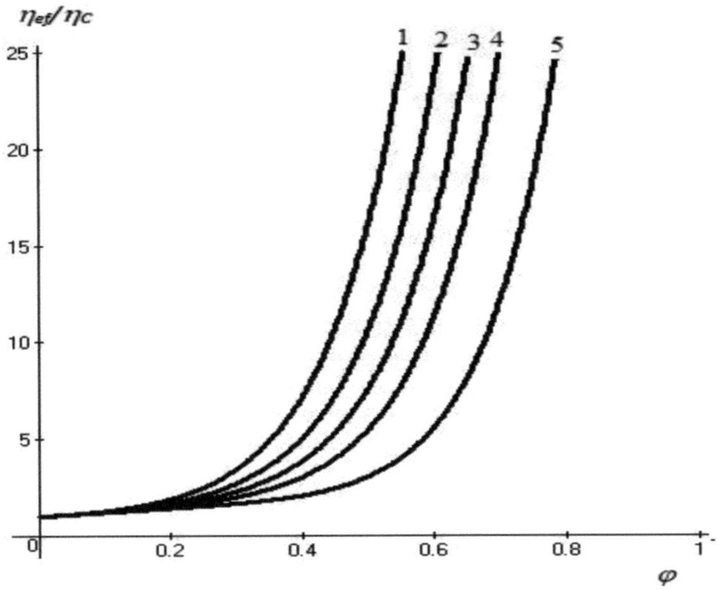

Figure 12.
The dependence of the viscosity of the oil emulsion on the water content: (1) highly concentrated emulsions, b = 7.3; (2) concentrated emulsions, b = 5.5; (3) for average emulsion concentrations, b = 4.5; (4) for diluted emulsions, b = 3.8; (5) for highly diluted emulsions, b = 3.0.

concentrated emulsions, b = 5.5 for concentrated emulsions, b = 4.5 for medium concentration emulsions, b = 3.8 for diluted emulsions, and b = 3.0 for very diluted emulsions. **Figure 12** shows the calculated curves of the dependence of the viscosity of the oil emulsion on the volumetric water content.

It is important to note that, in addition to the above factors, the viscosity of emulsions is associated with the presence of deformable drops and bubbles in them, and at high concentrations of drops with the formation of coagulation structures (flocculus), leading to rheological properties. The work [44] considers possible options for calculating the viscosity of emulsions taking into account structural changes. If we introduce the stress relaxation time in the form

$$\tau = \frac{\eta_C R}{\sigma} \frac{(2\lambda + 3)(19\lambda + 16)}{40(\lambda + 1)} \quad (68)$$

then the viscosity of the emulsions can be calculated by the formula

$$\eta_{ef} = \frac{\eta_C}{1 + (\tau\dot{\gamma}^2)} \left[1 + \frac{1 + 2.5\lambda}{1 + \lambda}\varphi + \left(1 + \varphi\frac{5(\lambda - 1)}{2\lambda + 3}((\tau\dot{\gamma}^2))\right)\right] \quad (69)$$

Here $\gamma = \eta_d/\eta_C$ and τ is the shear stress. For small quantities $\tau\dot{\gamma} < < 1$, this equation takes the following form

$$\frac{\eta_{ef}}{\eta_C} = \frac{1 + 2.5\lambda}{1 + \lambda}\varphi \quad (70)$$

and, when $\lambda \to \infty$, i.e., for particulate matter, $\eta_{ef}/\eta_C = 1 + 1.25\varphi$. **Figure 13** shows the visual nature of the change in the viscosity of emulsions depending on the shear stress and the volume fraction of drops. The following formula is given in [45]

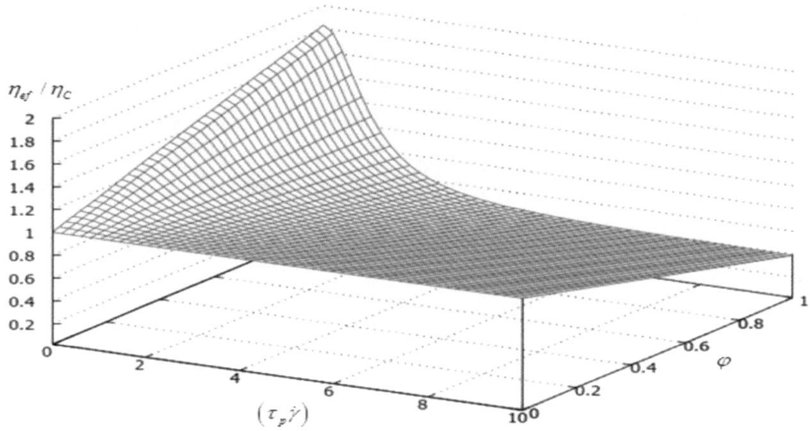

Figure 13.
Spatial interpretation of the nature of the change in viscosity of emulsions at $\lambda = 0.5$.

for calculating the viscosity of monodisperse emulsions depending on the droplet size and their volume fraction

$$\frac{\eta_{ef}}{\eta_C} = 1 + \frac{\eta_C + 2.5\eta_d + (\eta_{ds} + \eta_{di})/a}{\eta_C + \eta_d + 0.4(\eta_{ds} + \eta_{di})/a}\varphi \tag{71}$$

Here η_{ds} is the interfacial shear viscosity, η_{di} is the dilatant viscosity, and a is the droplet size.

3.2 The dependence of the effective viscosity of oil on the content asphaltenes

An experimental study of the effect of the content of asphaltenes and resins in oil on its rheological properties and viscosity was proposed in [46–48].

Using the results of these studies, it can be noted that the presence of asphaltenes, resins, and paraffins in oil, which change the properties of oil, significantly affects their movement and transport. First of all, this affects the stress and shear rate and the increase in viscosity of non-Newtonian oil. In **Figure 14**, the dependence of the effective viscosity of Iranian oil on shear rate by various rheological models is proposed [47].

The table below shows the values of the main coefficients included in these rheological models at various temperatures [47] (**Table 2**).

Of all the models, a satisfactory approximation to the experimental data gives the expression (T = 25°C)

$$\eta = 45.86\dot{\gamma}^{0.75}$$

Given this expression, a rheological dependence satisfying the experimental data can be represented as

$$\tau = \tau_0 + 45.76\dot{\gamma}^{1.75} \tag{72}$$

The dependence of the coefficient of consistency on temperature can be expressed by the following equation:

$$k = 399.2\exp(-0.081T)$$

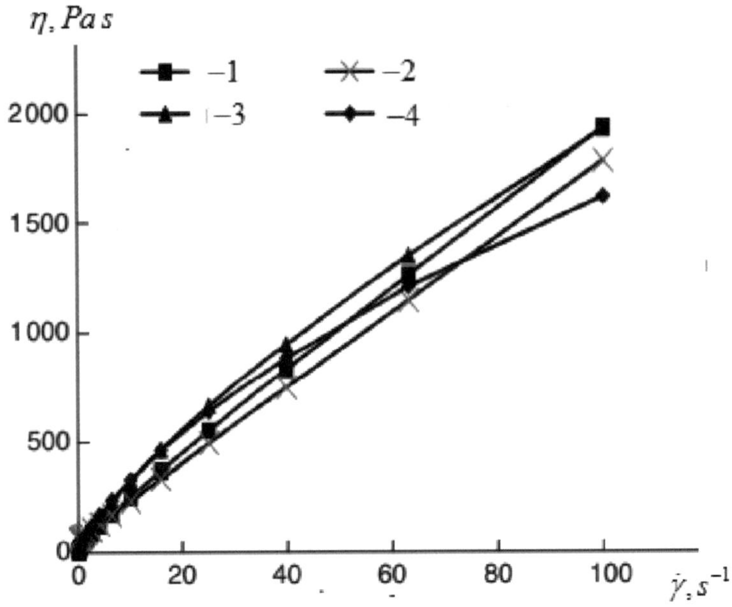

Figure 14.
Approximation of the dependence of viscosity on shear rate by various rheological models: (1) Casson model, $\tau = \left(\tau_0^{1/2} + k^{1/2}\dot{\gamma}^{1/2}\right)^2$; (2) Bingham model, $\tau = \tau_0 + \eta\dot{\gamma}$; (3) exponential function, $\tau = k\dot{\gamma}^n$; (4) experiment.

	Temperature								
		25°C			45°C			60°C	
Model	τ_0, Pa	k, Pas	n	τ_0, Pa	k, Pas	n	τ_0, Pa	k, Pas	n
Casson	8.13	4.11	–	0.57	2.2	–	0.15	1.53	–
Power law	–	54.65	0.77	–	9.26	0.88	–	3.86	0.9
Bingham	61	17.23	–	8.66	4.81	–	3.13	2.33	–

Table 2.
Coefficients of rheological models at T = 25, 45, and 60°C.

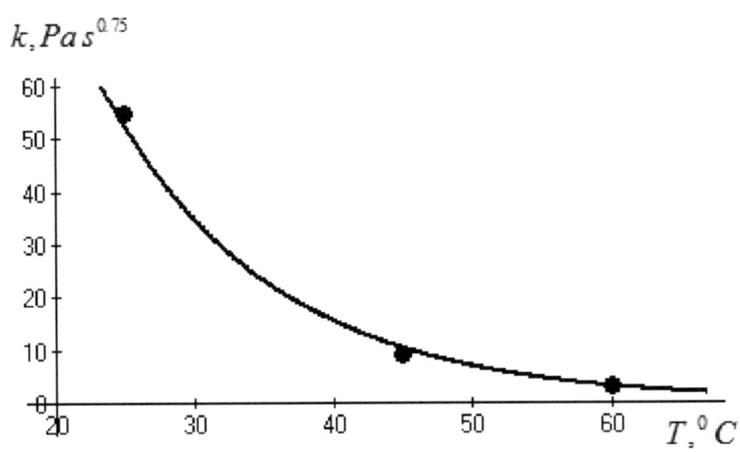

Figure 15.
The dependence of the coefficient of consistency on temperature.

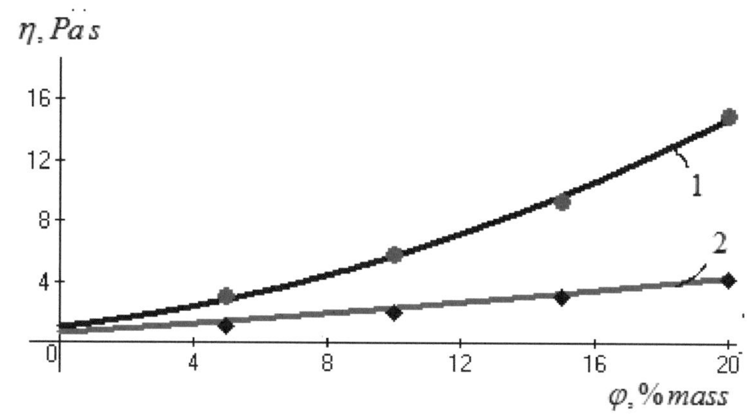

Figure 16.
Dependence of oil viscosity on the content of asphaltenes in it at temperatures: 1–25°C (k_0=0.022); 2–45°C (k_0=0.003).

Figure 15 shows the dependence of the coefficient of consistency on temperature.

The dependence of oil viscosity on the content of asphaltenes (% wt.) in oil using experimental data is expressed by the formula (**Figure 16**)

$$\eta = \eta_0\left(1 + 0.25\varphi + k_0\varphi^2\right) \tag{73}$$

Provided that $\varphi < 10\%$ this expression coincides with the Einstein formula.

In [49], similar studies were conducted for West Siberian oils for the concentration of asphaltenes in oil from 4 to 72% (mass.). This work presents experimental studies of the effective viscosity of non-Newtonian oil as a function of asphaltene content at various temperatures (**Figure 17**). As follows from **Figure 17**, the region of transition from Newtonian to non-Newtonian properties with an increase in the content of asphalt-resinous substances *I* is limited by an abrupt change in the viscosity of oil for all temperatures. Obviously, this is explained by the fact that when the content of asphaltenes is 38–46% (mass.) in West Siberian oil, an abrupt change in the effective viscosity of the oil, structural and mechanical strength, the temperature of the transition to the state of a non-Newtonian fluid, and molecular

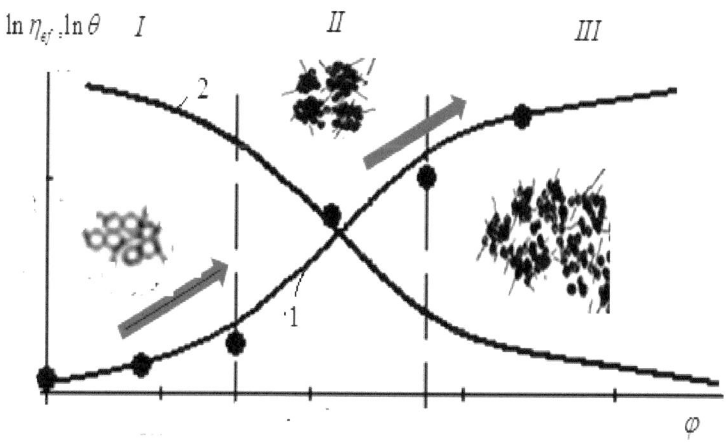

Figure 17.
Characteristic stages of structure formation in oil depending on the content of asphaltenes: I, dispersed oil; II, area of formation of structures; III, structured oil system, 1, viscosity; 2, fluidity.

weight occurs, which is due to the formation of coagulation structures, aggregates, up to the frame throughout the volume. A spasmodic change in viscosity during the period of structure formation (**Figure 17**) and destruction of the structure (**Figure 11**) is a characteristic feature of non-Newtonian oils, which complicates the character of the description of the entire viscosity and mobility curve of the oil system. The process of formation of coagulation structures is associated with an increase in the probability of interaction and collision of particles with an increase in their concentration in the volume. In the next section, problems of coagulation, coalescence of drops and bubbles, and many issues related to solving this problem will be described in detail.

As follows from **Figure 17**, as the structure formation and the concentration of asphaltenes increase, the mobility or fluidity of the oil system decreases, and the fluidity of the system is defined as

$$\ln\theta = \frac{\ln\eta_{\infty}}{\ln\eta_{ef}} \tag{74}$$

Figure 18 shows the experimental data on the change in viscosity of West Siberian oil depending on the asphaltene content [4].

The equation describing the experimental data on the viscosity of oil in large intervals of changes in the content of asphaltenes is presented in the form

$$\ln\mu_{ef} = \ln\eta_0 + b_0\varphi + b_1\delta(\varphi) + b_2\left(1 - \exp\left(-b_3\varphi^6\right)\right) \tag{75}$$

Here φ is the mass fraction of asphaltenes in oil; b_0–b_3 are the coefficients determined experimentally and depending on temperature; b_1 is the maximum value of the delta function; $\delta(\varphi)$ is the delta function, defined as

$$\delta(\varphi) = \frac{1}{\exp\left(72.5(\varphi - 0.45)\right) + \exp\left(-72.5(\varphi - 0.45)\right)} \tag{76}$$

and η_0 is the initial viscosity,

$$\eta_0 = 2.05x10^{-8}\exp\left(\frac{6075}{T + 273}\right) \tag{77}$$

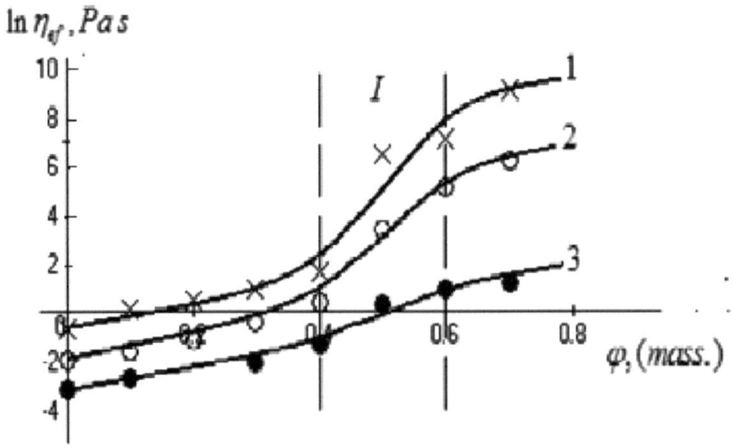

Figure 18.
The dependence of the effective viscosity on the content of the dispersed phase of tar-asphaltene at temperatures: 1–84°C; 2–112°C; 3–144°C. (I—Region of spasmodic structure formation).

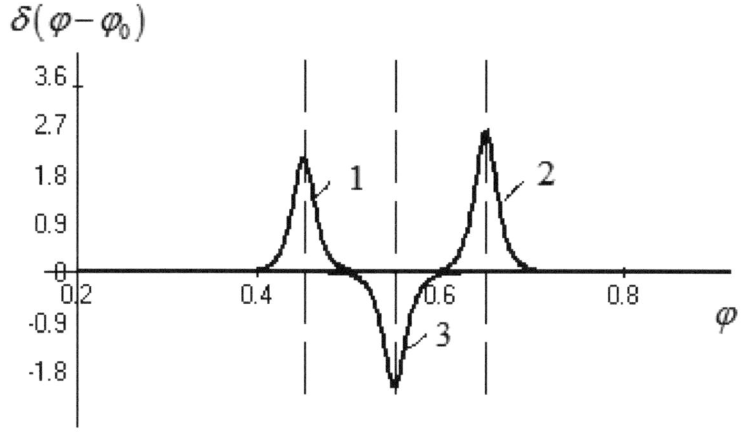

Figure 19.
Delta functions: 1 and 2, positive values of the function $\delta(\varphi) > 0$ *with centers* $\varphi = 0.45, 0.65$*; 3, negative values of the function* $\delta(\varphi) < 0$ *with center* $\varphi = 0.55$.

The value of the delta function characterizes the viscosity jump in the region of structure formation. In particular, the main property of the delta function is as follows

$$\delta(\varphi\text{-}\varphi_0) = \left\{ \begin{matrix} 0, & \varphi \neq \varphi_0 \\ \infty, & \varphi = \varphi_0 \end{matrix} \right\} \tag{78}$$

The expression of the partial approximation of the delta function can be represented

$$\delta(\varphi) = \frac{1}{\exp\left(b_1(\varphi\text{-}\varphi_0)\right) + \exp\left(-b_2(\varphi\text{-}\varphi_0)\right)} \tag{79}$$

Here b_1 and b_2 are the coefficients that determine the width of the base of the delta function, and φ_0 is the coordinate of the center of the jump. **Figure 19** shows various types of delta functions.

Thus, the use of the delta function allows one to describe all the spasmodic phenomena occurring during the formation and destruction of structures in non-Newtonian oil. At the same time, satisfactory results are obtained by using an exponential function of a higher order, which allows one to obtain a smoothing effect in the region of the jump.

The use of aromatic and other solvents partially dissolves asphaltenes, thereby reducing or eliminating the formation of coagulation structures, which improves the rheological properties of dispersed petroleum media. As follows from **Figure 18**, for a given oil, if the asphaltene content is less, the formation of coagulation structures is excluded, although there may be other conditions for different oil fields. An analysis of various studies on the influence of asphalt-resinous substances on the rheology of non-Newtonian oil of various fields leads to conflicting results, although in all cases there is an increase in viscosity as a result of structure formation. It should be noted that in addition to asphaltenes, the rheological properties of the oil disperse system are affected by the content of water and solid phase in it.

4. Evolution of the droplet distribution function in an oil emulsion

Coalescence and fragmentation of droplets significantly change the dispersion of oil emulsions, which is characterized by the evolution of the probability distribution function over time and size, described by the Boltzmann kinetic equation and the stochastic Fokker-Planck Equation [7, 8, 49, 50]. Changing the size and shape of water droplets in an oil emulsion as a result of their coalescence, deformation, and crushing significantly affects the rheological parameters, in particular, the effective viscosity of the emulsion. Coalescence and crushing of water droplets in emulsions can occur simultaneously. Then the rate of change in the number and size of particles per unit volume is determined by the rates of their coalescence and crushing

$$\frac{dN}{dt} = U_k - U_d \tag{80}$$

where N is the current number of drops in the volume and U_k and U_d are the rates of coalescence and fragmentation of the drops. At a fast droplet crushing rate, the particle distribution function is asymmetric with respect to the maximum and is characterized by a single maximum independent of shear rate, although with slow coagulation, the particle size distribution function can have several maxima and minima, i.e., be multimodal. Moreover, each maximum will characterize the primary, secondary, etc. coagulation of particles of a dispersed medium.

During slow coagulation of solid particles, it is important to construct the evolution of the distribution function over the residence time and size, which gives a complete picture of the change in the number and size of particles over time. In [1, 2], the Fokker-Plank equation is used to construct the evolution of the particle distribution function. The stochastic Fokker-Planck equation describes disperse systems with a continuous change in the properties of the medium and the size of dispersed inclusions. Although the processes of coalescence and fragmentation are characterized by an abrupt change in the properties of particles (sizes), in principle, for a sufficiently long period of time, a change in the average properties can be assumed to be quasicontinuous with an infinitely small jump. In particular, it can be assumed that the average size of droplets and bubbles varies continuously over time and obeys the equation of the change in the average particle mass over time:

$$\frac{dm}{dt} = \omega(a)m \tag{81}$$

Many experimental studies on the fragmentation and coagulation of particles in a turbulent flow show that the average particle size is set at the minimum or maximum level, which corresponds to the aggregative stability of a dispersed medium. Given the above, in Eq. (81) should be considered as the reduced mass relative to the extreme values of the particles, i.e., $m = \frac{\pi}{6}\rho_d(a\text{-}a_{min})^3$ for crushing and $m = \frac{\pi}{6}\rho_d(a\text{-}a_{max})^3$ for coalescence. In particular, based on Eq. (81), we obtain the expression for changing the size of the droplets when they are crushed in the form

$$\begin{aligned} &\frac{da}{dt} = -K(\omega, a)(a\text{-}a_{min}) = m_0 - m_1 a = f(a), m_0 = Ka_{min}, \\ &m_1 = K, t = 0, a = a_0 \end{aligned} \tag{82}$$

being a time-continuous process where $K(\omega, a) = \omega(a)/3 \approx \frac{C_1}{3}\varphi\left(\frac{k_0\dot{\gamma}^{n-1}}{a^2}\right)^{1/3}$ for a power non-Newtonian fluid and $K(\omega, a) = \frac{C_1}{3}\varphi\dot{\gamma}$ for a visco-plastic fluid.

Thus, considering the change in particle size as a continuous function, the Fokker-Planck equation in the simplest case, taking into account (82), can be written as [8, 49, 50].

$$\frac{\partial P(\mathrm{a,t})}{\partial t} = \frac{\partial y}{\partial \mathrm{a}}[P(\mathrm{a,t})(m_0 - m_1 a)] + \frac{B}{2}\frac{\partial^2 P(\mathrm{a,t})}{\partial a^2} \qquad (83)$$
$$t = 0, P(\mathrm{a},0) = P_0(\mathrm{a}); a \to 0, P(\mathrm{a,t}) \to 0$$

where B is the coefficient of stochastic diffusion.

The solution to this equation presents great difficulties associated with specifying the form of the function $f(a)$, although some particular analytical solutions of Eq. (83) depending on the nature of the function can be found in [8, 49, 50].

The solution of Eq. (83) by the method of separation of variables will be presented in the form

$$P(r,t) = r^{\theta} \exp\left(\frac{ka_0^2 r^2}{2B}\right) \sum_{n=0}^{\infty} C_n L_n^{(\alpha)}\left(\frac{ka_0^2 r^2}{2B}\right) \exp(-2knt) \qquad (84)$$

where $\theta = {m_R a_0^2}/_B$, $\alpha = \frac{m_R a_0^2 - B}{2B}$, $L_n^{(\alpha)}$ Laguerre functions, and

$$C_n = \frac{\theta^{\frac{\theta+1}{2}} \int_0^{\infty} P_0(r) L_n^{(\alpha)}\left(\frac{ka_0^2 r^2}{2B}\right) dr}{2^{\frac{\theta-1}{2}} \Gamma\left(n + \frac{\theta+1}{2}\right) m^{\frac{\theta+1}{\theta}} n!} \qquad (85)$$

Solutions (84) and (85) characterize the evolution of the probability density distribution function of droplets in size and in time. The asymptotic value of the distribution for i $t \to \infty$ s is obtained from solution (84), taking into account the properties of the Laguerre function, in the form

$$P_{\infty}(r) = C_R r^{\theta} \exp\left(-\frac{ka_0^2 r^2}{2B}\right) = C_{PR} a^{\theta} \exp\left(-ba^2\right) \qquad (86)$$

$$C_{PR} = 2a_0^{-\theta}\left(\frac{\theta}{2m}\right)^{\frac{\theta+1}{2}}, \quad b = {k}/_{2B}$$

Having introduced some simplifications taking into account the initial distribution in the form of a lognormal function $P_0(a) = A_0(a)\exp\left(-m_0(\ln a - \alpha_0)^2\right)$ and the limiting distribution (86) taking into account the experimental data for the family of distribution curves with a number m, with some assumptions in a more simplified form, we obtain

$$P(a,t) = \sum_{n=0}^{\infty} A_n(t) \exp\left[-m_n(t)(\ln a - \alpha_{sn})^2\right] \qquad (87)$$

where $\alpha_{sn} = \ln a_s$ is the parameter corresponding to the logarithm of the maximum value of each extremum.

Figure 20 shows the evolution of the distribution function of the fragmentation of a non-Newtonian viscoelastic drop (oil) in an aqueous medium.

The spectrum of large and small droplets is practically shifted relatively to each other [8, 49] (**Figure 20**).

It is important to note that the fluctuation of the distribution function on the left side of the curve indicates secondary, tertiary, etc. the nature of droplet crushing, and on the right side - about their multiple coalescence. However, after some time, when the resources of the large-droplet or small-droplet spectrum are exhausted,

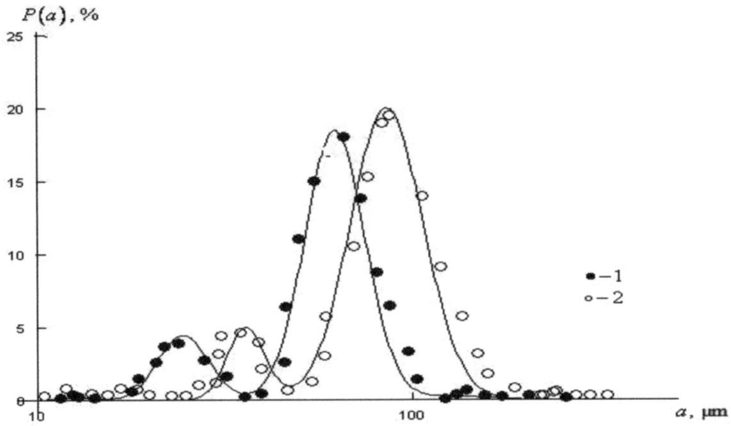

Figure 20.
The characteristic distribution of the distribution function during crushing drops in size and time equal to 1, 10 min., and 2, 20 minutes.

the spectrum begins to behave like a single-humped one. In practice, the behavior of multi-hump distributions in the model representation is confirmed when the distribution is represented by the sum of two or more distribution functions. The character of the evolution of the distribution function and the change in the coefficient of turbulent diffusion can also be significantly affected by the deposition of particles from the turbulent flow. The distribution spectrum varies significantly with a change in the droplet deposition rate. In conclusion, we note that the phenomena of coalescence and fragmentation of droplets are spasmodic. In the case of small jumps, such processes are satisfactorily described by the Fokker-Planck equation. Obviously, jumps should become smaller and more likely, so the diffusion process can always be approximated by a jump process, but not vice versa.

5. Discussion of results and conclusions

The content in the composition of crude oil of various particles of the dispersed phase significantly affects the rheological parameters of the liquid. The main phenomena in the processes of coalescence of water droplets in oil emulsions are the destruction of the adsorption film on the surface due to asphalt-resinous substances, the thinning and rupture of the interfacial film between the droplets, and the coalescence of droplets.

The formation and formation of the adsorption layer is described by Eq. (5), a comparison of which with experimental data gives satisfactory results. The equation for estimating the thickness of the adsorption layer is given in (4). To study the thinning of the interfacial film, Eqs. (17) and (18) are derived that take into account the presence of dynamic, capillary, proppant pressure and the Marangoni effect. Particular cases of solving proposed Eqs. (20)–(24) are presented. Comparison with the experimental data on the thinning of the interfacial film [38] for West Siberian oils (**Figure 5**) showed that for large values of the film thickness, Eq. (20) with coefficients equal to $b_3 = 1.2.10^{-3}$ is the most suitable, and coefficient β_1 is shown in **Table 3**.

For very thin films $\delta \leq \delta_{кр}$, expression (21) with a coefficient $b_3 = 0.098$ is suitable, and the change in surface tension is described by the formula $\sigma = (3.6 + (\sigma_0 - 3.6)\exp(-23.1C)) \times 10^{-3}, H/м$.

$C, g/l$	0,10	0,20	1,00	1,20
β_1	0.14	0.235	0.265	0.30

Table 3.
The dependence of the coefficient β_1 on the concentration demulsifier.

After reaching the critical value of the thickness $\delta \leq \delta_{\kappa p}$, spontaneous thinning and interfacial film breaking occur (**Figure 5**). As follows from formulas (17)–(23), a proppant pressure, inversely proportional to the film thickness and depending on the asphaltene content in oil and the concentration of demulsifier, plays an important role in thinning and rupture of an interfacial film.

The presence of two-dimensional pressures and the complexity of its distribution on the film surface, taking into account Eq. (14), show that, when it is thinned, the presence of the Marangoni effect to some extent helps to stabilize oil emulsions, i.e., has an inhibitory effect on tearing the film. As follows from Eq. (20) and the formula for determining the coefficient, the Marangoni effect contributes to the temporary stabilization of the interfacial film, since at any point where the film becomes thinner due to the influence of external forces, a local increase in surface tension occurs, which counteracts the thinning. The process of thinning and rupture of the film is random (spontaneous) in nature, and the probability of its rupture is inversely proportional to its thickness.

The main physical phenomena that occur in oil emulsions are the coalescence of droplets in the presence of asphalt-resinous substances in the oil, leading to structure formation. An analytical solution of the equation of diffusion transfer of droplets in an isotropic turbulent flow determines the coalescence and fragmentation frequencies of droplets (29–31).

The paper proposes many expressions for determining the structural viscosity of oil from the content of water droplets, as well as the empirical or semiempirical dependences of the oil viscosity on the content of asphalt-resinous substances (73) for Iranian oil and (81) for West Siberian oil. Theoretical and experimental studies have shown that the value of the structural viscosity of oil during structure formation sharply increases, and when the structure is destroyed, it sharply decreases (**Figure 11**).

Based on the Fokker-Planck equation, the evolution of the distribution function of water droplets in an oil emulsion as a function of size and time is studied (84) and (85).

The intensification of the processes of flow and separation of oil emulsions is associated primarily with the rheological properties of the oil emulsion and turbulization of the flow. High-frequency turbulent pulsations contribute to the mechanical weakening of the adsorption and interfacial film and intermolecular bonds between its components, a decrease in the strength and destruction of the film as a result of their deformation (tension, compression), and improvement of the conditions of mutual effective collision (increase in the collision frequency) and coalescence.

Acknowledgements

This work was supported by the Science Foundation of «SOCAR» under the grant project 04LR - AMEA (10/09/2019) at the Institute of Catalysis and Inorganic Chemistry named after Acad. M.F.Nagiyev.

Nomenclature

A	van der Waals-Hamaker constant;
b_1, b_2, b_3	coefficients in Eq. (18)
a	diameter of drops
C	concentration
c_P	heat capacity
D	molecular diffusion coefficient
D_T	droplet diffusion coefficient
d	pipe diameter
f	resistance coefficient in pipes
F	the force acting on the interfacial film
F_g	hypergeometric function
H	height of the intermediate layer
g	acceleration of gravity
I	mass flow to the surface of a drop per unit time
$P(a,t)$	size distribution function of the probability of droplets
R_K	interfacial film radius
R	drop radius
P	pressure
T	temperature
V_P	particle velocity
V	flow rate in the film
U	flow rate
$\overline{U}^2$	mean square velocity
t	time
Γ	the concentration of adsorbed matter
δ	film thickness
$\dot{\gamma}$	shear rate
δ_0	initial film thickness
Δ	the thickness of the adsorbed layer
ε	the porosity of the intermediate layer
ε_R	specific energy dissipation
ν_C	kinematic viscosity of the medium
η	film viscosity
η_c	dynamic viscosity of the medium
η_d	dynamic viscosity of a drop
η_{ef}	effective viscosity of emulsions
λ	coefficient of thermal conductivity
μ_P	the degree of entrainment of drops by a pulsating medium
μ	eigenvalues
σ	surface tension
Π	proppant pressure
ρ_C	medium density
ρ_d	droplet density
τ_P	relaxation time
τ	shear stress
φ	volume fraction of droplets in the stream
ω	collision frequency
$\mathrm{Mo} = \frac{g\eta_c^4}{\rho_c\sigma^3}\frac{\Delta\rho}{\rho_c}$	Morton's number
$\mathrm{Pe} = \frac{Ua_r}{D}$	Peclet number

$\mathrm{Re} = \frac{V_p d}{\nu_c}$	Reynolds number
$\mathrm{We} = \frac{\rho_c U^2 a}{\sigma}$	the Weber number

Indices:

0	initial conditions
p	particle
c	medium

Author details

Gudret Isfandiyar Kelbaliyev, Dilgam Babir Tagiyev and Manaf Rizvan Manafov*
Azerbaijan National Academy of Sciences, Nagiyev Institute of Catalysis and Inorganic Chemistry, Baku, Azerbaijan

*Address all correspondence to: mmanafov@gmail.com

IntechOpen

© 2020 The Author(s). Licensee IntechOpen. This chapter is distributed under the terms of the Creative Commons Attribution License (http://creativecommons.org/licenses/by/3.0), which permits unrestricted use, distribution, and reproduction in any medium, provided the original work is properly cited.

References

[1] Lissant L. Emulsion and Emulsion Technology. New York: Marsel Dekker; 1976. p. 211

[2] Sjoblom J, Urdahl O, Hoiland H, Christy AA, Johansen EJ. Water in crude oil emulsions formation, characterization and destabilization. Progress in Colloid and Polymer Science. 1990;**82**:131

[3] Pozdnyshev GN. Stabilization and Destruction of Oil Emulsions. Moscow: Nedra; 1982

[4] Tronov VP. The Destruction of Emulsions in Oil Production. Moscow: Nedra; 1974. p. 314

[5] Tirmizi NP, Raghurankan B, Wiencek J. Demulsification of water/oil/solid emulsions by hollow-fiber membranes. AICHE Journal. 2004; **42**(5):1263

[6] Danae D, Lee CH, Fane AG, Fell CJD. A fundamental study of the ultrafiltration of oil-water emulsions. Journal of Membrane Science. 1987;**36**: 161

[7] Kelbaliev GI, Rasulov SR. Hydrodynamics and Mass Transfer in Dispersed Media. ChemIzdat: St. Petersburg; 2014. p. 567

[8] Kelbaliyev GI, Tagiyev LB, Rasulov SR. Transport Phenomena in Dispersed Media. Boca Raton, London, New York: Taylor and Francis Group, CRC Press; 2019. p. 424

[9] Sarimeseli A, Kelbaliyev G. Modeling of the break-up of deformable particles in developed turbulent flow. Chemical Engineering Science. 2004;**59**(6): 1233-1240

[10] Kelbaliyev G, Sarimeseli A. Modeling of drop coalescence in isotropic turbulent flow. Journal of Dispersion Science and Technology. 2006;**27**:443

[11] Migashitani K, Yamauchi K, Mastuno Y. Coalescence of drop in viscous fluid. Journal of Chemical Engineering. 1985;**18**:299

[12] Colaloglou CA, Tavlarides II. Description of interaction process in agitated liquid-liquid dispersions. Chemical Engineering Science. 1977;**32**: 1289

[13] Soo SL. Fluid Dynamics of Multiphase Systems. London: Blaisdell Puiblishing; 1970

[14] Hirschberg A, DeJong NL, Schipper BA, Meijer JG. Influence of temperature and pressure on Asphaltene flocculation. Society of Petroleum Engineers. 1984;**24**(3):283

[15] Laux H, Rahiman I, Browarzik D. Flocculation of asphaltenes at high pressure. I. Experimental determination of the onset of flocculation. Petroleum Science and Technology. 2001;**19**(9/10): 1155

[16] Mulhins OC, Shey EY. Structures and Dynamics of Asphaltenes. New York: Plenum Press; 1998

[17] McLean J, Kilpatrick PK. Effects of asphaltene solvency on stability of water crude oil emulsions. Journal of Colloid and Interface Science. 1997;**189**(2):242

[18] Levich VG. Physicochemical Hydrodynamics. Moscow: Fizmatgiz; 1962

[19] Ermakov SA, Mordvinov AA. On the effect of asphaltenes on the stability of oil-water emulsions. Oil and Gas Business. 2007;**10**:1

[20] Wegener M, Fevre M, Wang Z, Paschedag A, Kraune M. Marangoni convection in single drop flow – Experimental investigation and 3D-simulation. In: 6th International Conference of Multiphase Flow. Leipzig, Germany; 2007. p. 9

[21] Fanton X, Cazabat AM, Quyru D. Thickness and shape of films driven by a Marangoni flow. Langmuir. 1996;**12**: 5875

[22] Leo LY, Matar OK, Perez de Ortir ES, Hewitt GF. A description of phase inversion behavior in agitated liquid-liquid dispersions under the of Marangoni effect. Chemical Engineering Science. 2002;**57**:3505

[23] Scheludko A. Thin liquid film. Advances in Colloid and Interface Science. 1967;**11**:391

[24] Chen JD, Slattery JC. Effects of London-van der Waals forces on the thinning of a dimpled liquid films as a small drop or bubble approaches a horizontal solid phase. AICHE Journal. 1990;**28**(6):955

[25] Petrov AA, Blatov SA. Study of the stability of hydrocarbon layers at the interface with aqueous solutions of demulsifiers. Chemistry and Technology of Fuels and Oils. 1969;**5**: 25-33

[26] Liao Y, Lucas D. A literature review of theoretical models for drop and bubble breakup in turbulent dispersions. Chemical Engineering Science. 2009;**64**(15):3389-3395

[27] Altunbas A, Kelbaliyev G, Ceylan K. Eddy diffusivity of particles in turbulent flow in rough channels. Journal of Aerosol Science. 2002;**33**:1075

[28] Wang T, Wang J, Jin Y. A novel theoretical breakup kernel function for bubbles/droplets in a turbulent flow. Chemical Engineering Science. 2003;**58**: 4629-4636

[29] Chatzi E. Analysis of interactions for liquid–liquid dispersions in agitated vessels. Industrial and Engineering Chemistry Research. 1987;**26**:2263-2272

[30] Chatzi E, Kiparissides C. Dynamic simulation of bimodal drop size distributions in low-coalescence batch dispersion systems. Chemical Engineering Science. 1992;**47**:445-456

[31] Alopaeus V. Simulation of the population balances for liquid–liquid systems in a nonideal stirred tank. Part 2: Parameter fitting and the use of the multiblock model for dense dispersions. Chemical Engineering Science. 2002;**57**: 1815-1826

[32] Lehr F, Milles M, Mewes D. Bubble-size distributions and flow fields in bubble columns. AICHE Journal. 2002; **48**:2426-2436

[33] Raymond F, Rozant JM. A numerical and experimental study of the terminal velocity and shape of bubbles in viscous fluids. Chemical Engineering Science. 2000;**57**:943-953

[34] Liu L, Yan H, Zhao G. Experimental studies on the shape and motion of air bubbles in viscous liquids. Experimental Thermal and Fluid Science. 2015;**62**: 109-121

[35] Batchelor GK. The effect of Brownian motion on the bulk stress in a suspension of spherical particles. Journal of Fluid Mechanics. 1977;**83**:97-117

[36] Krieger IM, Dougherty TJ. A mechanism for non-Newtonian flow in suspensions of rigid spheres. Transactions. Society of Rheology. 1959; **N3**:137-152

[37] Quemada D. Rheology of concentrated disperse systems and

minimum energy dissipation principle I. Viscosity-concentration relationship. Rheologica Acta. 1977;**16**:82-94

[38] Brownstein BI, Schegolev VV. Hydrodynamics, mass – and heat transfer in column apparatus. Moscow: Chemistry; 1988. 325p

[39] Khodakov GS. Rheology of suspensions. The theory of phase flow and its experimental justification. Ross Khim Zh. 2003;**XLVII**(2):33-41

[40] Vielma JC. Rheologocal Behavior of Oil-Water Dispersion flow in horizontal pipes. A thesis submitted in partial fulfillment of the requirements for the degree of Master of Science in the Discipline of Petroleum Engineering. The University of Tulsa; 2006

[41] Mewis J, Wagner NJ. Colloidal Suspension Rheology. Cambridge, UK: Cambridge University Press; 2012

[42] Kelbaliyev GI, Rasulov SR, Mustafayeva GR. Viscosity of structured disperse systems. Theoretical Foundations of Chemical Engineering. 2018;**52**(3):404-411

[43] Oil Emulsions. Available from: http://petrowiki.org/Oil emulsions

[44] Kroy K, Capron I, Djabourov M, Thermique P. ESPCI. Paris. France; 1999

[45] Krassimir D. Danov on the viscosity of dilute emulsions. Journal of Colloid and Interface Science. 2001;**235**:144-149

[46] Argillier JF, Coustet C, Hénaut I. Heavy oil rheology as a function of asphaltene and resin content and temperature. SPE/Petroleum Society of CIM/CHOA 79496, International Thermal Operations and Heavy Oil Symposuim and International Horizontal Well Technology Conference. 2002

[47] Davarpanah L, Vahabzadeh F, Dermanaki A. Structural study of Asphaltenes from Iranian heavy crude oil. Oil and Gas Science and Technology. 2015;**70**(6):1035-1049

[48] Mukhmedzyanova AA, Buduik VA, Alyabev AS, Khaybullin AA. Influence of temperature and asphaltenes concentration on rheological properties of disperse systems of the west Siberian oils tar. Bashkir Chemical Journal. 2012; **19**(4):1-4

[49] Sis H, Kelbaliyev G, Chander S. Kinetics of drop breakage in stirred vessels under turbulent conditions. Journal of Dispersion Science and Technology. 2005;**26**:565

[50] Gardiner CW. In: Haken H, editor. Handbook of Stochastic Methods for Physics, Chemistry and the Natural Sciences. New York: Springer; 1985

Chapter 8

Aggregation of Partially Hydrophilic Silica Nanoparticles in Porous Media: Quantitative and Qualitative Analysis

Siti Rohaida Mohd Shafian, Ismail M. Saaid, Norzafirah Razali, Ahmad Fadhil Jahari and Sonny Irawan

Abstract

In this experimental work, the adsorption of partially hydrophilic silica nanoparticles, SiO_2 has been investigated to determine the degree of silica nanoparticle aggregation in the porous media. An integrated quantitative and qualitative method was used by flowing silica nanoparticles into Buff Berea cores and glass micromodel. Water wet Buff Berea cores were flooded with 5 pore volumes of 0.05% silica nanoparticles solution followed by 10 pore volumes of brine post flush subjected to 30 and 60°C. The pressure drops increased rapidly at the initial stage of silica nanoparticles injection indicated the adsorption had taken place. Pressure drops reached the maximum value of ~3.1 psi and between 26.6–82.6 psi at 30 and 60°C respectively. Pressure drops gradually declined and stabilized in between ~0.4 and ~0.7 psi after couple of pore volumes of brine post flush, suggesting complete reversible and irreversible adsorption. Micromodel test provide qualitative information where the straining or log-jamming observed in the form of gelled-like suspension when silica nanoparticles in contact with brine. The adsorption is considered reversible when the suspension decreased after post flooded with brine. Silica nanoparticles used in this experimental work shows minimal aggregation that can be beneficial as improved oil recovery agent.

Keywords: nanotechnology, nanoparticles, silica nanoparticles, aggregation, adsorption, porous media, core flooding, micromodels, permeability impairment

1. Introduction

The advancement of nanotechnology attract researchers interest for its application in oil and gas that include the application for enhanced oil recovery, exploration, drilling, completion, well logging, chemical stabilizer, conformance control, heavy oil, stimulation and fines migration control [1–13]. The unique properties of nanoparticles comprises of extremely high surface area compared to their small sizes, thermally stable, high potential to alter the wettability of the reservoir formations, modify rock surface charges and associated impact on the rheological properties of suspensions [14] that showed potentials to enhance extraction of hydrocarbons. Silica nanoparticles, SiO_2 for example, can be found in most non-toxic inorganic materials which also the main component of sandstone rock, and is more environmental friendly compared to chemical based materials. Nanoparticles have showed remarkable performance in fixing the formation fines during fracturing activities [12]. Several studies suggested the nanoparticles has the effect of strengthening the attractive forces with regards to the repulsive forces and prevent the detachment of fines particles from the pore walls [15].

Nanoparticles are very small in nature with size range between 1 and 100 nm [16] which permits this tiny particles to flow in the porous media and show distinctive behavior which fascinating from petroleum engineering perspective. During nanoparticles transport in porous media, the physicochemical attraction between particles and the pore walls can lead to adsorption or retention that occurs as reversible and irreversible [17, 18]. Adsorption in porous media can create major issue and need to be control to avoid significant formation damage. Abdelfatah described; three different mechanisms were taken place when nanoparticles interact in the pores. These interactions are surfaces deposition, mono-particle plugging and multi-particles plugging [19]. The surface deposition interactions are dominated by five type of forces; the attractive potential force of Van der Waals, repulsion force of electric double layers, Born repulsion, acid–base interaction, and hydrodynamics [20]. The adsorption of nanoparticles and the pore walls will occur when the total force is negative, where the attraction is larger than repulsion between nanoparticles and pore walls.

The mono-particle plugging or screening or mechanical entrapment occur when larger particle block at the narrow pores. Injecting large volume of nanoparticles can lead to mono-particle plugging. Multi-particles plugging or log-jamming mechanism is similar to mono-particle plugging but the blocking occurs at pore channel larger than nanoparticles size. Log-jamming happen when nanoparticles flow from pores to narrow pore throat. Nanoparticles interaction between the particles itself can cause aggregation and gelation and the significantly block the pore throat if the aggregate size much bigger than pore throat. The adsorption of nanoparticle on the pore walls also depends on the type and pH of nanoparticles, rock clay content as well as the rock wettability [21]. The advantage of nanoparticles adsorption, instead, it contributed to the alteration of rock wettability that is desirable for

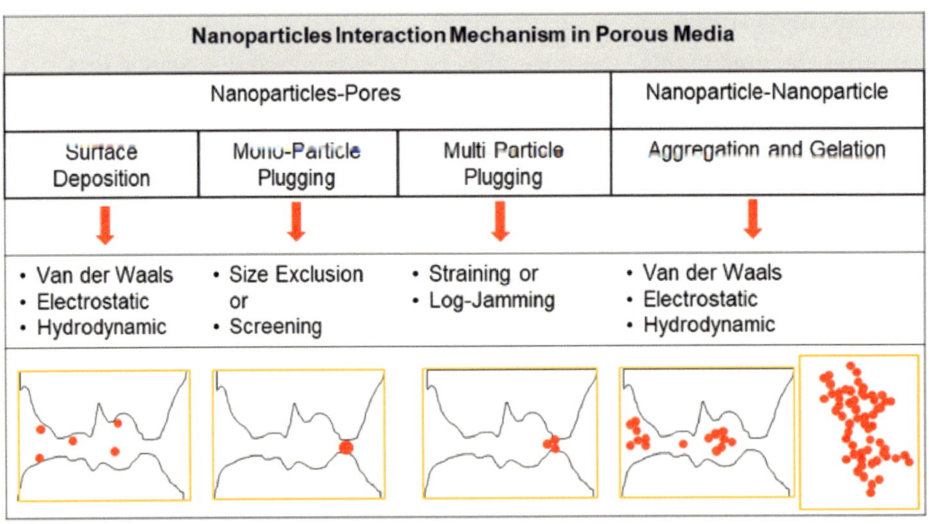

Figure 1.
Nanoparticles interactions mechanisms in porous media [19].

enhanced oil recovery [22–25]. Nanoparticles specifically silica nanoparticles on the other hand, are not stable in salts water and aggregates at elevated temperature, high concentration and at high injection rates that can lead to substantial permeability impairment [17, 24, 26–28]. **Figure 1** shows the illustration of nanoparticles interactions mechanisms in porous media.

This experimental work investigates the aggregation of partially hydrophilic silica nanoparticles, SiO_2 in porous media. The standard method for silica nanoparticles concentration measurement using UV-Vis spectrophotometer is not suitable, and hence more reliable quantitative and qualitative methods were developed. Core flooding pressure drops and particles size analysis of treated Buff Berea cores provide quantitative information supported by qualitative measurement of Field Emission Scanning Electron Microscope (FESEM) and micromodel test. The pressure drops value showed closed agreements with particles size during silica nanoparticles injection and brine post flush, visualization of silica nanoparticles in micromodel. FESEM analysis suggested the partially hydrophilic silica nanoparticles used in this experimental work showed minimal aggregation with insignificant permeability impairment.

2. Materials and methods

2.1 Materials for core flooding

2.1.1 Nanofluids

Partially hydrophilic silica nanoparticles (SiO_2) supplied by commercial nanomaterials company using code name NPN-ST. This nanoparticles was selected based the requirement of this research work in terms of size and solubility in water and selected solvent. NPN-ST supplied at 30% active concentration with average size of 12 nm and pH 5. NPN-ST was diluted in mutual solvent at 0.05% concentration and the solution undergoes sonication in ultrasonic bath for at least 40 minutes.

NPN-ST stability in the carrier fluid before and after 24 hours aged at room temperature and 60°C was determined through visual observation, turbidity test and particle size distribution measurement. The particle size of NPN-ST slightly increased from 24 nm to ~27 nm and 35 nm after kept for 24 hours at room temperature and at 60°C respectively. The incremental of particle size is minor which is within the accepted size required for this study.

The turbidity reading is in the low range between 0.95 and 1.98 NTU. **Figure 2** shows the particles size distribution and visual observation of NPN-ST after 24 hours sustained as clear solution and did not show any forms of precipitation. **Figure 3** shows the Transmission Electron Microscopy (TEM) image of NPN-ST solution at 20 and 100 nm scale which comparable with most common silica nanoparticles materials.

2.1.2 Fluid samples

Formation brine used in this study is mixture of major ion salts prepared in deionized water. $CaCl_2$, $MgCl_2$, KCl and NaCl salts were mixed in the appropriate proportions to make up 1.5 wt% formation water salinity. Brine sample was filtered with the Millipore vacuum filter through a 47 mm, 0.45 micron nominal pore opening cellulose filter. **Table 1** shows the brine composition of synthetic formation water.

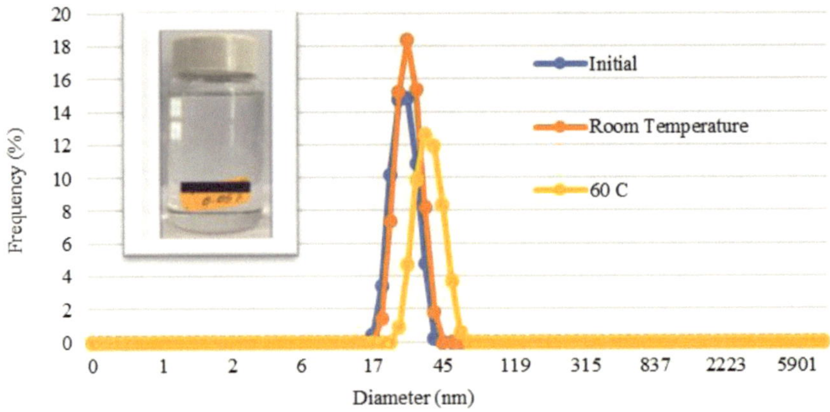

Figure 2.
Particle size and visual observation of NPN-ST at initial and after 24 hours aged at room temperature and 60°C.

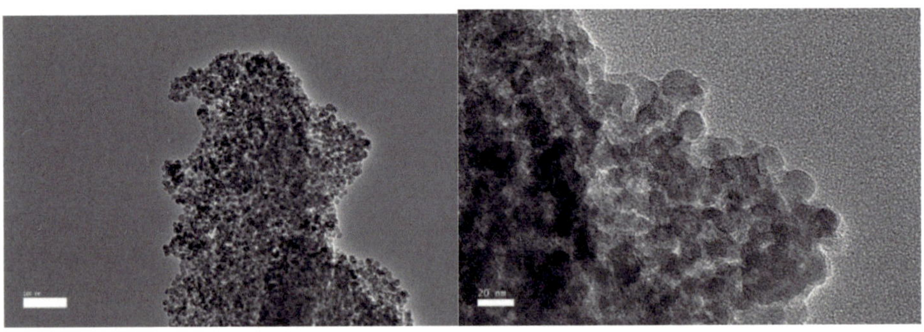

Figure 3.
Image of 0.05% NPN-ST under transmission electron microscopy (TEM): (a) at 100 nm scale and (b) at 20 nm scale.

Salts	Weight for 1 L (g)
NaCl	20.92
KCl	0.31
$MgCl_2.6H_2O$	0.08
$CaCl_2$	0.10

Table 1.
Salt composition for formation brine.

2.1.3 Core samples

Buff Berea cores of 3.8 cm in diameter and 7.5 cm in length (and 2 sets of core with 14.0 cm in length), permeability range between 200 and 400 mD that contained mixture of clays were used in this study. Five sets of core flood tests were conducted and details of core properties assigned for each experiment are listed in **Table 2**. **Table 3** shows the Buff Berea core detail mineralogy measured by X-Ray Diffraction (XRD) test.

Core ID	Diameter (cm)	Length (cm)	Porosity (%)	Air permeability (md)	Pore volumes (ml)	Test temperatures (°C)
B1–10	3.84	7.40	23.35	386.79	20.10	30
B3–21	3.84	7.44	23.20	328.89	20.02	30
L1	3.84	14.18	N.D.[1]	N.D.[1]	37.90	30
B7-16	3.84	7.44	23.50	325.42	19.82	60
L2	3.84	14.55	N.D.[1]	N.D.[1]	38.89	60

[1]*Not determine.*

Table 2.
Buff Berea core properties.

Core	Calculated whole rock composition (weight %)						
	Quartz	Plagioclase	K-Feldspar	Calcite	Dolomite	Siderite	Pyrite
Buff Berea	79.2	4.3	1.9	0.4	1.1	0.9	1.0
	Clay fraction Clay fraction (clay typing, weight %)						
	Kaolinite	Chlorite	Illite	Mixed layer (I/S)	Smectite	Total clay	
	36.2	19.7	33.2	7.9	2.5	10.7	

Table 3.
Buff Berea core X-ray diffraction (XRD) data.

2.2 Core flooding procedure

The dry weight of the core was measured before brine saturation. Core was saturated in desiccator with formation brine until all air trapped were removed. The core was then put in saturator for further saturation at 2000 psi for 24 hours. The saturated weight of the core was measured after saturation to calculate the core pore volume (PV) by gravimetric method. The core was carefully unloaded from saturator, into core holder and subject to 1500 psi confining pressure applied with mineral oil using automatic confining pressure pump. The back pressure was set at 200 psi and temperature set at 30 and 60°C. The core was flooded with brine for at least 2 pore volumes or until pressure stabilize at 0.5, 1.0 and 1.5 ml/min. The derived pressure drops data were used to calculate absolute permeability to water using Darcy's Law. The core flooding test was conducted using Formation Response Test (FRT) equipment model 3100. Core flooding equipment consists of:

- 12-inch core holder (1.5-inch diameter)
- Backpressure regulator
- 3 accumulators (1000 ml volume)
- A system of valves operated pneumatically via a computer
- An injection system, incorporating an electronically-controlled Quizix pump

- Automated auto sampler
- A balance to a data logger

Figure 4 shows the schematic of core flooding equipment.

After brine injection, 5 pore volumes of 0.05% SiO_2 NPN-ST was injected into Buff Berea core at 0.5 ml/min and aged for 24 hours. The core was flooded with brine for 10 pore volumes at 0.5 ml/min or until stable pressure drops is obtained. Finally, core is subjected to 2 pore volumes of brine at 0.5, 1.0 and 1.5 ml/min to determine the final permeability to water. The effluent during NPN-ST and brine post flush injection were collected every 5 ml per tube and analyzed for particle size using light scattering method. After completion of core flooding test, each of the treated Buff Berea cores were dried and cut into three sections (inlet, middle and outlet) for Field Scanning Electron Microscope (FESEM) analysis. The attachment and aggregation of silica nanoparticles under FESEM were determined by comparing the photomicrographs of untreated core (obtained from same core cut with treated cores).

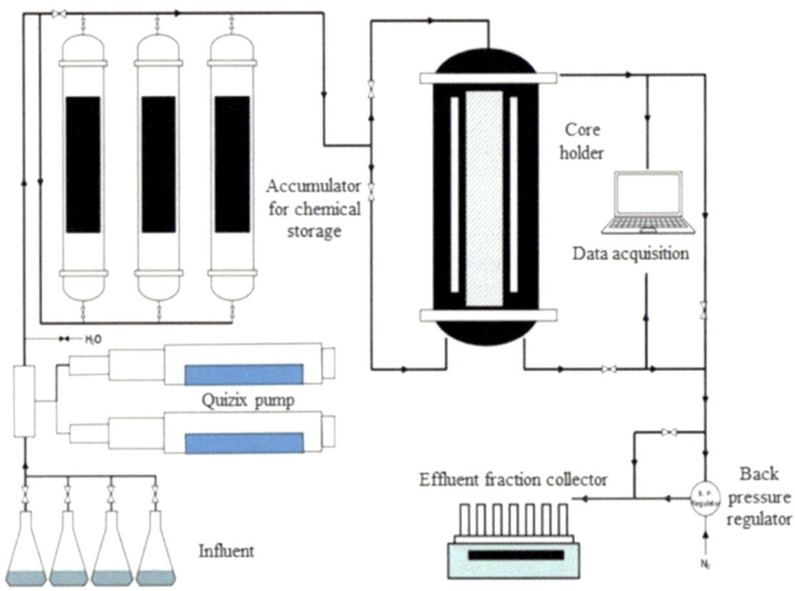

Figure 4.
Schematic of core flooding equipment.

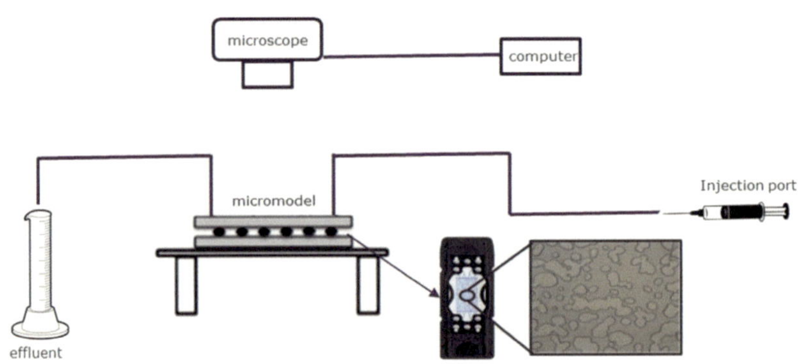

Figure 5.
Schematic of micromodel system.

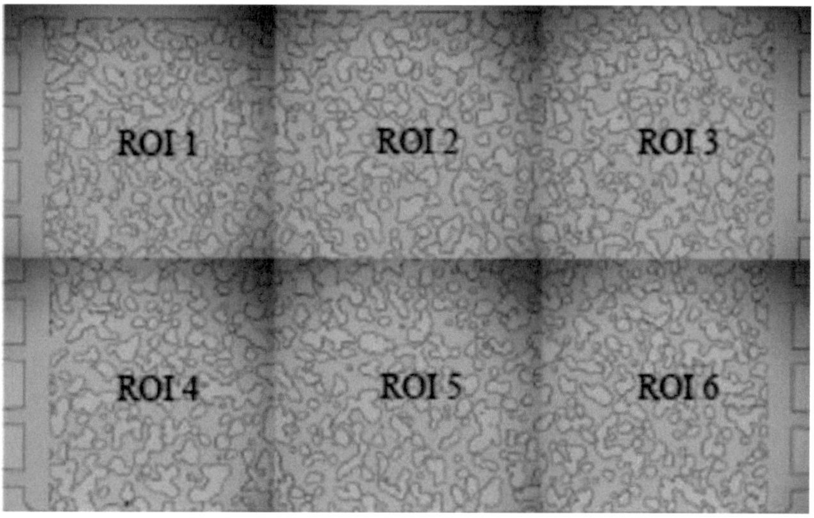

Figure 6.
Region of interest (ROI) at inlet, middle and outlet of the micromodel porous network.

Properties	Fine	Medium	Coarse
Pore size (μm)	36.33–87.76	90.3–191.4	205.37–441.46
Grain size (μm)	110.27–186.08	209.82–305.02	387.13–705.90

Table 4.
Micromodel pore and grain size.

2.3 Micromodel test

Figure 5 illustrates the micromodel experimental set up that comprised of 3 main components; the injection port and lines, that include the differential pressure set up (bypassed for this study), a flow cell represents as porous network (45 mm × 15 mm dimension) with 2.5 Darcy permeability that made of borosilicate glass and the slide made of polypropylene. The flow cell is placed under NIS-Element AR microscope which has 2X, 4X, 8X and 20X zoom lenses connected to a computer for image viewing. Six region of interest (ROI) have been identified at inlet, middle and outlet site of the micromodel. The images were taken by using microscope at 2X resolution.

Figure 6 shows the ROIs used for this micromodel experiment. The pore and grain size of micromodel is categorized as fine, medium and coarse. The pore and grain size output indicate the overall ROIs studies. **Table 4** shows the micromodel pore and grain size determined by using Annotations and Measurement tool on microscope software. 30 ml of 0.05% NPN-ST was injected at 0.001 ml/min followed by 40 ml of 1.5 wt% brine at 0.1 ml/min into the glass micromodel and aged for 1 week. After 1 week, 30 ml of brine was injected and the micromodel image of each ROI was analyzed.

3. Results and discussion

3.1 Core flooding test

For this study, 0.05% NPN-ST concentration was selected based on gravity-assisted flow (GAF) reported in previous work [29]. Injection rate was fixed at

0.5 ml/min throughout the injection to eliminate the permeability impairment caused by nanoparticles injection at high rates [27]. The recorded pressure drops during initial brine, NPN-ST and brine post flush injection enable the interpretation of silica nanoparticles adsorption or plugging inside the porous media. **Figure 7** shows the pressure drop profiles of water wet Buff Berea core; B1–10, B3–21 and L1 when injected with 0.05% NPN-ST at 30°C. B1–10 core flood results showed rapid increased in pressure drops from ~0.28 psi to maximum ~1.09 psi after 2.6 pore volumes of NPN-ST injection. The rapid increased of pressure drops at initial stage of silica nanoparticles injection caused by multilayer adsorption and gradual straining effects [17, 18]. After 2.6 pore volumes, the pressure drops gradually declined to ~0.87 psi that indicates the adsorption process had completed. The pressure drops start to increase rapidly to maximum ~1.16 psi during brine post flush which confirmed the NPN-ST multilayers adsorption. The pressure drops gradually declined after 2.4 pore volumes brine post flush and stabilized and reached steady state at 0.37 psi after six pore volumes that indicate no further detachment and straining of NPN-ST.

B3–21 and L1 core generated slightly higher pressure drops at initial stage and during post flush but with similar trend with B1–10 core. The pressure drops of L1 core increased rapidly from ~0.5 psi to maximum ~2.3 psi. After 1.56 pore volumes of NPN-ST injection, the pressure drops declined and stabilized at ~1.9 psi and further declined during brine post flush and stabilized at ~0.77 psi. Multilayer adsorption and gradual straining effects of B3–21 generated the highest pressure drops from ~0.27 to maximum 3.11 psi compared to B1–10 and L1 core. Nevertheless, B3–21 reached steady state at 0.4 psi, which slightly higher compared to B1–10 core. **Figure 8** shows the pressure drop profiles of Buff Berea core B7–16 and L2 when injected with 0.05% NPC-ST at 60°C. After brine injection, sharp increase in pressure drop from ~0.20–0.24 psi to maximum ~ 0.9–1.53 psi was observed. After 2.7 pore volumes of NPC-ST injection, the pressure drop temporary decline until sharp increase in pressure drop to maximum value of 82.61 and 26.61 psi for B7–16 and L2 core respectively. The maximum pressure drops observation occurred for less than 1 pore of NPN-ST injection until the pressure drop gradually declined and stabilized at ~ 0.28–0.30 psi. Pressure drop at 60°C showed more rapid increasing in pressure

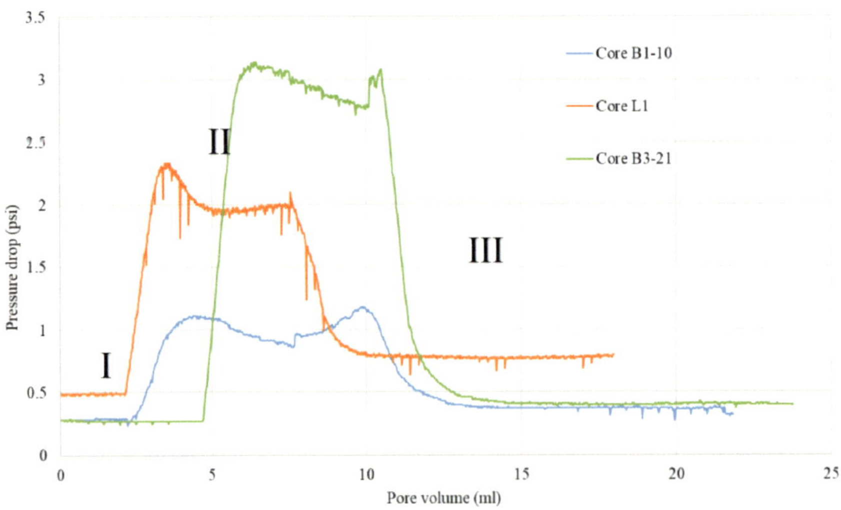

Figure 7.
Pressure drops of buff Berea Core B1–10, B3–21 and L1 during (I) initial brine injection, (II) 0.05% NPN-ST injection and (III) brine post flush at 30°C.

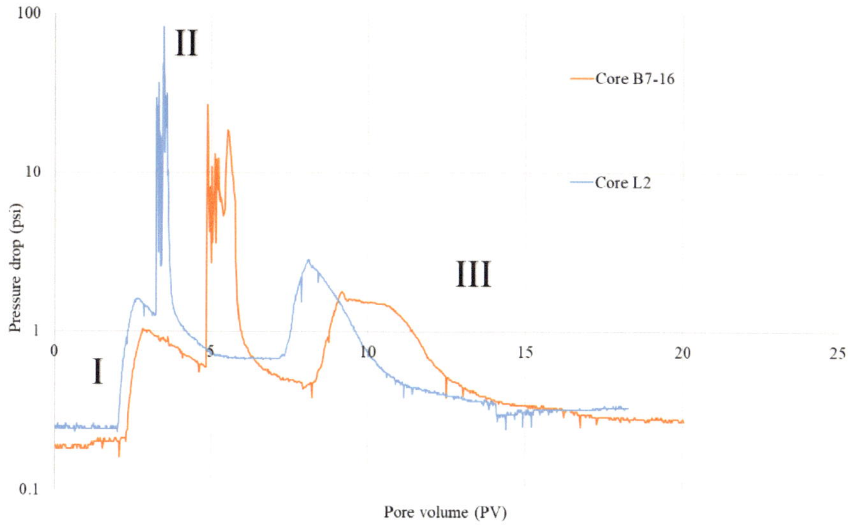

Figure 8.
Pressure drops of buff Berea Core B7–16 and L2 (I) initial brine injection, (II) 0.05% NPN-ST injection and (III) brine post flush at 60°C.

drops in comparison with 30°C during NPC-ST injection, but the permeability impairment is slightly lower at 60°C.

The permeability before and after silica nanoparticles injection were calculated using the pressure drops data during brine injection and calculated using Darcy's law.

$$k = \frac{Q\mu L}{A\Delta P} \tag{1}$$

where $k\ (D)$, $Q\ (cm^3/sec)$, $\mu\ (cP)$, $L\ (cm)$, $A\ (cm^2)$ and $\Delta P\ (atm)$ is permeability, flow rate, water viscosity, core length, core area and pressure drops respectively.

Table 4 shows the calculated permeability impairment of Buff Berea core B1–10, B3–21, L1, B7–16 and L2 after NPN-ST injection. The permeability impairment of each treated cores were calculated using the following equation:

$$Permeability\ impairment, k_{imp} = \left[\frac{(kw_i - kw_f)}{kw_i}\right] x\ 100\% \tag{2}$$

where k_{imp}, k_{wi} and k_{wf} is permeability impairment, initial permeability and final permeability respectively.

The calculated permeability impairment for B1–10, B3–21, L1, B7–16 and L2 are 28.6, 30.3 and 26.2% for 30°C and 19.6 and 16.4% at 60°C respectively as shown in **Table 5**. The permeability impairment between cores at designated temperature showed close values and slightly lower compared with other silica nanoparticles investigated in previous study [25–27]. Permeability impairment at 60°C is lower compared to 30°C indicated the silica nanoparticles used in this study is suitable for high temperature application.

3.2 Field scanning electron microscope (FESEM) analysis

FESEM photomicrographs of untreated core and cores injected with NPN-ST were compared to confirm the silica nanoparticles adsorption on core surface. At 500 nm magnification, untreated core displays as uniform surface as shown in **Figure 9**. Spherical shape of silica nanoparticles were detected on surface of B3–21

Core ID	Test temperature (°C)	Initial core permeability, k_{wi} (mD)	Final core permeability, k_{wf} (mD)	Permeability impairment, k_{imp} (%)
B1–10	30	247.8	176.8	28.6
B3–21	30	229.3	159.9	30.3
L1	30	234.8	173.3	26.2
B7–16	60	193.9	155.9	19.6
L2	60	253.5	211.9	16.4

Table 5.
Permeability impairment of buff Berea core B1–10, B3–21, L1, B7–16 and L2.

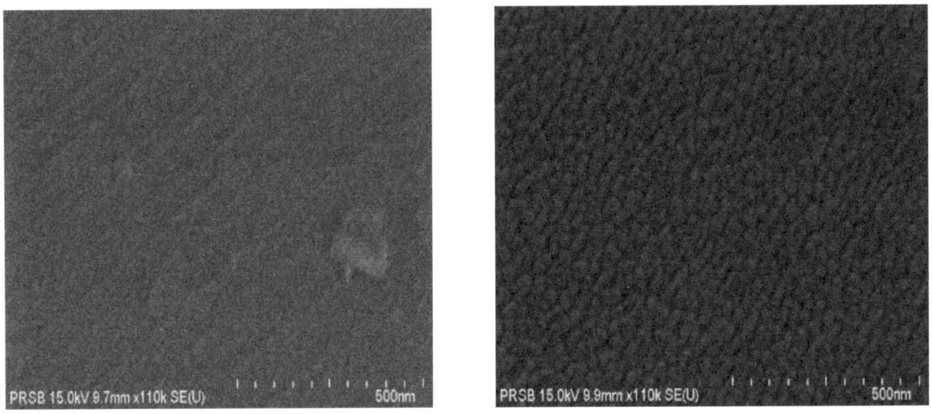

Figure 9.
FESEM photomicrographs of untreated buff Berea core at 500 nm magnification.

core with average particle size between 30 and 36 nm. Some aggregation of silica nanoparticles was observed at the inlet and middle core section and can be consider as minimal aggregation. Clear image of spherical silica nanoparticles adsorbed on the surface of L1 core observed at the inlet, middle and outlet section which also consider minimal aggregation. For both B1–10 and L1 core, most of the spherical particles was observed at the outlet section of the core where the non-adsorb silica nanoparticles was flushed out during post brine injection. **Figures 10** and **11** shows the FESEM photomicrographs at inlet, middle and outlet section of B1–10 and L1 core at 500 nm magnification.

On the other hand, no clear silica nanoparticles image detected for B7–16 and L2 core at inlet and middle section. Most of the spherical shape which also formed as aggregates observed at the outlet core section but the high charging during FESEM analysis caused unclear photomicrographs image as shown in **Figures 12** and **13**. Further analysis of aggregation of silica nanoparticles inside the porous media showed the aggregation could be substantial when in contact with residual water in the core. High aggregation can cause serious pore plugging and ultimately reduce the permeability. The silica nanoparticles spherical shape attached with each other and formed aggregates as shown in **Figure 14**.

3.3 Particle size of core flood effluents

The particles size of silica nanoparticles and post flush effluents provide indirect relationship with silica nanoparticles aggregation in the porous media. The

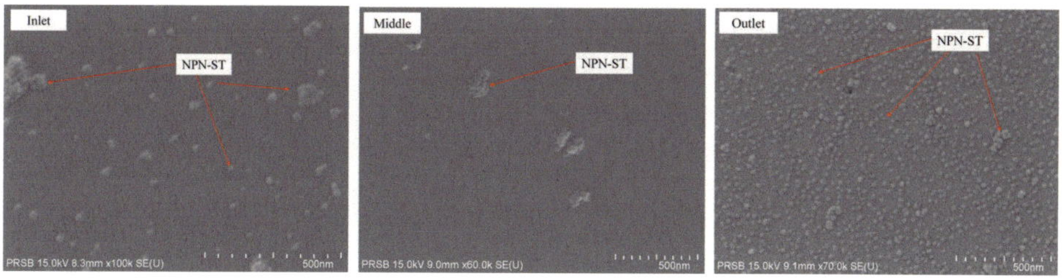

Figure 10.
FESEM photomicrographs of buff Berea core B1–10 treated with NPN-ST.

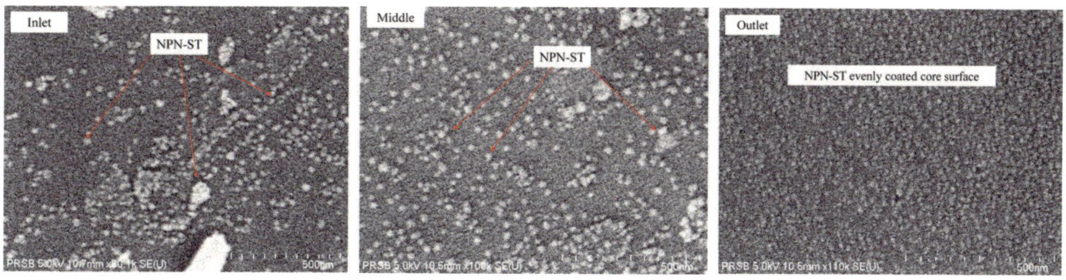

Figure 11.
FESEM photomicrographs of buff Berea core L1 treated with NPN-ST.

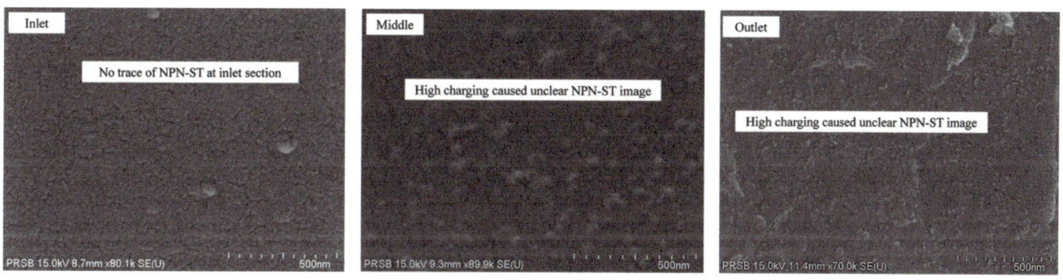

Figure 12.
FESEM photomicrographs of buff Berea core B7–16 treated with NPN-ST.

measured effluent particle size during NPN-ST is smaller compared to brine post flush as shown in blue line in **Figures 15–17**. Most of silica nanoparticles aggregates were flushed out, while the majority of larger particles size was detected during brine post flush as shown in orange line in **Figures 15–17**. The measurement of particles size provides useful information for this experimental work where the larger particles size corresponds with high pressure drops and vice-versa.

3.4 Micromodel test

The qualitative method using glass micromodel flooding test allow the in-situ visualization during silica nanoparticles injection and brine injection that enable the image capture for aggregation analysis. The micromodel porous network before fluid injection is shown **Figure 18**. Silica nanoparticles particles propagate in the porous media that captured at the respective ROIs marked in red circle as shown in **Figure 19**. Gelled liked suspension was observed in the porous network when the silica nanoparticles in contact with brine that indicate aggregation marked in red arrow as shown in **Figure 20**. The size of aggregation at respective ROIs was measured according to fine, medium and coarse.

The aggregation phenomena associated with the sharp increase in pressure drops observed during core flooding test when silica nanoparticles injected into water

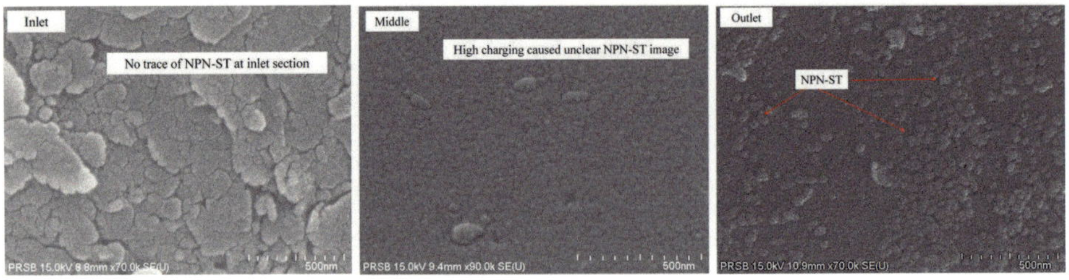

Figure 13.
FESEM photomicrographs of buff Berea core L2 treated with NPN-ST.

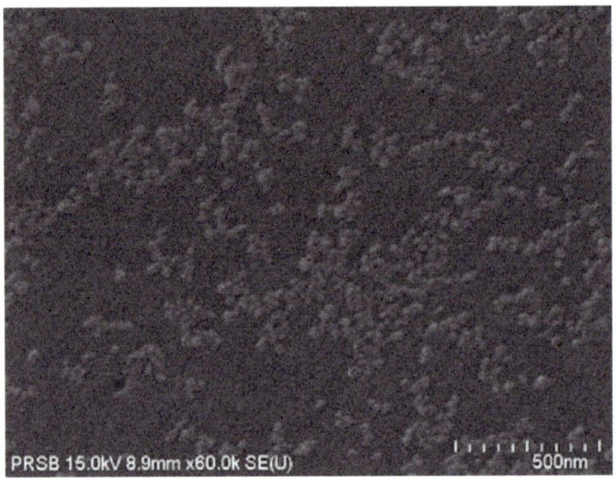

Figure 14.
FESEM photomicrographs of silica nanoparticles aggregation in the outlet section of buff Berea core.

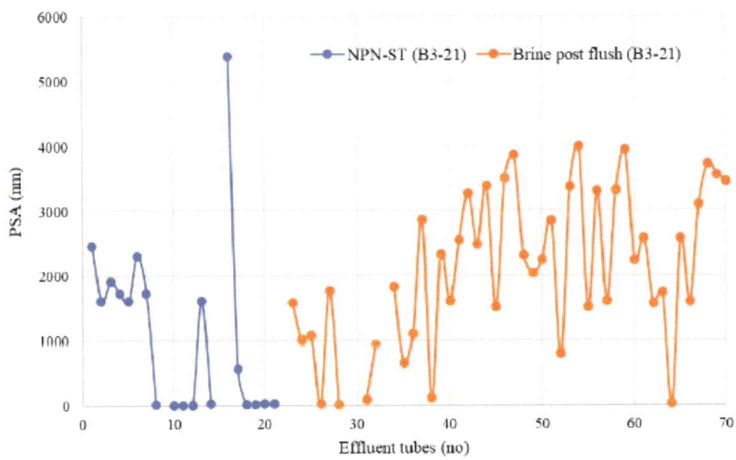

Figure 15.
B3–21 core effluent particles size during NPN-ST injection and brine post flush.

wet Buff Berea core. The treated micromodel was aged for 1 week to investigate the degree of aggregation. Post brine injection flushed out some of the silica nanoparticles suspension as shown in **Figure 21**. The size of aggregation size at respective ROIs was measured to compare with the initial stage of brine injection. The reduction of gelled-size aggregates results corresponds with the declined in pressure drops during brine post flush injection. Gel-liked suspension remains adsorbed in some parts of the porous network and strained on the pore walls. In relation, during

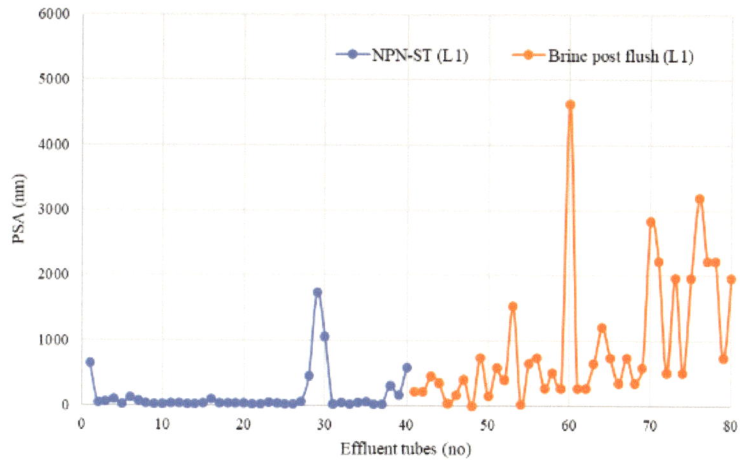

Figure 16.
L1 core effluent particles size during NPN-ST injection and brine post flush.

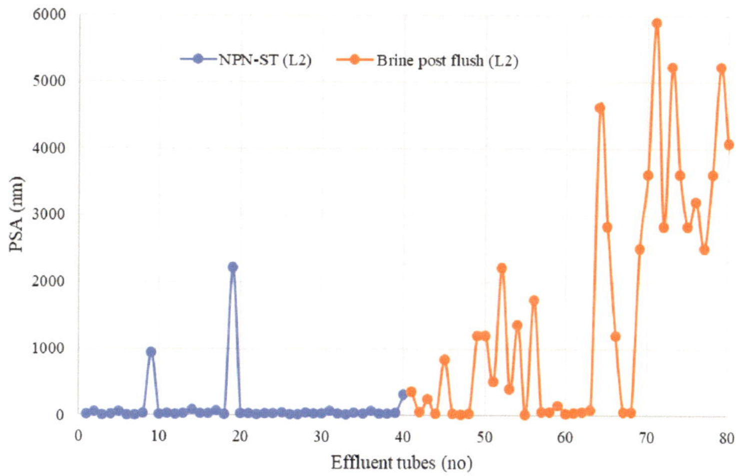

Figure 17.
L2 core effluent particles size during NPN-ST injection and brine post flush.

core flooding test, silica nanoparticles adsorption and straining will reduce the core permeability and block the fluid pathways.

The size of aggregation during initial brine and post flush is shown in **Figure 22**. Overall the aggregation size is reduced during brine post flush but some part formed bigger aggregates that possibly occurred when brine keep in contact with nanoparticles blocked in the porous network. Significant aggregates appeared after 1st and 2nd stage of brine injection at specified ROIs (ROI 1, ROI 2, ROI 3, ROI 4, ROI 5 and ROI 6), classified into fine, medium and coarse aggregation size. At initial stage, fine aggregates size during 1st and 2nd brine injection at each ROIs was not significant from one another. Since their size are relatively small, they are found abundantly in suspension mode (unattached to wall) which prone to propagate in the porous network. Medium aggregates size during 1st and 2nd brine injection indicate size reduction from the front (ROI 1/ROI 4) to end (ROI 3/ROI 4). After a week, the aggregates size at each ROIs decreased at about 5% and below. The medium size range during 1st and 2nd brine injection was insignificant which fall between 100 and 170 μm and 60–180 μm. Coarse aggregates size during 1st and 2nd

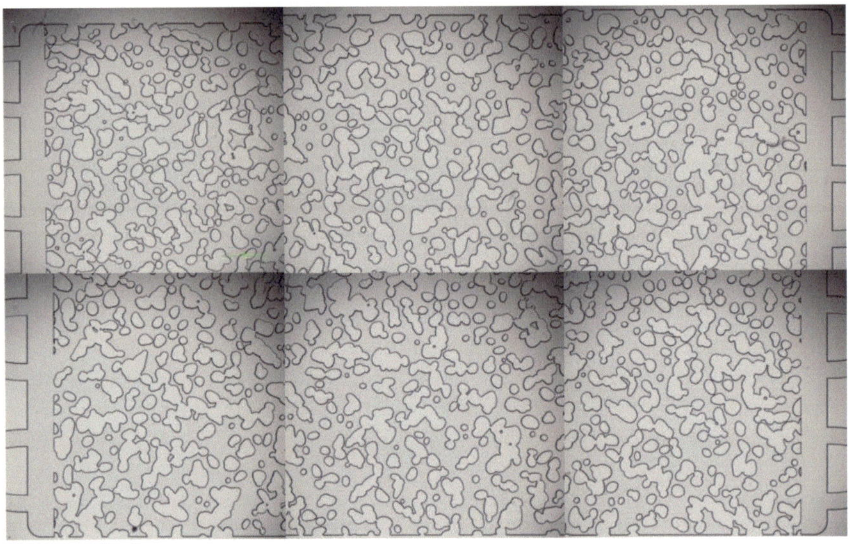

Figure 18.
Micromodel porous network before fluid injection.

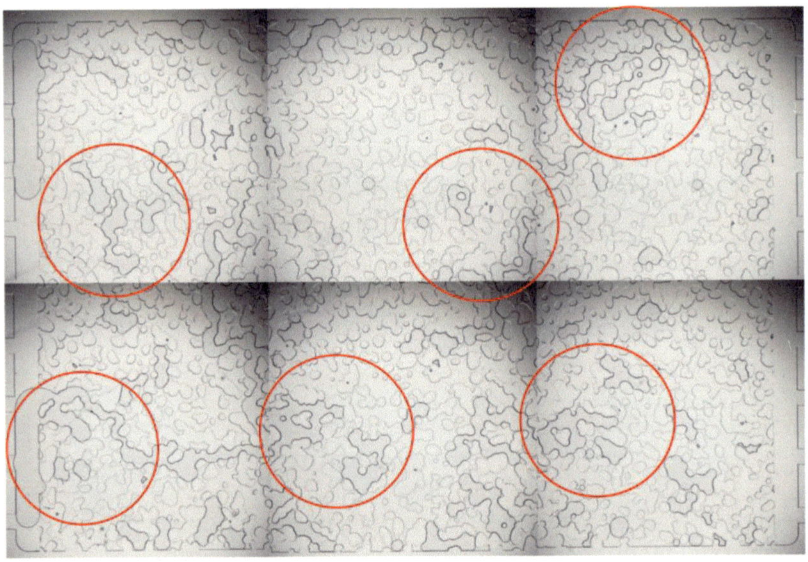

Figure 19.
Micromodel porous network during silica nanoparticles injection. Silica nanoparticles flowed through porous media marked in red circle at ROI 1, ROI 2, ROI 3, ROI 4, ROI 5 and ROI 6.

brine injection indicate size reduction from the front (ROI 1/ ROI 4) to end (ROI 3/ ROI6). After one week aging, the aggregates size decreased at about 10% and below at ROI 3/ROI 5 for 1st brine injection, then decreased at ROI 1, ROI 3 and ROI 5 for 2nd brine injection. The coarse size range during 1st/2nd brine injection are significant which fall between 190 and 340 μm and 160–430 μm.

4. Conclusions

In this study, partially hydrophilic silica nanoparticles adsorption and aggregation in porous media has been demonstrated through quantitative and qualitative

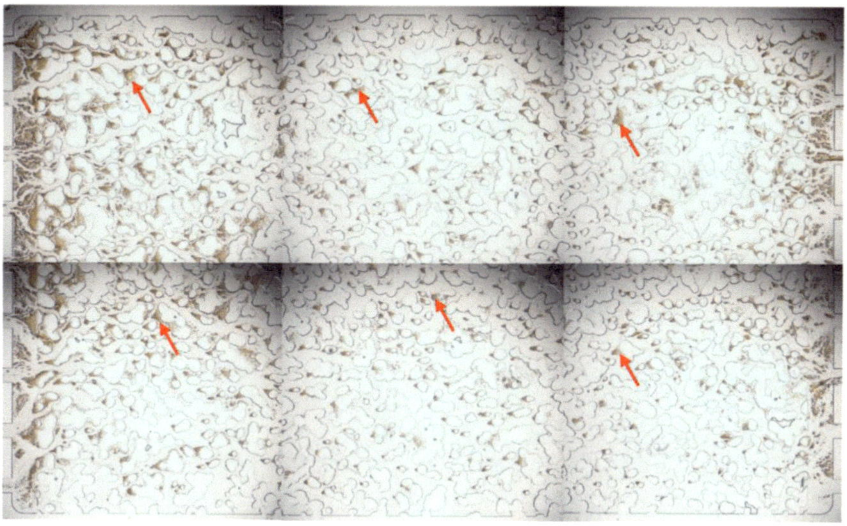

Figure 20.
Micromodel porous network during brine injection and in contact with silica nanoparticles. Gelled-like suspension formed at most of the porous area marked in red arrow.

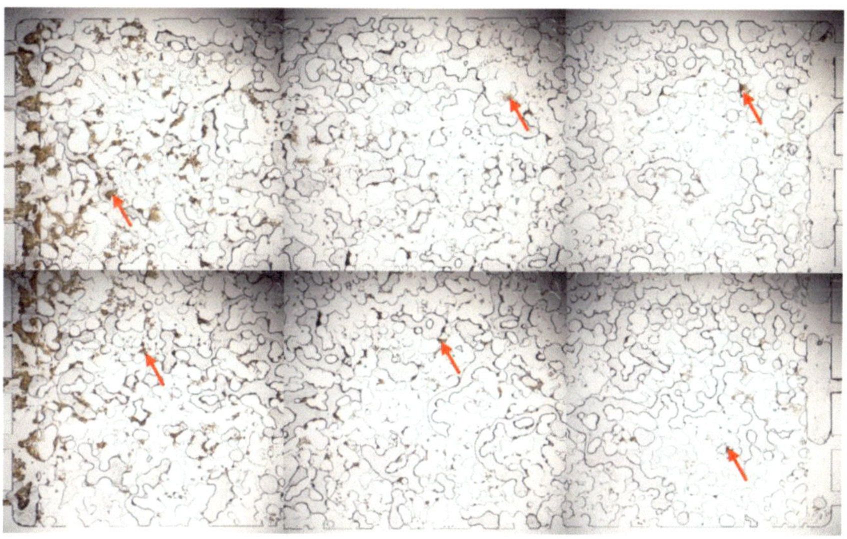

Figure 21.
Micromodel porous network during brine injection (after 1 week ageing). Most of the gelled like suspension pushed out from the porous network. Some adsorbed silica nanoparticles strained inside the porous network.

analysis. Four water wet Buff Berea cores treated with 0.05% silica nanoparticles at 30 and 60°C were evaluated. Micromodel added qualitative information through visualization of silica nanoparticles aggregation in the porous network. The results derived from the experimental work concluded as follows:

- The permeability impairment of treated core at 60°C is slightly lower compared to 30°C. The sharp increase in pressure drops at 60°C during initial silica nanoparticles provided important information of potential log-jamming effect that caused by aggregation of nanoparticles when in contact with water.

Fine: 32.36 Medium: 164.24 Coarse: 242.25	Fine: 19.88 Medium: 100.76 Coarse: 194.96	Fine: 20.71 Medium: 161.61 Coarse: 337.49
Fine: 26.29 Medium: 131.67 Coarse: 330.68	Fine: 17.6 Medium: 131.67 Coarse: 199.04	Fine: 25.66 Medium: 101.02 Coarse: 271.74

(a)

Fine: 29.69 Medium: 164.84 Coarse: 425.77	Fine: 22.13 Medium: 82.34 Coarse: 193.53	Fine: 18.35 Medium: 67.29 Coarse: 166.83
Fine: 25.8 Medium: 173.7 Coarse: 423.6	Fine: 27.7 Medium: 131.01 Coarse: 207.92	Fine: 22.83 Medium: 89.92 Coarse: 106.46

(b)

Figure 22.
The average size of silica nanoparticles at fine, medium and coarse classification (a) during initial brine injection (b) brine post flush after 1 week aging.

- From FESEM photomicrographs, most of the silica nanoparticles aggregates observed at the outer section of the treated core that has been pushed out during brine post flush and some remains adsorbed inside the core showed as spherical shape with little aggregates.

- The particles size of core flooding effluents during silica nanoparticles are smaller that supported the high pressure drops value. In contrast, the particles size is much larger during brine post flush supported with low pressure drops value.

- In general, the permeability impairment after silica nanoparticles injection is insignificant and the silica nanoparticles concentration can be further optimized that can be beneficial as improved oil recovery agent with minimum risk of formation damage.

- Micromodel test enable the visualization of silica nanoparticles aggregation in the porous network when in contact with brine. This observation supported the high pressure drops value during core flood when nanoparticles in contact with in-situ brine. Most of the aggregates at coarse section of micromodel network flushed out during brine post flush.

Acknowledgements

The author would like to thank Wan Shah Rizal Abdullah, Ms. Fatin Najihah Jasni, Ms. Nurul Syuhada M Sobri and Mr. Zulkarnain Harom, Ms. Afidah Sastro for their assistance in the laboratory. The use of equipment facilities at PETRONAS Research Sdn Bhd (under allocation E.025.JRD.02017.401) and support by Nazarbayev University (research funding ID: 080420FD1911) is gratefully acknowledged.

Conflict of interest

The authors declare no conflict of interest.

Author details

Siti Rohaida Mohd Shafian[1,2]*, Ismail M. Saaid[2], Norzafirah Razali[1], Ahmad Fadhil Jahari[2] and Sonny Irawan[3]

1 PETRONAS Research Sdn Bhd, Kajang, Selangor, Malaysia

2 Petroleum Engineering Department, Universiti Teknologi PETRONAS, Tronoh, Perak, Malaysia

3 School of Mining and Geosciences, Nazarbayev University, Kazakhstan

*Address all correspondence to: rohaidashafian@petronas.com.my

IntechOpen

© 2020 The Author(s). Licensee IntechOpen. This chapter is distributed under the terms of the Creative Commons Attribution License (http://creativecommons.org/licenses/by/3.0), which permits unrestricted use, distribution, and reproduction in any medium, provided the original work is properly cited.

References

[1] Ponmani S, Nagarajan R, Sangwai J. Applications of nanotechnology for upstream oil and gas industry. Journal of Nano Research. 2013;**24**:7-15

[2] Negin C, Ali S, Xie Q. Application of nanotechnology for enhancing oil recovery – A review. Petroleum. 2016;**2**(4):324-333

[3] Sun X, Zhang Y, Chen G, Gai Z. Application of nanoparticles in enhanced oil recovery: A critical review of recent progress. Energies. 2017;**10**(3):1-33

[4] Fakoya MF, Pateh H, Shan SN. Nanotechnology: Innovative applications in the oil and gas industry. International Journal of Global Advanced Materials and Nanotechnology. 2018;**1**(1):16-30

[5] Nazari N, Tsau JS, Barati R. CO_2 foam stability improvement using polyelectrolyte complex nanoparticles prepared in produced water. Energies. 2017;**10**(4):1-16

[6] Najafiazar B, Wessel-Berg D, Bergmo PE, Simon CR, Yang J, Torsæter O, et al. Polymer gels made with functionalized organo-silica nanomaterials for conformance control. Energies. 2019;**2**(19):1-25

[7] Lu T, Li Z, Zhou Y. Flow behavior and displacement mechanisms of nanoparticle stabilized foam flooding for enhanced heavy oil recovery. Energies. 2017;**10**(4):1-21

[8] Irfan SA, Shafie A, Yahya N, Zainuddin N. Mathematical modeling and simulation of nanoparticle-assisted enhanced oil recovery – A review. Energies. 2019;**12**(8):1-19

[9] Lau ZY, Lee KC, Soleimani H, Beh HG. Experimental study of electromagnetic-assisted rare-earth doped yttrium iron garnet (YIG) nanofluids on wettability and interfacial tension alteration. Energies. 2019;**12**:1-9

[10] Wang X, Xiao S, Zhang Z, He J. Effect of nanoparticles on spontaneous imbibition of water into ultraconfined reservoir capillary by molecular dynamics simulation. Energies. 2017;**10**(4):1-14

[11] Taborda EA, Franco CA, Alvarado V, Cortes FB. A new model for describing the rheological behavior of heavy and extra heavy crude oils in the presence of nanoparticles. Energies. 2017;**10**(12):1-13

[12] Huang T, Evans BA, Crews JB. Field Case Study on Formation Fines Control with Nanoparticles in Offshore Applications, SPE-13508-MS. Florence, Italy: SPE Annual Technical Conference and Exhibition; 2010

[13] Khan I, Saeed K, Khan I. Nanoparticles: Properties, applications and toxicities. Arabian Journal of Chemistry. 2019;**12**(7):908-931

[14] Agista M, Guo K, Yu Z. A state-of-the-art review of nanoparticles application in petroleum with a focus on enhanced oil recovery. Applied Sciences. 2018;**8**(6):871

[15] Yuan B, Moghanloo RG, Zheng D. Analytical evaluation of nanoparticle application to mitigate fines migration in porous media, SPE-174192-PA. SPE Journal. 2016;**21**(06):2317-2332

[16] Krishnamoorti R. Extracting the benefits for the oil industry. Journal of Petroleum Technology. 2006;**58**:24-26

[17] Zhang T, Murphy M, Yu H, Bagaria HG, Yoon KY, Nielson BM, et al. Investigation of nanoparticles adsorption during transport in porous media. SPE Journal. 2014;**20**:667-677

[18] Yuan B, Wang W, Moghanloo RG, Su Y, Wang K, Jiang M. Permeability reduction of Berea cores owing to nanoparticle adsorption onto the pore surface: Mechanistic modelling and experimental work. Energy & Fuels. 2017;**31**(1):795-804

[19] Abdelfatah E. Multiscale modeling of nanoparticles transport, aggregation and in-situ gelation in porous media [PhD]. Norman, Oklahoma: University of Oklahoma; 2017

[20] Khilar KC, Fogler HS. Migrations of Fines in Porous Media, Xiii. Dordrecht, The Netherlands: Kluwer Academic Publishers; 1998

[21] Agi A, Junin R, Gbadamosi A. Mechanism governing nanoparticle flow behaviour in porous media: Insight for enhanced oil recovery applications. International Nano Letters. 2018;**8**(2):49-77

[22] Giraldo J, Benjumea P, Lopera S, Cortés FB, Ruiz MA. Wettability alteration of sandstone cores by alumina-based nanofluids. Energy & Fuels. 2013;**27**:3659-3665

[23] Hendraningrat L, Li S, Torsæter O. Effect of some parameters influencing enhanced oil recovery process using silica nanoparticles: An experimental investigation. In: Proceedings of the SPE Reservoir Characterization and Simulation Conference and Exhibition. Abu Dhabi, UAE, Richardson, TX, USA: Society of Petroleum Engineers; 16-18 September 2013

[24] Li S, Torsæter O. The impact of adsorption and transport on wettability alteration of water wet Berea sandstone. In: Proceeding of the SPE/IATMI Asia Pacific Oil & Gas Conference and Exhibition. Nusa Dua, Bali, Indonesia, Richardson, TX, USA: Society of Petroleum Engineers; 20-22 October 2015

[25] Erfani Gahrooei HR, Ghazanfari MH. Application of a water based nanofluid for wettability alteration of sandstone reservoir rocks to preferentially gas wetting condition. Journal of Molecular Liquids. 2017;**232**:351-360

[26] DamgaardTS. Experimental investigation of nanoparticle adsorption and pore blockage in intermediate wet Berea sandstone [MSc]. Norwegian University of Science and Technology; 2017

[27] Hendraningrat L, Engest B, Suwarno S, Li S, Torsæter O. Laboratory investigation of porosity and permeability in Berea sandstones due to hydrophilic nanoparticles retention. In: Proceedings of the International Symposium of the Society of Core Analysts. Napa Velley, California, USA; 16-19 September 2013

[28] Hendraningrat L, Li S, Torsæter O. Improved oil recovery by hydrophilic silica nanoparticles suspension: 2-Phase flow experimental studies. In: Proceedings of the International Petroleum Technology Conference. Beijing, China, Richardson, TX, USA; 26-28 March 2013

[29] Mohd Shafian SR, Jahari AF, Razali N, Irawan S, Ibrahim JM, Salleh IK. Controlling fines migration by enhancing fines attachment using silica nanoparticles. International Journal of Advanced Science and Technology. 2020;**29**(1):318-331

Section 3

Nano- and Micro-Emulsions: Formulations and Applications

Chapter 9

Microemulsion Formulation of Botanical Oils as an Efficient Tool to Provide Sustainable Agricultural Pest Management

Abhishek Sharma, Saurabh Dubey and Nusrat Iqbal

Abstract

Microemulsion formulation is among the most suitable carrier for the delivery of bioactive and, therefore, has excellent potential for industrial applications. The microemulsion system is thermodynamically and kinetically stable. Due to the smaller droplet size of the microemulsion system, the bioactive covers a larger surface of the target pest. Botanicals and essential oils, in particular, are green options to control various soil and seed-borne pathogens. Each oil contains several bioactive constituents that practically avoid microbe-resistance against it. Nevertheless, to improve the handling and shelf-life of botanicals, microemulsion formulation is the best option available. The current chapter provides the insight of a microemulsion system and explores the possibility of botanical oil-based biopesticides for a sustainable agro-ecosystem. We believe that botanical oil microemulsion could be a better alternative to synthetic pesticides and opens a new corridor for the promotion of the greener way of plant protection in India and across the globe.

Keywords: botanicals, essential oil, microemulsion, pathogen, formulation

1. Introduction

Essential oils from aromatic plants are a competent source of pesticides that have a diverse role in pest management like insecticides, fungicides, growth-regulators, deterrent, and repellent activities [1]. Essential oils' role in pharmacology or therapeutic activities and cosmetics is quite known. In recent years, the essential oil is being used in pest management applications and regularly used by the farmers to promote organic farming in an environmentally friendly way [2]. Essential oils of aromatic plants are rich in bioactive compounds viz., terpenes, terpenoids, flavonoids, phenolics, etc. These constituents have different physicochemical properties and stability, but their utilization in pure form is not feasible. Hence, a suitable delivery system is needed to enhance its bio-efficacy and stability during the application.

Various formulations of bioactive compounds are available in the market, but they have certain limitations like un-stability, high in cost, complex compositions, non-targeted delivery, and post-application wastage. It is, therefore, compelling to look upon the carrier system that overcomes the limitations mentioned above. In recent years, researchers have reported that microemulsion (ME) formulation is the

IntechOpen

most suitable carrier for the delivery of bioactive constituents of essential oils and has excellent potential for industrial applications. The microemulsion system is not only thermodynamically and kinetically stable but also possesses a small droplet size (preferably below 100 nm). It means the formulation can incorporate a large amount of bioactive essential oil in the disperse phase. Due to these characteristic features, essential oil-based ME favors a stabilized and intelligent approach for the delivery of their active ingredients into the targeted site and results in enhanced bio-efficacy. In this chapter, we will discuss the essential oil-based ME and their role in pest management.

2. Microemulsion systems: a brief background about the origin and characteristic features

Hoar and Schulman gave the concept of microemulsion in the 1940s. They prepared the first microemulsion by dispersing oil in an aqueous solution of surfactants and co-surfactants, which finally provides a transparent solution [3].

The microemulsion, as defined by Danielsson and Lindman, in 1981 [4]. The definition was as given below:

> *"a microemulsion is a system of water, oil, and an amphiphile which is a single optically isotropic and thermodynamically stable liquid solution."*

In microemulsion systems, surfactants and co-surfactant play an essential role, which stabilized the system by reducing the interfacial surface tension between two immiscible liquids and compensates the dispersion entropy and make the system thermodynamically stable.

2.1 Types of microemulsion systems

After the 5 years of microemulsion concept, Winsor studied the phase behavior of water, oil, and surfactant and classified microemulsion system in different phases, also known as Winsor phases as shown in **Figure 1**:

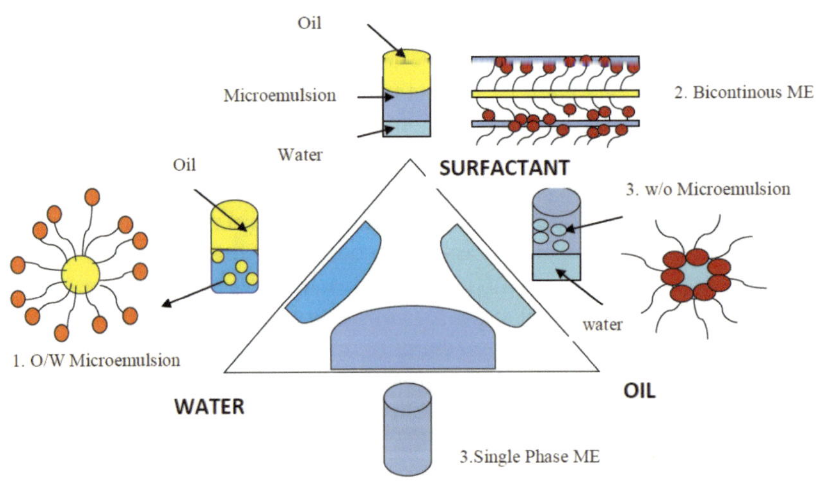

Figure 1.
Phases of the microemulsion system.

a. Oil in water (o/w) microemulsion: In this system, oil is dispersed in a water medium, and the surfactant is in high concentration in water medium and low surfactant concentration in oil medium.

b. Water in oil (w/o) microemulsion: In this system, water is dispersed in oil medium. The surfactant is a high concentration in the oil phase and surfactant-low in the aqueous phase (Winsor II).

c. Bicontinuousmicroemulsion (transition state from o/w to w/o): A three-phase system where a surfactant-rich middle-phase coexists with both water and surfactant (Winsor III or middle-phase microemulsion).

d. Single-phase homogeneous mixture: single-phase isotropic micelle solution

2.2 Characteristics features of ME

The microemulsion system is a competent and stabilized carrier system for all types of active constituents. The characteristic features of microemulsion are:

- Thermodynamically stable
- Isotropic
- Transparent colloidal system
- Easily penetrate
- Long shelf-life
- Zero interfacial tension
- Easy to prepare
- Droplet size is tiny, i.e., 1–100 nm

2.3 Theories of micro emulsion formation

Three theories explain the microemulsion formation and stability.

i. **Interfacial or Mixed film theory**: According to this theory, the microemulsion is formed due to the formation of oil and water complex interface reduction by surfactant and co-surfactants. This theory depends on the reduction of interfacial tension and expressed as [Eq. (1)]:

$$\Upsilon_i = \Upsilon_{o/w} - \psi \tag{1}$$

Ψ = spreading pressure; Υ_i = interfacial tension; $\Upsilon_{o/w}$ = interfacial tension between oil and water.
Interfacial of oil and water reduced to zero and increases the spreading pressure.

ii. **Solubilization theory:** According to this theory, oil or water reverse micelle structures solubilized and form the monophasic system.

iii. **Thermodynamic theory:** According to this theory, microemulsion formation is a spontaneous process that depends upon the lowering of interfacial tension on the addition of surfactants and co-surfactants, and mixing of one

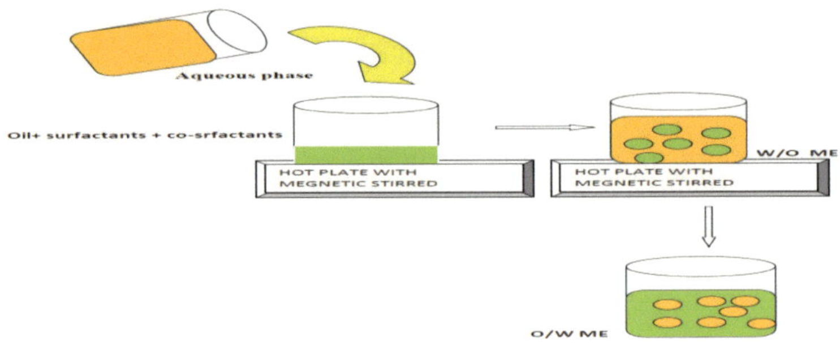

Figure 2.
Diagrammatic representation of the phase inversion method of microemulsion.

phase to another contributes in enhancing the entropy which results into reduction of droplet size. The following thermodynamic equation expresses this theory as (Eq. (2):

$$\Delta G_f = \gamma \Delta A - T \Delta S \tag{2}$$

ΔG_f = free energy of formation; γ = surface tension of the oil–water interface; ΔA = change in the interfacial area after microemulsion; ΔS = change in entropy of the system after mixing; T = is the temperature.

2.4 Preparation methods

There are two methods to develop a microemulsion system of very low interfacial tension at the correct ratio of surfactants and co-surfactants. There are two methods of microemulsion preparation:

I. **Phase inversion method**. In this method, phase inversion occurs after the addition of excess dispersed phase in the surfactant system under temperature control. During phase inversion, the particle size of any drug or agrochemical reduced, which results in active release kinetics. This method is also called the phase inversion temperature method. Because after the cooling phase, inversion will occur from w/o to o/w. short chains of surfactants promote this inversion (**Figure 2**).

II. **Phase titration method**. This method is also known as a spontaneous emulsification method and can represent with the help of phase diagrams. The phase diagram is handy in studying the various interactions that occur while mixing different components of the microemulsion. The phase diagram is constructed to find out the zones of the microemulsion, and each corner represents 100% of each element. The phase diagram is built at fixed surfactant and co-surfactant weight ratios and titrated with water at room temperature. The formation of the transparent monobasic system is established by physical appearance (**Figure 3**).

3. Factor affecting the particle size of active entity (drug or agrochemical) in microemulsion

The microcavities in microemulsion by surface-active agents causes a cage-like effect and check the particle agglomeration [5]. The stability of microemulsion drops depends upon the following factors.

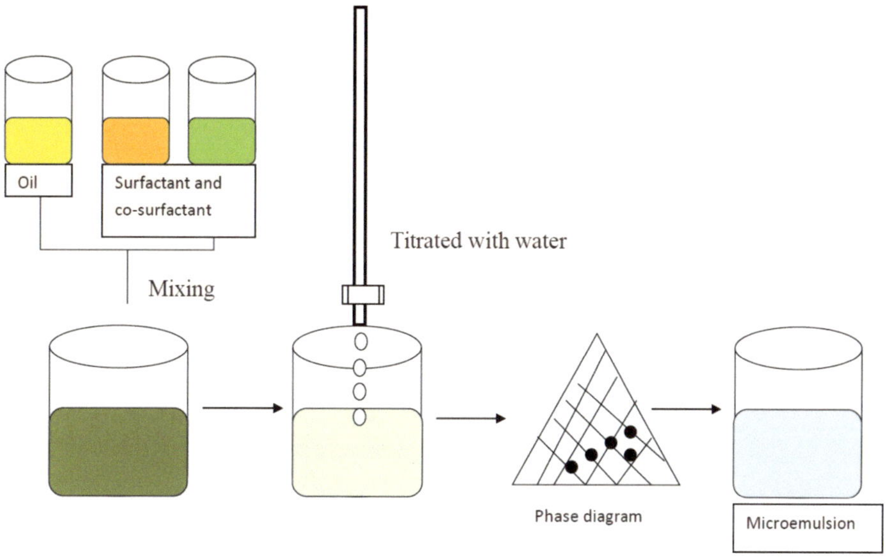

Figure 3.
Diagrammatic representation of the titration method of microemulsion.

I. **The viscosity of the microemulsion**: The size of particle in a microemulsion is depended upon the viscosity of the mixture after adding all the surface-active agents and water and expressed by the following equation [Eq. (3)]:

$$\eta_r = \eta/\eta_o = 1 + 5/2\varphi \tag{3}$$

where, η_r = relative viscosity; η = viscosity of the dispersion; η_o = solvent viscosity; φ = volume of droplets.

In the microemulsion system, breaking up of droplets gives droplet volume fractions up to 0.2, the expected relative maximum viscosity is 1.5, which results in droplet interactions and destabilizes the microemulsion system [5].

II. **The ratio of water to surface-active agents:** The water level inside the spherical micelles gives the radius measurement by the following expression [Eq. (4)] and **Figure 4**.

$$r = 3\ Vm/s \tag{4}$$

where, Vm is the dispersed volume of water; s is the interfacial area by surfactant molecules.

As the water level is high, it lowers the stability due to less capability of surface-active agents to protect the more substantial drop — consequently, particles undergo coagulation and flocculation. Therefore, the size of the droplet depends upon the ration of water to surface-active agents (ώ).

III. **Nature of surface-active agents and concentration of aqueous reactants**: An increase in surface-active agents decreases the particle size. The surface-active agents stabilized the microemulsion by reducing the ration of water to surface-active agents (ώ). Therefore, surface-active agents control the droplet size as well as provide stability to the microemulsion system.

IV. **Temperature**: Temperature plays a significant role in droplet size reduction. As temperature decreases, the viscosity of the microemulsion increases, which results in particle agglomeration. Elevated temperature decreases the solubility

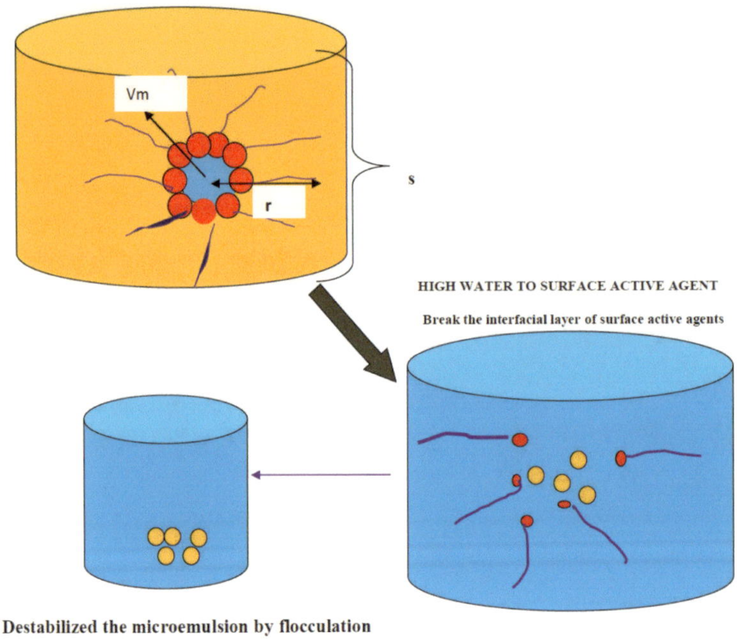

Figure 4.
Diagrammatic representation of the effect of water on the surface-active agent on the stability of the microemulsion.

of non-ionic surfactants due to de-hydration of hydrophilic groups at high temperature. In the oil phase, on the other hand, active agents' solubility increases in the oil phase. Therefore temperature optimization is critical in droplet size reduction and microemulsion stabilization.

4. Microemulsion evaluation parameters

4.1 Physical appearance

For Physical appearance, microemulsion can be checked visually by the fluidity, optical clarity, and uniform appearance.

4.2 Transmittance test

Transparency of microemulsion is the first sign of the microemulsion system. The percent transmittance is measured by UV–visible spectroscopy.

4.3 Scattering Techniques

Microemulsion structures can be studied by scattering of x-ray radiations. This technique identifies the nature of microemulsions weather; it is a diluted monodispersed or polydispersed system.

4.4 Droplet size

The droplet size of the microemulsion is measured by dynamic light scattering experiments or electron microscopy. Along with droplet size, it also gives polydispersity values of the microemulsion system.

4.5 Active ingredient stability

The active ingredient stability is quantified by suitable analytical techniques like HPLC, GC–MS, LC–MS, and others. According to the active constituents after formulation development. The active constituent's stability is crucial after formulation development.

4.6 Viscosity measurement

Viscosity is the fundamental property of the microemulsion system. If any type of viscosity change occurs, it will destabilize the microemulsion and leads to flocculation or phase separation.

4.7 Electrical conductivity

The electrical conductivity of formulated samples in microemulsion form was checked after adding a surfactant, oil, and water components. A conductometer does this measurement at ambient temperature and 1 Hz frequency.

4.8 In-vitro drug release

The bioactive content release study was carried out in Franz diffusion cell of volume 20 ml. Two compartments are present- one is a receptor compartment, and the other is the donor compartment. Receptor compartment is filled with buffer, and the donor compartment is filled with a microemulsion sample and covered by a cellophane membrane. At certain intervals of time the donor compartment is analyzed for active ingredient content.

4.9 Advantages

- Solubilize water-insoluble active constituents
- Enhanced bio-efficacy
- Slow-release delivery system
- Effective in both contact as well as systemic delivery
- Easy to form
- Smell masking of unpleasant active ingredients
- Easy to develop
- Protect the active constituents from hydrolysis and oxidation.

4.10 Disadvantages

- Use of high amount of surfactants and co-surfactants
- Limiting solubilizing capacity for high melting active constituents
- Microemulsion stability influenced by temperature and ph.

5. Applications of microemulsion

Microemulsion are being used in many areas.

a. **Drug delivery**: Microemulsion formulation has been extensively used in drug delivery. From the last few decades, the microemulsion system has been used in a variety of drug delivery systems like oral, topical, parenteral, and oral.

b. **Analytical applications**: The microemulsion system is the suitable solubilizing medium for hydrophobic constituents and then can be analyzed for various constituent detection.

c. **Biotechnology applications**: Enzymatic reaction, immobilization of proteins, and bioseparation can be done successfully in microemulsion systems.

d. **Oil recovery**: The microemulsion system also helps in the improvement of oil due to the high amount of surfactants.

Besides, the applications mentioned above, microemulsion formulation also find its applications in the following fields:

- Cosmetics
- Coating of Textiles
- Detergents
- Environmental Remediation
- Agrochemicals
- Food

6. Botanical oil microemulsion in crop protection with emphasis on essential oil

Several botanicals sources of phytochemicals offer great promise for insect pest control. Six plant families with several representative species, Asteraceae, Cladophoraceae, Labiatae, Meliaceae, Oocystaceae, and Rutaceae, appear to have the most significant potential for providing future insect control in crops [6].

A most crucial source of phytochemical compounds against insect pests is the essential oil. Essential oil is the mixture of volatile compounds generally produced by Plant as secondary metabolites, constituted by hydrocarbons (terpenes and sesquiterpenes) and oxygenated compounds (alcohols, esters, ethers, aldehydes, ketones, lactones, and phenols) [7]. Bioactive chemical compounds of essential oils have repellent properties against mosquitoes. Previous studies revealed that terpenoid groups are biologically active compounds for mosquito repellency. There are 20 active terpenoids with a functional group of negatively charged and containing ester/ether bonds or an ethanol hydroxyl group and other positively charged end containing alkane groups [8]. These bio-active chemicals have several properties, which are categorized as repellents, feeding deterrents, toxins, and growth regulators. Five major categories of bioactive compounds are (1) nitrogen compounds (primarily alkaloids), (2) terpenoids, (3) phenolics, (4) proteinase inhibitors, and (5) growth regulators [9].

Many bioactive compounds (phytochemicals) have been discovered by the researchers who have good repellent activity against insect pests [10]. These botanical-based repellents not only have excellent repellency but also influences the physiology of insect. These botanical bioactive agents (phytochemicals) can effectively replace the presently available synthetic pesticides against the mosquito.

6.1 Issues with essential oils in agriculture

Essentials are potent pesticides. But still, exploitation of them in pure form is not encouragable in the agriculture because of the following reasons:

a. **Water solubility:** Essential oils are water-insoluble due to fatty acids and cannot be dispersed uniformly in water before application [11]. Non-uniformity during use creates the problem of dispersion over the applied areas. It is the main ineffectiveness of essential oil application.

b. **Penetration:** Essential oils in a pure form not penetrate in the targeted area and wash off by rain or evaporated quickly by air [12].

c. **Shelf life:** In the pure form, shelf life of essential oil decreases and their constituents starts degrading in the open atmosphere by light, pH, temperature variations, etc. [13].

6.2 Microemulsion system: a practical approach to solve the inefficiencies of essential oil in crop protection

Microemulsions are the thermodynamically stable isotropic solution of nanodispersions of size 10–200 nm. These are highly stabilized solutions with surfactants and co-surfactants [14, 15]. These microemulsion systems provide effective delivery systems, give extended shelf life, easy to prepare, and can easily scalable by low input of energy [16].

In microemulsion physio-chemical parameters of essential oil changes like improvement insolubilization, better bioavailability, and enhance the rate of penetration in targeted sites without any wastage [14, 17] in addition to this essential oil bio-constituents spreading capacity in aqueous solution improves and gives uniform dispersion on targeted sites after application [18] and provide good bio-efficacy [19]. Moreover, in microemulsion formulation, essential oil active ingredient degradation rate decreases and enhances their shelf life for an extended period [20]. Further, due to the smaller droplet size in microemulsion also enhances wetting, spreading, and permeability and uniformly deposited over leaf surfaces [21, 22]. Characteristic features of essential oil microemulsion have been highlighted in **Figure 5**.

6.3 Available essential oil microemulsions and targeted pest

Microemulsions can incorporate the natural oil or essential oil in a high amount in water without any destabilization of active constituents. Essential oil gives a superstability performance in microemulsion form as compared to emulsion forms [23]. The essential oil has many potential active ingredients that give very good bioefficacy in insect pests. Hence, essential oil could be a better alternative to

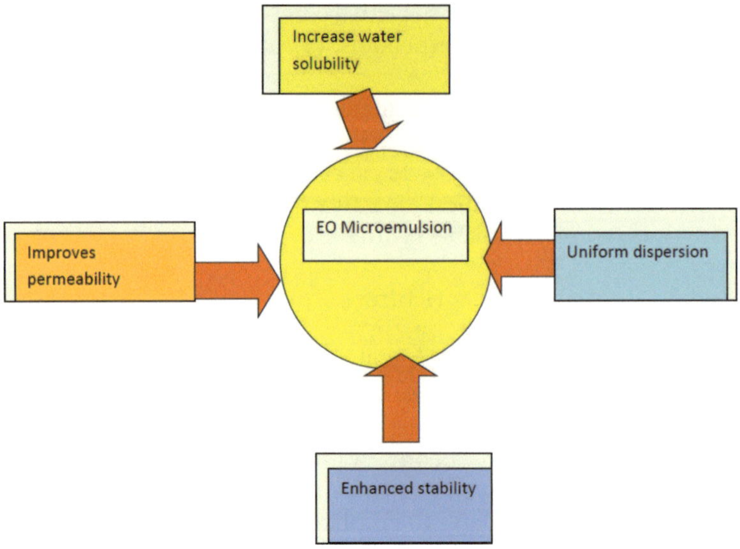

Figure 5.
Characteristics of essential oil microemulsion.

synthetic pesticides. In microemulsion systems, essential oil active constituents are protected in micelles and give a useful model of the delivery system against different pest populations.

In the microemulsion system, droplet size is very small, i.e., in the range of 10–100 nm. So, the translocation through vascular tissues is very easy in systemic, and due to good adherence and spreadability, it gives equally good results in the non-systemic mode of action. **Table 1** shows the available microemulsions in crop protection.

Cinnamon (CM) essential has been reported as a potential alternative to chemical fungicides. In CM microemulsion formulation rate of control of gray mold was increased up to 20% with 500ug L-1 in comparison with the non-microemulsion formulation. CM microemulsion postponed the ascorbic acid loss and cause no significant influence on pear qualities such as color and taste [24].

The microemulsion system, along with stabilizers and surfactants, gives stable physicochemical characteristics and excellent stability. Insecticidal bioassay indicated that the acute LC50 to P. xylostella was 12.477mg/L. It will be environment-friendly and shows potential alternative features to synthetic pesticide against P. xylostella [25].

Neem, along with Karanja oil, has been termed as a natural pesticide microemulsion system. This combination has been proven economical as well as the stabilized formulation for an extended period and gives good bioefficacy against different types of crop pest populations [26].

Essential oils give combinatory properties along with synthetic pesticides. Along with stability, it also enhances the bio-efficacy against different insect pests.

Neem oil microemulsion by using biodiesel waste as co-solvent has been developed as an effective delivery system against different pests. These microemulsions are eco-friendly, economical, and safe for non-targets. The developed microemulsions highly stabilized and efficient at a low dose [27].

Lemongrass oil has been proved a right stabilizer as well as a dispersant in the neem oil microemulsion system. The primary specialty of this formulation is that these Neem ME formulations are free from any co-solvents. In the presence of lemongrass stability of active ingredient, i.e., azadirachtin also increased, and HPLC data shows a very less degradation after 14 days of storage at 54°C [28].

S.No.	Essential oil	Active constituents	Mode of action	Insect pest	References
1.	Cinnamon oil	Cinnamaldehyde Cinnamyl Acetate Caryophyllene Linalool Eugenol Cinnamaldehyde (3-phenyl-2-propanal)	Fungicide	Gray mold of pears	[24]
2.	Castor Oil	Ricinoleicacid	Herbicide	*Convolvulus arvensis*	[23]
	Camphor Oil	Pinene Camphene Limonene 1,8-Cineole p-Cymene	Herbicide	*Convolvulus arvensis*	[23]
	Peppermint Oil	Menthol Menthone 1,8-Cineole Menthyl acetate Isovalerate Pinene Limonene	Herbicide	*Convolvulus arvensis*	[23]
	Jojoba Oil	Gondoic acid	Herbicide	*Convolvulus arvensis*	[23]
3	Peppermint Oil	Menthol Menthone 1,8-Cineole Menthyl acetate Isovalerate Pinene Limonene	Insecticide	*Sitophilus oryzae*	[29]
4.	Thyme oil	Borneol Carvacrol Linalool Thymol Tannin Saponins Triterpenic Acids	Fungicide	*Geotrichum citri* (citrus sour rot)	[30]
5.	Eucalyptus oil	Eucalyptol or 1,8-cineol	Insecticide	*Sitophilus oryzae* (L.) and *Tribolium castaneum* (Herbst)	[31]
6.	Neem oil	Azadirachtin	Acaricides	*Tetranychus urticae*	[32]
7.	Neem oil + lemon grass oil	Myrcene Citral Citronellal Geranyl Acetate Nerol Geraniol Limonene	Insecticides	—	[28]
8.	Natural pyrethrin	Pyrethrin I Pyrethrin II Cinerin I Cinerin II Jasmolin I Jasmolin II	Insecticides	*Aphis gossypii*	[33]

S.No.	Essential oil	Active constituents	Mode of action	Insect pest	References
9.	Betel leaf (*Piper betle* L.) essential oil	Cadinene Sesquiterpene Chavicol Geraniol A-Thujene Terpinolene Chavibetol Phenyl Propane Trans B-Ocimene Safrole Caryophyllene Cineole Cadinol Eugenol Camphene Limonene Pinene Eugenyl Acetate	Fungicide	*Aspergillus* species	[34]
10.	Chlorpyrifos + jatropha and karanj oil	Karanjin Pongamol Oleic Acid	Insecticides	Stored Grain Pest	[35]
11.	Clove and lemongrass oil	Myrcene Citral Citronellal acetyl eugenol beta-caryophyllene vanillin crategolic acid tannins Flavinoids	Fungicide	*Fusarium oxysporum*	[36]
12.	Eucalyptus oil	Eucalyptol or 1,8-cineol	Insecticides	*Tribolium castaneum*	[37]

Table 1.
Literature survey on essential oil microemulsion for crop protection.

Natural oil microemulsion along with botanical synergist (*Prosopis juliflora*) have been proved the stability of active constituents in ME formulation. The HPLC data showed that botanical synergist lowers the degradation rate of active components of natural oil. Further, the bioefficacy results showed a prominent biocontrol against Spodopteralitura at 400 PPM [38].

Clove (CO) and lemongrass oil (LGO) ME showed potential antifungal agents against *Fusarium oxysporum* f.sp. *lycopersici* (FOL) without showing any sign of phytotoxicity in tomato plants [36].

Eukalyptus (*Eucalyptus globules*) oil ME was developed along with Karanja (Pongamiaglabra) and jatropha cakes (*Jatropha curcas*) to enhance the bioefficacy against Triboliumcastaneum, a stored grain pest. The mortality data shows that Eucalyptus oil ME with Karanja and jatropha cakes extract gives LC50 at 50 ppm, and without extract, it LC50 at 100 PPM. The GC-ms data shows that degradation % of a marker compound, i.e., 1, 8-cineole, also reduced in filtrate based ME. So, this study discovered that essential oil stability and bioefficacy could be improved in microemulsion by using these types of botanical extracts [37].

Previous studies revealed that essential oil microemulsion formulation with optimum surfactants and botanical synergists or stabilizers could improve the

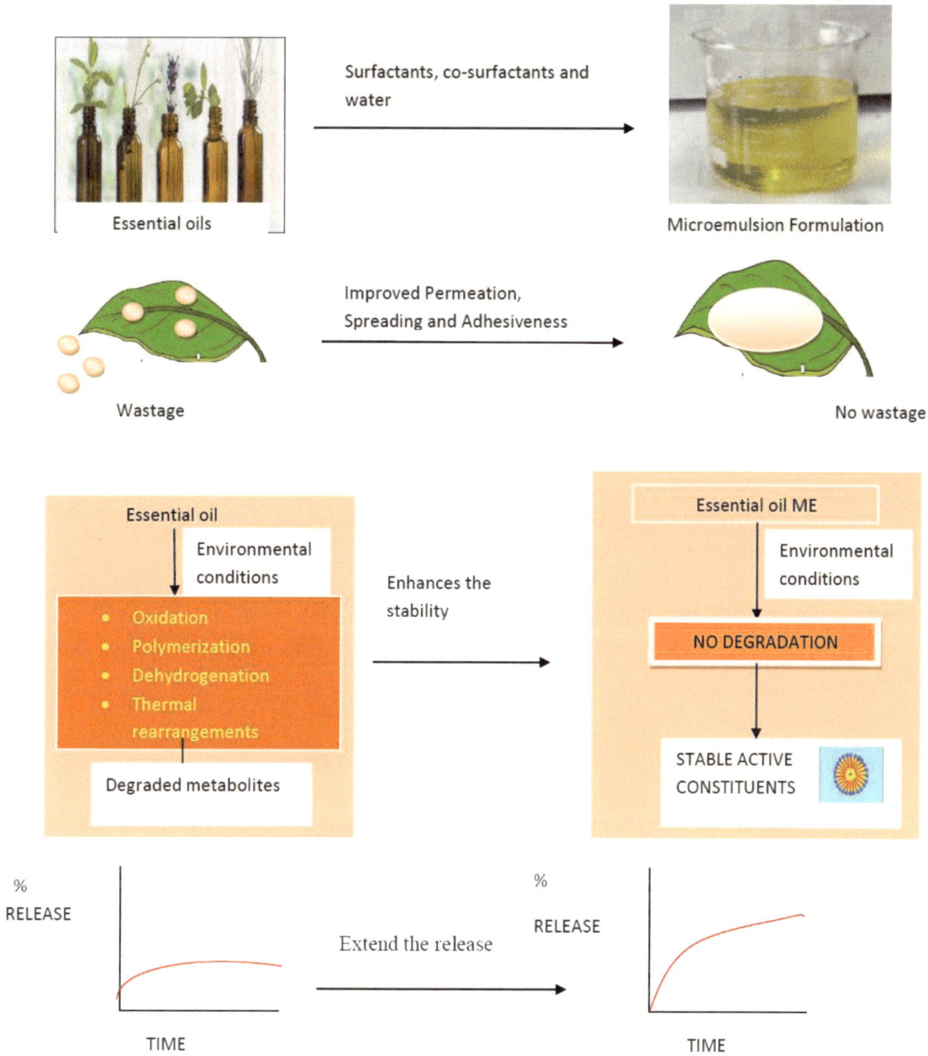

Figure 6.
Advanced features of essential oil ME formulations over essential oil.

stability as well as bioactivity against different crop pests. Therefore essential oil ME could be the safest mode of a delivery system shortly. Advanced features of essential oil microemulsion are depicted in **Figure 6**.

6.4 Scope of work in promoting essential oil microemulsion in crop protection

Essential oil based microemulsion formulation is a promising tool for the biocontrol of the pests of economic importance. However, there are still some areas of improvement that should be focused upon in order to promote oil based microemulsion system in the agriculture sector.

1. **The need for combinatory botanicals or synergists**: Essential oil ME in pure form requires a higher rate of application for controlling pest species, which will increase the cost of formulation and limits its usage. So, there is an urgent need for discovering new combinatory or synergistic constituents, which will be very helpful in promoting essential oil ME.

2. **Extraction and refinement of active components**: There are many active components present in the essential oils, and each gives some specific property. So, many research studies are required to extract, isolate, and identify these constituents. After refinement of most active components, Microemulsion formulation will be straightforward and give much fold of efficacy against various insect pests in an economical way.

3. **Regulatory approval:** The developed essential oil ME with high efficiency shouldbe approved by regulatory systems so that the commercialization will be easy and successfully used by the farmers.

4. **Availability of raw material:** Essential oil plant or tree sources should be cultivated so that enough amount of raw material is available to scale up the essential oil ME formulation.

5. **Needs awareness:** As we know, people are very used to synthetic pesticides and less aware of these types of formulations due to lack of knowledge about these formulations.

All these advanced formulations are only up-to the lab level. So, a proper system of endorsement and awareness is required for the promotion of essential oil ME formulation.

7. Conclusion

Microemulsion formulation is the most suitable thermodynamically stable formulation for essential oils. Essential oils give maximum stability in microemulsions with optimized surfactants and co-surfactants. Various essential oil microemulsions have been formulated and found very useful for controlling multiple agricultural pests. Many studies revealed that essential oil stability and bio-efficacy could be further improved by using eco-friendly stabilizers and botanical synergists. Essential oil microemulsion could be a better alternative to synthetic pesticides and opens a new corridor for the promotion of the greener way of plant protection in India and across the globe.

Acknowledgements

The first author gratefully acknowledges the founder president of Amity University, Dr. Ashok K Chauhan, for his kind support and motivation.

Conflict of interest

The authors declare no conflict of interest.

Appendix and nomenclature

O/W	oil in water
w/o	water in oil
Υ_i	interfacial tension
ΔG_f	free energy of formation

η_r	relative viscosity
HPLC	high pressure liquid chromatography
GC-MS	gas chromatography-mass spectrophotometer
LC-MS	liquid chromatography-mass spectrophotometer

Author details

Abhishek Sharma[1]*, Saurabh Dubey[2] and Nusrat Iqbal[3]

1 Amity Food and Agriculture Foundation, Amity University Uttar Pradesh, Noida, India

2 RS Formulation Development and Consultant, Bhiwadi, India

3 Institute of Pesticide Formulation Technology, Ministry of Chemicals and Fertilizer, Government of India Sec-20, Gurugram, Haryana, India

*Address all correspondence to: asharma5@amity.edu

IntechOpen

© 2020 The Author(s). Licensee IntechOpen. This chapter is distributed under the terms of the Creative Commons Attribution License (http://creativecommons.org/licenses/by/3.0), which permits unrestricted use, distribution, and reproduction in any medium, provided the original work is properly cited. CC BY

References

[1] Sharifi-Rad J, Sureda A, Tenore GC, Daglia M, Sharifi-Rad M, Valussi M, et al. Biological activities of essential oils: From plant chemoecology to traditional healing systems. Molecules. 2017;**22**:1-55. DOI: 10.3390/molecules22010070

[2] Alejandro U, Rocío S, Javier E, Carolina V, Sara M. Insecticidal properties of *Peumus boldus* Mol. essential oil on the house Fly, *Musca domestica* L. PALACIOS2 & Yanina ROSSI Boletín Latinoamericano y del Caribe de Plantas Medicinales y Aromáticas. 2010;**9**:465-469

[3] Hoar TP, Schulman JH. Transparent water-in-oil dispersions: The oleopathic hydro-micelle. Nature. 1943;**152**: 102-103. DOI: 10.1038/152102a0

[4] Danielsson I, Lindman B. The definition of microemulsion. Colloids and Surfaces. B, Biointerfaces. 1981;**3**: 391-392

[5] Lade M. On the nanoparticle synthesis in microemulsions: Detailed characterization of an applied reaction mixture. Colloids and Surfaces A: Physicochemical and Engineering Aspects. 2000;**163**:3-15. DOI: 10.1016/S0927-7757(99)00425-2

[6] Bakkali F, Averbeck S, Averbeck D, Idaomar M. Biological effects of essential oils-a review. Food Chemical Toxicolology. 2008;**46**:446-475. DOI: 10.1016/j.fct.2007.09.106

[7] Dhifi W, Bellili S, Jazi S, Bahloul N, Mnif W. Essential oil's chemical characterization and investigation of some biological activities: A critical review. Medicine. 2016;**25**:1-16. DOI: 10.3390/medicines3040025

[8] Sheila PM, Helder FT, Ádley ANL, Valdir FVJ, Letícia SK. Essential oils and isolated terpenes in nanosystems designed for topical administration: A review. Biomolecules. 2019;**9**:1-19. DOI: 10.3390/biom9040138

[9] Marta FM, Sarah JM. Plant-based insect repellents: A review of their efficacy, development and testing. Malaria Journal. 2011;**10**:1-14. DOI: 10.1186/1475-2875-10-S1-S11

[10] Muller-Riebau F, Berger B, Yegen O. Chemical composition and fungitoxic properties to phytopathogenic fungi of essential oils of selected aromatic plants growing wild in Turkey. Journal of Agriculture and Food Chemistry. 1995;**43**:2262-2266. DOI: 10.1021/jf00056a055

[11] Terrance G, Lawrence GD. Solubilities of terpenic essentile oil components in aqueous solutions. Journal of Chemical & Engineering Data. 1980;**25**:150-152

[12] Wang J, Zhu F, Zhou XM, Niu CY, Lei CL. Repellent and fumigant activity of essential oil from *Artemisia vulgaris* to *Tribolium castaneum* (Herbst) (Coleoptera: Tenebrionidae). Journal of Stored Products Research. 2006;**42**: 339-347. DOI: 10.1016/j.jspr.2005.06.001

[13] Turek C, Stintzing FC. Stability of essential oils: A review. Comprehensive Reviews in Food Science and Food Safety. 2013;**12**:40-53. DOI: 10.1111/1541-4337.12006

[14] Giulia B, Marco C, Monica MF, Giovanni FP. Colloidal soft matter as drug delivery system. Journal of Pharmaceutical Sciences. 2009;**98**:11-42. DOI: 10.1002/jps.21423

[15] Lawrence MJ, Rees GD. Microemulsion-based media as novel drug delivery systems. Advanced Drug Delivery Reviews. 2000;**45**:89-121. DOI: 10.1016/S0169-409X(00)00103-4

[16] David JM. Nanoemulsions versus microemulsions: Terminology, differences, and similarities. Soft Matter. 2012;**8**:1719-1729. DOI: 10.1016/S0169-409X(00)00103-4

[17] Gupta S, Moulik SPJ. Biocompatible microemulsions and their prospective uses in drug delivery. Journal of Pharmaceutical Sciences. 2008;**97**:22-45. DOI: 10.1002/jps.21177

[18] Abeer H, Abdulaziz AA, Ramalingam R, Al-Bandari FA, Horiah AA, Dilfuza E, et al. Arbuscular mycorrhizal fungi regulate the oxidative system, hormones and ionic equilibrium to trigger salt stress tolerance in Cucumis sativus L. Saudi Journal of Biological Sciences. 2018;**25**:1102-1114. DOI: 10.1016/j.sjbs.2018.03.009

[19] Sakulku U, Nuchuchua O, Uawongyart N, Puttipipatkhachorn S, Soottitantawat A, Ruktanonchai U. Characterization and mosquito repellent activity of citronella oil nanoemulsion. International Journal of Pharmaceutics. 2009;**372**:105-111. DOI: 10.1016/j.ijpharm.2008.12.029

[20] Tadros T, Izquierdo P, Esquena J, Solans C. Formation and stability of nano-emulsions. Advances in Colloid and Interface Science. 2004;**20**:108-109. DOI: 10.1016/j.cis.2003.10.023

[21] Flanagan J, Singh H. Microemulsions: A potential delivery system for bioactives in food. Critical Reviews in Food Science and Nutrition. 2006;**46**:221-237. DOI: 10.1080/10408690590956710

[22] Du Z, Wang C, Tai X, Wang G, Liu X. Optimization and characterization of biocompatible oil-in-water nanoemulsion for pesticide delivery. ACS Sustainable Chemistry & Engineering. 2016;**4**:983-991

[23] Balah MA. Formulation of prospective plant oils derived micro-emulsions for herbicidal activity. Mansoura Plant Protection and Pathalogy. 2013;**4**:911-926

[24] Wang Y, Zhao R, Yu L, Zhang Y, He Y, Yao J. Evaluation of cinnamon essential oil microemulsion and its vapor phase for controlling postharvest gray mold of pears (*Pyrus pyrifolia*). Journal of the Science of Food and Agriculture. 2014;**30**:1000-1004. DOI: 10.1002/jsfa.6360

[25] Shao H, Xi N, Zhang Y. Microemulsion formulation of a new biopesticide to control the diamondback moth (Lepidoptera: Plutellidae). Scientific Reports. 2018;**8**:1-9

[26] Xavier-Junior FH, Vauthier C, Morais ARV, Alencar EN, Egito EST. Microemulsion systems containing bioactive natural oils: An overview on state of the art. Drug Development and Industrial Pharmacy. 2017;**4**:1-59. DOI: 10.1080/03639045.2016.1235186

[27] Iqbal N, Pant M, Dubey S, Sogan N, Patanjali N, Naik SN. Preparation of neem oil microemulsion using biodiesel waste for larvae control. International Journal of Mosquito Research. 2019; **6**(1):104-108

[28] Iqbal N, Kumar N, Agrawal A, Kumar J. Development of highly stabilized neem oil microemulsion system: A green approach. World Journal of Pharmaceutical Research. Microemulsion Formulation of Botanical Oils as an Efficient Tool to Provide Sustainable. 2019;**8**: 1507-1517. DOI: 10.20959/wjpr20193-14435

[29] Massoud A, Manal MA, Osman AZ, Magdy IEM, Abdel-Rheim KH. Eco-friendly Nano-emulsion formulation of *Mentha piperita* against stored product pest *Sitophilus oryzae* Magdy. Advances in Crop Science and Technology. 2018;**6**: 1-6

[30] Liu X, Wang LP, Li YC, Li HY, Yu T, Zheng XD. Antifungal activity of thyme oil against geotrichum citri-aurantii in vitro and in vivo. Journal of Applied Microbiology. 2009;**10**: 1450-1456. DOI: 10.1111/j.1365-2672.2009.04328.x

[31] Adak T, Barik N, Patil NB, Rath PC. Nanoemulsion of eucalyptus oil: An alternative to synthetic pesticides against two major storage insects (*Sitophilus oryzae* (L.) and *Tribolium castaneum* (Herbst)) of rice. Industrial Crops and Products. 2019;**143**:111849. DOI: 10.1016/j.indcrop.2019.111849

[32] Jiao X, Fan QJ, Yin ZQ, Li XT, DuYH JRY, Wang KY, et al. The preparation of neem oil microemulsion (*Azadirachta indica*) and the comparison of acaricidal time between neem oil microemulsion and other formulations in vitro. Veterinary Parasitology. 2010;**169**:399-403. DOI: 10.1016/j.vetpar.2010.01.016

[33] Nikos EP, Kalaitzaki A, Filitsa K, Michaelakis A, Papadimitriou V, Dourtoglou V, et al. Nano-formulation enhances insecticidal activity of natural pyrethrins against *Aphis gossypii* (Hemiptera: Aphididae) and retains their harmless effect to non-target predators. Environmental Science and Pollution Research. 2018;**25**: 10243-10249. DOI: 10.1007/s11356-017-8596-2

[34] Basak S, Guha P. Use of a predictive model to describe sporicidal and cell viability efficacy of betel leaf (*Piper betle* L.) essential oil on *Aspergillus flavus* and *Penicillium expansum* and its antifungal activity in raw apple juice. Food Science and Technology. 2017;**80**:510-516. DOI: 10.1016/j.lwt.2017.03.024

[35] Kumara N, Pant M, Singh OP, Dubey S, Naik SN, Sharma S, et al. Bioefficacy and stabilization of hydrolytically unstable pesticide in water based microemulsion against *Periplaneta americana*. International Journal of Advanced Research, IT and Engineering. 2016;**5**:9-25

[36] Sharma A, Sehra G, Sabnis P, Kamra A, Sharma S. Development of clove oil based nanoformulation against *Fusarium oxysporum*. Indian Phytopathalogy. 2016;**69**:313-315

[37] Pant M, Dubey S, Patanjali PK, Naik SN, Sharma S. Insecticidal activity of eucalyptus Patanjali oil nanoemulsion with karanja and jatropha aqueous filtrates. International Biodeterioration and Biodegradation. 2014;**91**:119-127. DOI: 10.1016/j.ibiod.2013.11.019

[38] Sharma R, Kumari A, Sarat SN, Singh MK, Dubey S, Iqbal N, et al. Development and stability enhancement of neem oil based microemulsion formulation using botanical synergist. Journal of Molecular Liquids. 2019;**296**: 112012. DOI: 10.1016/j.molliq.2019.112012